Study Guide for

McCance & Huether's Pathophysiology

The Biologic Basis for Disease in Adults and Children

Study Guide for

McCance & Huether's Pathophysiology

The Biologic Basis for Disease in Adults and Children

Ninth Edition

Julia L. Rogers

Prepared by:

Linda Felver, PhD, RN
Associate Professor
School of Nursing
Oregon Health & Science University
Portland, Oregon

ELSEVIER

Elsevier
3251 Riverport Lane
St. Louis, Missouri 63043

STUDY GUIDE FOR MCCANCE & HUETHER'S PATHOPHYSIOLOGY: THE BIOLOGIC
BASIS FOR DISEASE IN ADULTS AND CHILDREN, NINTH EDITION   ISBN: 978-0-323-87498-4

Copyright © 2024 by Elsevier, Inc. All Rights Reserved.

No part of this publication may be reproduced or transmitted in any form or by any means, electronic or mechanical,
including photocopying, recording, or any information storage and retrieval system, without permission in writing
from the publisher, except that, until further notice, instructors requiring their students to purchase Study Guide for
McCance & Huether's Pathophysiology by Julia L. Rogers, may reproduce the contents or parts thereof for instructional
purposes, provided each copy contains a proper copyright notice as follows: Copyright © 2024 by Elsevier Inc.

Details on how to seek permission, further information about the Publisher's permissions policies and our
arrangements with organizations such as the Copyright Clearance Center and the Copyright Licensing Agency, can be
found at our website: www.elsevier.com/permissions.

This book and the individual contributions contained in it are protected under copyright by the Publisher (other than as
may be noted herein).

Notice

Practitioners and researchers must always rely on their own experience and knowledge in evaluating and using
any information, methods, compounds or experiments described herein. Because of rapid advances in the medical
sciences, in particular, independent verification of diagnoses and drug dosages should be made. To the fullest
extent of the law, no responsibility is assumed by Elsevier, authors, editors or contributors for any injury and/
or damage to persons or property as a matter of products liability, negligence or otherwise, or from any use or
operation of any methods, products, instructions, or ideas contained in the material herein.

Previous editions copyrighted **2019, 2015, 2010, 2006, 2002, and 1998.**

Content Strategist: Sonya Seigafuse
Director, Content Development: Laurie K. Gower
Publishing Services Manager: Deepthi Unni
Project Manager: Sheik Mohideen K
Cover Designer: Gopalakrishnan Venkatraman

Printed in the United States of America

Last digit is the print number: 9 8 7 6 5 4 3 2 1

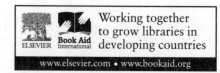

Working together
to grow libraries in
developing countries

www.elsevier.com • www.bookaid.org

Preface

The study of pathophysiology can be an exciting process. What happens in the tissues to cause the redness and swelling of inflammation? What happens in the heart during a heart attack? Why do people who have a specific disease display characteristic signs and symptoms? How might the same disease process be different in children, adults, and older adults?

This study guide is written to accompany the ninth edition of *McCance & Huether's Pathophysiology: The Biologic Basis for Disease in Adults and Children* by Julia L. Rogers. In a logical progression, the textbook begins with the central concepts of pathophysiology at the cellular and tissue levels, followed by pathophysiologic processes at the organ and system levels. This study guide follows that logical progression. For example, it assists with building a working knowledge of what happens in the tissues during inflammation before addressing questions regarding heart attacks and other disease processes at the organ and system levels.

The study guide follows the organization of the textbook, with 49 chapters. Each chapter contains a variety of activities that develop several cognitive skills, moving from the basic skills of learning definitions and acquiring knowledge to the higher-level skills of explaining, application, and integration of knowledge. Here are examples of these activities:

- **Match the Definitions:** A clear understanding of definitions provides the foundation for higher-level knowledge.
- **Puzzle Out the Technical Terms:** Occasional crossword puzzles assist with learning technical terms.
- **Circle the Correct Words:** Recognizing the correct word that belongs in a sentence reinforces basic knowledge acquisition.

- **Complete the Sentences:** Filling in the blanks requires more knowledge than simply recognizing words.
- **Draw Your Answers:** Explaining a concept or process by drawing it requires mental processing of ideas that enables people to remember them for future use.
- **Order the Steps:** Putting the parts of a pathophysiologic process into their correct sequence facilitates learning to explain them, a higher order skill.
- **Explain the Pictures:** Directed toward visual learners, these questions build explaining and integrating skills.
- **Categorize:** Choosing the category into which items belong requires understanding them and assists with differentiating between them.
- **Describe the Differences:** These questions build the skill of comparing and contrasting, an excellent way to learn about similar items without confusing them.
- **Teach People about Pathophysiology:** Unique to this study guide, these teaching activities provide the opportunity to learn pathophysiology at the level of explaining rather than rote recall.
- **Clinical Scenarios:** Patient examples with questions assist with application and integration of knowledge in real-world settings.

As a whole, the activities in each study guide chapter build a sequence of cognitive skills that facilitate mastery of pathophysiology at the application level needed for clinical practice.

Working with people at Elsevier has been delightful. I appreciate their receptiveness to my ideas and their enthusiasm for this project.

I dedicate this study guide to my past, present, and future students.

Linda Felver

Contents

Cellular Biology

IDENTIFY CELLULAR STRUCTURES AND THEIR FUNCTIONS

Identify the structures and match their cellular functions with their location in the picture.

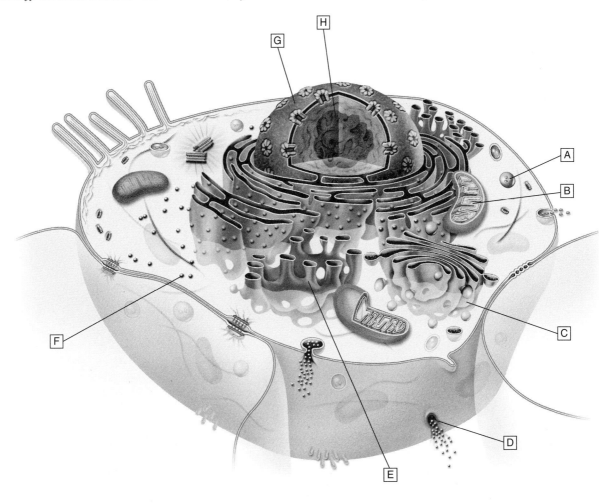

_____ 1. This structure generates ATP by oxidative phosphorylation; it is a _____.

_____ 2. This structure synthesizes proteins; it is a _____.

_____ 3. This structure processes and packages proteins for delivery; it is the _____ _____.

_____ 4. This structure serves as a repository of genetic information; it is the _____.

Copyright © 2024 by Elsevier, Inc. All Rights Reserved.

1

_____ 5. This structure synthesizes steroid hormones and folds proteins; it is the _____ _____.

_____ 6. This structure synthesizes ribosomes; it is the _____.

_____ 7. This structure delivers proteins that are secreted to their destinations; it is a secretory _____.

_____ 8. This structure contains digestive enzymes; it is a _____.

DESCRIBE THE DIFFERENCES

Describe the difference between each pair of terms.

9. What is the difference between a eukaryote and a prokaryote?

10. What is the difference between the nucleolus and the nucleus?

11. What is the difference between microtubules and microfilaments?

12. What is the difference between hydrophilic and hydrophobic?

13. What is the difference between a lysosome and a peroxisome?

COMPLETE THE SENTENCES

Write one word in each blank to complete these sentences.

14. Proteins in the nucleus that bind DNA and help regulate its activity are called _____.

15. Cells such as neutrophils that use hydrogen peroxide as a defensive weapon synthesize it in their _____.

16. A section of a membrane that is rich in cholesterol and helps organize membrane proteins is called a lipid _____.

17. The cells that secrete the extracellular matrix are called _____.

18. The mechanical force of water pushing against cellular membranes is called _____ pressure.

19. An _____ solution has the same osmolality as normal body fluids.

Copyright © 2024 by Elsevier, Inc. All Rights Reserved.

20. In a simple epithelium, the epithelial cells are in contact with a _____ membrane that provides support.

21. _____ tissue is characterized by only a few cells surrounded by a lot of extracellular matrix.

22. A myocyte is a _____ cell.

ORDER THE STEPS

Sequence the events that occur during each of these processes.

23. Write the letters here in the correct order of the events that occur during a neuronal action potential:
    _____
    A. Sodium ions move into the cell.
    B. Potassium ions leave the cell.
    C. Sodium permeability increases.
    D. Resting membrane potential is reestablished.
    E. Potassium permeability increases.

24. Write the letters here in the correct order of the phases of the normal cell cycle, beginning with the phase that precedes DNA synthesis: _____
    A. M phase
    B. S phase
    C. G_1 phase
    D. G_2 phase

CIRCLE THE CORRECT WORDS

Circle the correct word from the choices provided to complete these sentences.

25. The main difference between cells that divide rapidly and those that divide slowly is the amount of time they spend in the (S, G_1) phase of the cell cycle.

26. Cells develop specialized functions through the process of (differentiation, proteostasis).

27. A particle that is dissolved is called a (substrate, solute).

28. Mitochondria need a lot of (glucose, oxygen) to function normally.

29. During osmosis, (particles, water molecules) move across the plasma membrane.

30. (Autocrine, Paracrine) signals act on nearby cells by (diffusion, active transport) through interstitial fluid.

31. A cell that has an insufficient oxygen supply will not be able to perform the chemistry of (the citric acid cycle, glycolysis).

32. (Active transport, Diffusion) can move substances against their concentration gradients.

33. Receptors are (proteins, lipids) that bind specific small molecules.

34. An ion that has a negative charge is called (a cation, an anion).

Copyright © 2024 by Elsevier, Inc. All Rights Reserved.

Test your understanding by defining each term using your own words.

35. Ligand

36. Caveolae

37. Glycocalyx

38. Amphipathic molecule

39. Endocytosis

CHOOSE THE DIRECTION

For each situation, choose the direction in which the items will move. Choose A or B from the figure.

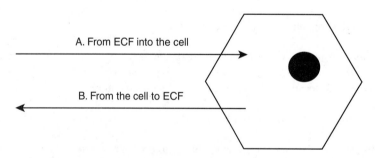

_____ 40. If the ECF becomes hypotonic, in which direction will water move?

_____ 41. If the concentration of substance X in the ECF is higher than its concentration inside the cell, in which direction will active transport move substance X?

_____ 42. If the glucose concentration in the ECF is higher than its concentration inside the cell, in which direction will facilitated diffusion move glucose?

_____ 43. In which direction does Na^1, K^1-ATPase move sodium ions?

_____ 44. In which direction does Na^+, K^+-ATPase move potassium ions?

Copyright © 2024 by Elsevier, Inc. All Rights Reserved.

Use appropriate technical terms to explain these events, as if you are talking to another health professional.

45. Explain to a nurse in a cardiac intensive care unit how the presence of gap junctions in cardiac muscle facilitates cardiac function.

46. Explain to physician assistant why intracellular receptors do not use second messengers, but many cell surface receptors do.

47. Explain to a nurse practitioner what happens during the interphase portion of the cell cycle and why those events are important.

Copyright © 2024 by Elsevier, Inc. All Rights Reserved.

2 Altered Cellular and Tissue Biology: Environmental Agents

MATCH THE DEFINITIONS

Match the word on the right with its definition on the left.

_____ 1. Stiffening of skeletal muscles after death

_____ 2. Unintentional decrease of core body temperature below 35°C (95°F)

_____ 3. A type of cellular housekeeping in which a cell digests some of its own components

_____ 4. Area of cell death in which dead cells disintegrate, but the debris is not digested completely by enzymes

_____ 5. Area of cell death in which denatured proteins appear firm and opaque

_____ 6. An atom or group of atoms having an unpaired electron

_____ 7. Purple discoloration of dependent tissues after death

_____ 8. Cell death that involves orderly dismantling of cell components and packaging the remainders in vesicles

A. Apoptosis

B. Free radical

C. Livor mortis

D. Accidental hypothermia

E. Rigor mortis

F. Coagulative necrosis

G. Autophagy

H. Caseous necrosis

CATEGORIZE THE CLINICAL EXAMPLES

Write the type of cellular adaptation beside its clinical example. Choices: atrophy, hypertrophy, hyperplasia, metaplasia.

_____ 9. Lining of uterus thickens after ovulation because of increased amounts of estrogen.

_____ 10. A man who lifts weights regularly develops larger biceps.

_____ 11. The thymus gland decreases in size during childhood.

_____ 12. Columnar epithelium in the bronchi of a cigarette smoker is replaced by stratified squamous epithelium.

_____ 13. A shot put champion has larger shoulder muscles on right than left.

_____ 14. The left calf is smaller than the right calf when cast is removed from it.

_____ 15. The liver regenerates after surgical removal of damaged portion.

Copyright © 2024 by Elsevier, Inc. All Rights Reserved.

CIRCLE THE CORRECT WORDS

Circle the correct word from the choices provided to complete these sentences.

16. Cell death by (necrosis, apoptosis) causes inflammation, but cell death by (necrosis, apoptosis) does not.

17. Dysplasia also is called (normal, atypical) hyperplasia.

18. Release of (potassium, calcium) ions from intracellular stores into the cytoplasm during ischemia damages the cell.

19. Compared with normal aerobic metabolism, cells that use anaerobic metabolism produce (more, less) ATP and (more, less) lactic acid.

20. The most important way to prevent medication-related poisoning deaths in children is safe (storage, prescribing) of medications.

21. Reactive oxygen species, such as (superoxide radicals, superoxide dismutase), damage cells by attacking their (potassium, membranes).

22. Postmortem changes (involve, do not involve) the inflammatory response.

23. Liquefactive necrosis occurs most commonly in the (brain, heart) because the cells there are rich in (lipases, hydrolases).

24. Gangrene occurs when cells die of (hypoxia, trauma) and (poisoning, bacterial invasion).

DESCRIBE THE DIFFERENCES

Describe the difference between each pair of terms.

25. What is the difference between hypertrophy and hyperplasia?

26. What is the difference between suffocation and strangulation?

27. What is the difference between an abrasion and a laceration?

28. What is the difference between dystrophic calcification and metastatic calcification?

29. What is the difference between a penetrating gunshot wound and a perforating gunshot wound?

7

Copyright © 2024 by Elsevier, Inc. All Rights Reserved.

ORDER THE STEPS

Beginning with the acute obstruction of a coronary artery, sequence the events that occur during necrosis of a myocardial cell.

30. Write the letters here in the correct order of the steps: _____
    A. ATP supply decreases within the cell.
    B. Acute obstruction of coronary artery cuts off arterial blood supply to myocardium.
    C. Cell runs on anaerobic metabolism because of lack of oxygen.
    D. Cell bursts and spills its contents into the interstitial fluid.
    E. Active transport of ions across the cell membrane slows.
    F. Lysosomal enzymes destroy components of their own cell.
    G. Osmosis causes cell swelling, and calcium accumulates in the cell.
    H. Organelles, including lysosomes, swell and rupture.

COMPLETE THE SENTENCES

Write one word in each blank to complete these sentences.

31. Active enzymes that dismantle the cellular components during apoptosis are called _____.

32. Acute cellular swelling during ischemia is reversible if _____ is supplied quickly.

33. Active tuberculosis disease is characterized by _____ necrosis, whereas death of brain cells is characterized by _____ necrosis.

34. During apoptosis, cell contents are contained in vesicles called _____ _____, which are removed by _____.

35. Liver enzymes metabolize most blood ethanol to _____, which damages tissues.

36. When excessive reactive oxygen species overwhelm the endogenous antioxidant systems, _____ _____ occurs.

37. Death of the entire person is called _____ death.

38. Melanin is synthesized by epidermal cells called _____ and accumulates in epidermal cells called _____.

39. Gases such as carbon dioxide, methane, and fluorinated gases are called _____ gases because they trap _____ in the atmosphere.

RESPOND TO CLINICAL SITUATIONS

Place yourself in these situations and write your responses in the spaces provided.

40. Mr. Turino had severe crushing injuries of both lower extremities when his house collapsed on him during an earthquake. Among other abnormal values, his laboratory tests show elevated creatine kinase in his blood. Why is his blood creatine kinase high?

Copyright © 2024 by Elsevier, Inc. All Rights Reserved.

41. Mrs. Montoya died peacefully in her sleep at home while lying prone. When her relatives discovered her body and rolled her over, they saw purple discoloration of half of her face and of her abdomen. They are very concerned that she might have been beaten the night before she died. What factual information do they need to relieve their concern?

42. The entire Berg family was in the hospital room when Mrs. Berg died quietly from terminal cancer. As the family is preparing to leave, Kevin Berg, age 10, says to his mother, "I think grandma is not really dead. She is just sleeping. Dead people are stiff as boards. I saw that on TV. Grandma's hands are cold, but her arms are not stiff." His mother looks at the nurse for help. In addition to addressing the emotional issues, what factual information should be provided?

43. Two of your colleagues are discussing the effects of reactive oxygen species (ROS) on cells. "Too many ROS cause necrosis," says one. "But I read that too many ROS cause apoptosis," says the other. What information should be explained to them to clarify that both are correct?

DRAW YOUR ANSWERS

Read the questions and draw your answers.

These are normal cells that are capable of cell division and normally receive basal levels of hormonal stimulation.

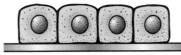

Normal

(From Lewis SM, Heitkemper MM, Dirksen SR: *Medical-surgical nursing: assessment and management of clinical problems*, ed 6, St Louis, 2004, Mosby.)

44. Draw what these cells would look like after their hormonal stimulation has been reduced substantially for several weeks.

45. Draw what these cells would look like after receiving excessive hormonal stimulation for several weeks.

Copyright © 2024 by Elsevier, Inc. All Rights Reserved.

IDENTIFY THE CHARACTERISTICS

Choose the characteristics of apoptosis. You may select more than one answer. Choose all that apply.

46. Write the letters of your choice(s) here: _____
    A. Cell is damaged by its own lysosomal enzymes.
    B. Cell shrinks when its cytoskeleton is dismantled.
    C. The cell injury is reversible if nutrients are restored in time.
    D. Process causes inflammation.
    E. Sections of the cell bud off into vesicles.
    F. Cell swells when osmosis occurs.
    G. Process occurs when caspases are inactivated.

TEACH PEOPLE ABOUT PATHOPHYSIOLOGY

Write your response to each situation in the space provided.

47. Kenesha Francis, age 9, broke her arm 6 weeks ago, and the cast will be removed today. Before the cast is removed, teach her about the expected appearance of her arm in words appropriate to her age.

48. "The doctor said my heart enlarged because my blood pressure is high," says Mr. Hendricks. "Please explain that!"

49. Mr. Bax has diabetes and will have amputation of toes shown in the photograph.

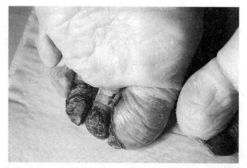

(From Damjanov I: *Pathology for the health professions,* ed 4, Philadelphia, 2012, Saunders.)

He asks, "Why did my toes get black and hard rather than swollen and mushy like my dad's toes did before surgery?"

Chapter **2** **Altered Cellular and Tissue Biology: Environmental Agents**   Copyright © 2024 by Elsevier, Inc. All Rights Reserved.

Clinical Scenario:

Kevin Jackson, age 17, spent most of his free time on a skateboard. His left foot developed a callus where his shoe rubbed it. He started working out at a gym to build his strength for a skateboard competition. Kevin's shoulders and biceps increased in size as he continued his workouts.

One day when he was practicing a new skateboard move on a ramp he had constructed on the sidewalk, Kevin crashed and broke his left arm. He soon figured out how to skateboard with a cast on his arm and continued his workouts at the gym, using his right arm only. After 6 weeks, the cast was removed. To his dismay, Kevin discovered that his left upper arm looked shrunken when compared with his right arm.

Several cellular adaptations, but fewer than five, are illustrated in the clinical scenario. Write the contributing factors for the adaptations illustrated in the scenario. If the adaptation is not illustrated, write "Not applicable".

50. Atrophy _____

51. Hypertrophy _____

52. Hyperplasia _____

53. Metaplasia _____

54. Dysplasia _____

Copyright © 2024 by Elsevier, Inc. All Rights Reserved.

PUZZLE OUT THESE TECHNICAL TERMS

Use the clues to complete the puzzle, demonstrating your knowledge of important technical terms.

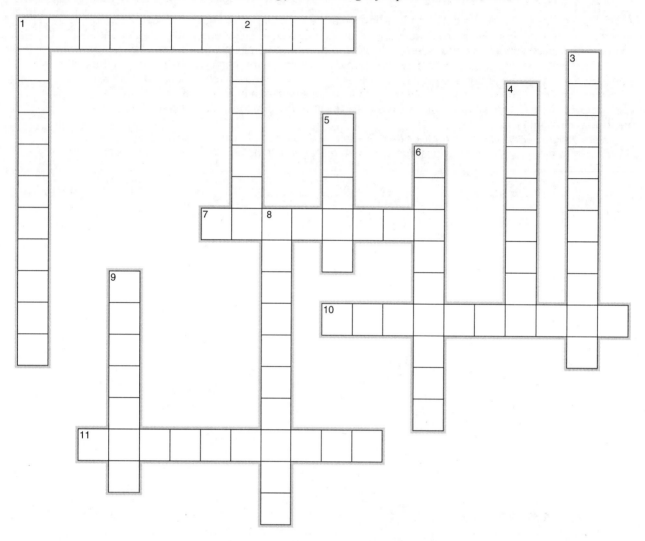

Across

1. Adaptive increase in the number of cells
7. Shrunken nucleus appearing as a small, dense mass
10. Adaptive replacement of one mature cell type by another normal cell type
11. Yellow-brown age pigment

Down

1. Adaptive increase in cell size
2. Adaptive decrease in cell size
3. Loss of skeletal muscle mass and strength
4. Lack of oxygen to tissues caused by insufficient blood supply
5. Goes with mortis to denote postmortem reduction of body temperature
6. Abnormal change in size, shape, and organization of mature tissue cells
8. Nuclear dissolution and lysis of chromatin
9. Partial deprivation of oxygen

Copyright © 2024 by Elsevier, Inc. All Rights Reserved.

3 The Cellular Environment: Fluids and Electrolytes, Acids and Bases

MATCH THE DEFINITIONS

Match each word on the right with its definition on the left.

_____ 1. Excessive carbon dioxide in the blood

_____ 2. Elevated sodium concentration in the blood

_____ 3. Fluid accumulation in interstitial spaces

_____ 4. Fluid accumulation in the peritoneal cavity

_____ 5. Decreased pH of the blood

_____ 6. Elevated potassium concentration in the blood

A. Edema

B. Ascites

C. Acidosis

D. Hypercapnia

E. Hyperkalemia

F. Hypernatremia

CIRCLE THE CORRECT WORDS

Circle the correct word from the choices provided to complete these sentences.

7. The osmolality of the intracellular fluid normally is (higher than, the same as, lower than) the extracellular fluid because water crosses cell membranes (with difficulty, freely) through aquaporins.

8. (Sodium, Albumin) is primarily responsible for the plasma oncotic pressure.

9. Thirst prompts fluid intake through action of (baroreceptors, osmoreceptors) located in the (hypothalamus, posterior pituitary).

10. Isotonic fluid excess causes (hypernatremia, hypervolemia).

11. Renal compensation for an acid-base balance is (fast, slow); pulmonary compensation for an acid-base balance is (fast, slow).

12. Fluid moves out of capillaries by (osmosis, filtration) and into or out of cells by (osmosis, filtration).

13. Hypercapnia means an excess of (metabolic acid, carbon dioxide) in the blood.

14. The most dangerous effect of hyperkalemia is its action on the (kidneys, heart).

CATEGORIZE THE CAUSES OF EDEMA

Write the major cause of the edema beside each clinical situation. Choices: increased capillary hydrostatic pressure, decreased plasma oncotic pressure, increased capillary permeability, lymphatic obstruction.

_____ 15. Tumor grows in lymph node

_____ 16. Right heart failure

Copyright © 2024 by Elsevier, Inc. All Rights Reserved.

_____ 17. Infected wound

_____ 18. Clot in a vein

_____ 19. Protein malnutrition

_____ 20. Bee sting

_____ 21. End-stage kidney disease

SELECT THE GREATER

Consider the pairs and select the one that is greater.

22. Who has a greater percentage of body weight as water: a lean woman or an obese woman?

23. Who has a greater percentage of body weight as water: an infant or an adolescent?

24. Who has a greater percentage of body weight as water if both people weigh the same: a woman or a man?

25. Who has a greater percentage of body weight as water if both people weigh the same: a 56-year-old man or a 78-year-old man?

26. Where is the potassium ion concentration greater: extracellular fluid or intracellular fluid?

27. Where is the sodium ion concentration greater: extracellular fluid or intracellular fluid?

28. Which is greater: the pH of an acid solution or the pH of an alkaline solution?

29. Which is greater: the respiratory rate during metabolic acidosis or the respiratory rate during metabolic alkalosis?

EXPLAIN THE PICTURES

Examine the pictures and answer the questions about them.

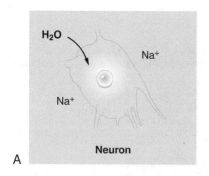
A

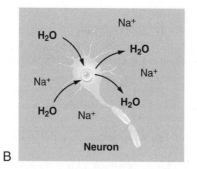
B

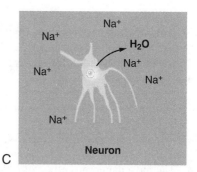
C

30. Compare the sodium concentration in panels A, B, and C. Panel B shows isotonic fluid, so the fluid in A is _____, and the fluid in C is _____.

Chapter **3** **The Cellular Environment: Fluids and Electrolytes, Acids and Bases**

Copyright © 2024 by Elsevier, Inc. All Rights Reserved.

31. Why did the neuron in panel A swell?

32. What cerebral clinical manifestations occur when neurons swell as in panel A?

33. Why are the cerebral clinical manifestations of the situation in panel C similar to those in panel A?

CHARACTERIZE THE HORMONES

Write one letter and one number by each hormone in the left column to indicate the stimuli that increase its secretion and its physiologic effects when secreted.

Hormone	Choose the Stimuli that Increase Secretion of the Hormone	Choose the Physiologic Effects of the Hormone
_____ 34. Aldosterone	A. High plasma calcium	1. Increases renal sodium and water excretion
_____ 35. Parathyroid hormone	B. Increased plasma osmolality, substantially decreased arterial blood pressure	2. Increases renal sodium and water reabsorption; increases renal excretion of potassium and hydrogen ions
_____ 36. Atrial natriuretic peptide	C. Low plasma calcium	3. Increases resorption of bone; stimulates renal reabsorption of calcium; inhibits renal reabsorption of phosphate
_____ 37. Calcitonin	D. Increased volume in the cardiac atria	
_____ 38. Antidiuretic hormone	E. Angiotensin II, increased plasma potassium	4. Increases renal water reabsorption, vasoconstriction
		5. Inhibits osteoclasts in bone

DESCRIBE THE DIFFERENCES

Describe the difference between each pair of terms.

39. What is the difference between interstitial fluid and extracellular fluid?

40. What is the difference between a volatile acid and a nonvolatile acid?

Copyright © 2024 by Elsevier, Inc. All Rights Reserved.

41. What is the difference between acidemia and acidosis?

42. With regard to an acid-base imbalance, what is the difference between correction and compensation?

COMPLETE THE SENTENCES

Write one word in each blank to complete these sentences.

43. One-third of body water is in the _____ fluid, and two-thirds is in the _____ fluid.

44. A standard 70-kg man has _____ liters of total body water.

45. Excessive fluid within the interstitial space is called _____.

46. An _____ fluid has the same concentration of solute as the plasma.

47. A person who has a lung disease may develop a primary _____ acid–base imbalance, but a person who has a kidney disease may develop a primary _____ acid–base imbalance.

48. When the blood pH is 7.40, the bicarbonate-to-carbonic acid ratio is _____.

49. A buffer pair is a weak _____ and its _____ _____.

50. Calculating the anion gap may help to distinguish between different causes of metabolic _____.

51. Overuse of phosphate-containing, over-the-counter enemas can cause _____, which in turn will _____ the plasma calcium concentration.

WORK WITH THESE PATIENTS

For each patient situation, select the imbalance(s) for which that patient has high risk and the assessment findings for the imbalance(s).

52. Mrs. Singh takes glucocorticoids for a chronic disease. She has highest risk for _____(1)_____, which would be evidenced by _____(2)_____.

Options for 1	Options for 2
Isotonic fluid deficit, hypokalemia, metabolic alkalosis	Dependent edema, weight gain, distended neck veins when upright, skeletal muscle weakness, constipation, abdominal distention
Isotonic fluid excess and hypokalemia	Fatigue, weakness, anorexia, constipation, lethargy
Hypercalcemia	Tachycardia; rapid weight loss; decreased urine output; skeletal muscle weakness; slow, shallow respirations; lethargy

Copyright © 2024 by Elsevier, Inc. All Rights Reserved.

53. Mr. Wiggins has been sobbing and breathing deeply and rapidly for an hour since his wife died. He has highest risk for _____(1)_____, which would be evidenced by _____(2)_____.

Options for 1	Options for 2
Respiratory acidosis	Paresthesias of fingers, lightheadedness, confusion
Respiratory alkalosis	Slow, shallow respirations; blood pH less than 7.35; blood Pa_{CO_2} increased

54. Mr. Jenkins is comatose from a heroin overdose. He has highest risk for _____(1)_____, which would be evidenced by _____(2)_____.

Options for 1	Options for 2
Respiratory acidosis	Paresthesias of fingers, lightheadedness, confusion
Respiratory alkalosis	Slow, shallow respirations; blood pH less than 7.35; blood Pa_{CO_2} increased

55. Baby Maria has repeated vomiting from pyloric stenosis. She has highest risk for _____(1)_____, which would be evidenced by _____(2)_____.

Options for 1	Options for 2
Isotonic fluid deficit, hypokalemia, metabolic alkalosis	Dependent edema, weight gain, distended neck veins when upright, skeletal muscle weakness, constipation, abdominal distention
Isotonic fluid excess and hypokalemia	Fatigue, weakness, anorexia, constipation, lethargy
Hypercalcemia	Tachycardia; rapid weight loss; decreased urine output; skeletal muscle weakness; slow, shallow respirations; lethargy

56. Mx. Smythe has hyperparathyroidism. They have highest risk for _____(1)_____, which would be evidenced by _____(2)_____.

Options for 1	Options for 2
Isotonic fluid deficit, hypokalemia, metabolic alkalosis	Dependent edema, weight gain, distended neck veins when upright, skeletal muscle weakness, constipation, abdominal distention
Isotonic fluid excess and hypokalemia	Fatigue, weakness, anorexia, constipation, lethargy
Hypercalcemia	Tachycardia; rapid weight loss; decreased urine output; skeletal muscle weakness; slow, shallow respirations; lethargy

Copyright © 2024 by Elsevier, Inc. All Rights Reserved.

CHOOSE THE DIRECTION

For each situation, choose the direction that the items will move. Choose A or B from the figure.

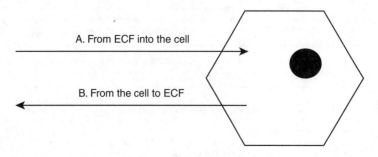

A. From ECF into the cell

B. From the cell to ECF

_____ 57. In which direction does insulin move potassium ions?

_____ 58. In which direction does epinephrine move potassium ions?

_____ 59. In which direction does alkalosis move potassium ions?

_____ 60. In which direction does hypernatremia move water?

TEACH PEOPLE ABOUT PATHOPHYSIOLOGY

Write your response to each situation in the space provided.

61. Mr. Sheehan has bilateral ankle edema from right heart failure. "Are my ankles inflamed?" he asks. "I know that inflammation causes swelling."

62. Mrs. Kiley, who is taking care of her husband at home after his hospitalization for a stroke, was told to call the doctor if Mr. Kiley develops dependent edema. She says, "I know what edema looks like, but where is dependent edema located?"

63. Mr. Janus, who is having his first renal dialysis session, says, "I know that my failed kidneys cannot excrete acids, but I did not eat any acids, so why did I get metabolic acidosis?"

64. Ms. Winsom, age 16, has diabetic ketoacidosis. "Why is she breathing so fast?" asks her father. "Does she have pneumonia as well as diabetic ketoacidosis?"

Copyright © 2024 by Elsevier, Inc. All Rights Reserved.

65. "Tell me the most common fluid, electrolyte, and acid-base imbalances in oliguric end-stage kidney disease patients," says a nurse. "I am being sent to help on the renal unit this morning."

CLINICAL SCENARIO

Read the clinical scenario and answer the questions to explore your understanding of fluid, electrolyte, and acid-base imbalances.

Mrs. Tanaka, age 76, was brought to an urgent care facility because she fell when she stood up after sitting all afternoon in her apartment, where she lives alone. Although slow to answer questions, Mrs. Tanaka states she has muscle weakness, muscle cramping, and constipation. She has had diarrhea for 3 weeks. Physical examination with Mrs. Tanaka supine revealed flat neck veins, HR 102, pulse regular but weak, BP 90/56, respirations 20 breaths/min and deep. The on-site clinical laboratory provided these results: serum sodium 142 mEq/L, potassium 2.8 mEq/L.

66. What fluid imbalance does Mrs. Tanaka have? _____ What data support that?

67. What imbalance is indicated by her laboratory results? _____ What other clinical manifestations are consistent with that imbalance?

68. What additional electrolyte imbalance(s) might Mrs. Tanaka have? Provide supporting data.

69. Mrs. Tanaka may have an acid-base imbalance. Which one? _____ What aspects of her history and clinical presentation support that?

70. Mrs. Tanaka was given intravenous isotonic sodium chloride, with appropriate electrolytes in it. What was the purpose of administering that particular fluid?

Copyright © 2024 by Elsevier, Inc. All Rights Reserved. Chapter **3 The Cellular Environment: Fluids and Electrolytes, Acids and Bases**

4 Genes and Genetic Diseases

MATCH THE DEFINITIONS

Match the words on the right with the definitions on the left.

_____ 1. Different version of a paired gene

_____ 2. Substance that alters genetic material (DNA)

_____ 3. Chromosome that is not a sex chromosome

_____ 4. Segment of DNA that is the basic unit of inheritance

_____ 5. Sequence of three nitrogenous bases that specifies a particular amino acid

_____ 6. Noncoding segment spliced out of mRNA

_____ 7. Alteration of DNA capable of being passed to offspring

_____ 8. Segment of mRNA that codes for proteins

_____ 9. Strand of condensed chromatin visible right before cell division

A. Codon

B. Intron

C. Exon

D. Mutation

E. Mutagen

F. Gene

G. Chromosome

H. Autosome

I. Allele

COMPLETE THE SENTENCES

Write one word in each blank to complete these sentences.

10. A display of chromosomes ordered according to length and centromere location is called a _____.

11. A somatic cell has _____ pairs of chromosomes.

12. A _____ mutation of DNA involves addition or deletion of a number of base pairs that is not a multiple of three and thus alters all of the codons downstream from the site of insertion or deletion.

13. A _____ gene will be expressed only if it is present in two copies.

14. Persons who have Down syndrome have high risk for developing _____ disease because of involvement of chromosome 21.

15. Persons who have the 47,XXY karyotype have _____ syndrome.

16. Interchanging of genetic material between nonhomologous chromosomes is called _____.

Copyright © 2024 by Elsevier, Inc. All Rights Reserved.

INTERPRET A PEDIGREE CHART

Examine the pedigree chart and answer the questions about it.

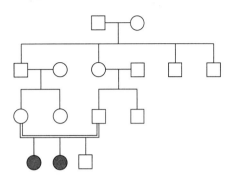

17. How many boys in this family have the genetic disorder? _____

18. What does the double line between the parents of the children with the disorder indicate? _____
    _____

19. The mother of the affected children has a sister. What symbol would be used if the mother and her sister were identical twins? _____

DESCRIBE THE DIFFERENCES

Describe the difference between each pair of terms.

20. What is the difference between heterozygous and homozygous?

21. What is the difference between monosomy and trisomy?

22. What is the difference between genotype and phenotype?

23. What is the difference between mitosis and meiosis?

Copyright © 2024 by Elsevier, Inc. All Rights Reserved.

ORDER THE STEPS

Sequence the events that occur during synthesis of a protein.

24. Write the letters here in the correct order of the steps: _____
    A. Translation
    B. Transcription
    C. mRNA leaves the nucleus
    D. RNA polymerase binds to DNA promoter region
    E. mRNA is spliced to remove noncoding sections

CATEGORIZE THE CLINICAL EXAMPLES

Write the type of genetic disorder beside its clinical example. Choices: chromosomal disorder, single-gene disorder.

_____ 25. Huntington's disease

_____ 26. Turner syndrome

_____ 27. Down syndrome

_____ 28. Fragile X syndrome

_____ 29. Cystic fibrosis

_____ 30. Klinefelter syndrome

_____ 31. Duchenne muscular dystrophy

CIRCLE THE CORRECT WORDS

Circle the correct word from the choices provided to complete these sentences.

32. A somatic cell that has 46 chromosomes in its nucleus is called a (diploid cell, gamete).

33. Genetic diseases caused by (single genes, multiple genes) usually are autosomal dominant, autosomal recessive, or X-linked recessive.

34. X-linked recessive diseases are seen much more often in (females, males) than in (females, males).

35. The structure of (mRNA, DNA) is a double helix.

36. Proteins are made of a sequence of (amino acids, nucleotides).

37. If the cells have three copies of each chromosome, (triploidy, trisomy) is present.

38. (Gain, Loss) of chromosomal material has more serious consequences than duplication of chromosomal material.

39. A Barr body is an inactivated (X, Y) chromosome that is seen in normal (male, female) cells.

Copyright © 2024 by Elsevier, Inc. All Rights Reserved.

Examine the Punnett square and determine what mode of inheritance it depicts.

		Normal parent	
		d	d
Affected parent	D	Dd Heterozygous affected	Dd Heterozygous affected
	d	dd Homozygous normal	dd Homozygous normal

40. This Punnett square represents what type of genetic condition?
    A. Autosomal dominant
    B. Autosomal recessive with two heterozygous carriers
    C. X-linked recessive with normal male and female carriers

WRITE YOUR DEFINITIONS

Test your understanding by defining each term using your own words.

41. Haploid cell

42. Homologous chromosomes

43. Polyploidy

44. Nondisjunction

45. Carrier

Copyright © 2024 by Elsevier, Inc. All Rights Reserved.

Write your response to each question in the space provided.

46. Mr. and Mrs. Medlow's infant, Kira, has phenylketonuria (PKU), an autosomal recessive disorder. "Tell me how Kira could inherit PKU from us when neither of us has it," says Mr. Medlow. "I remember what genes are, but if we both have the PKU gene, why don't we have the disease like Kira does?"

47. "What does autosomal mean?" asks Mr. Medlow.

48. "I know a child who has cystic fibrosis," says Mrs. Medlow. "That is genetic too, isn't it?"

49. "If cystic fibrosis is autosomal recessive like PKU, why can't they manage it by diet like we do for Kira's PKU?" asks Mrs. Medlow.

 Copyright © 2024 by Elsevier, Inc. All Rights Reserved.

5 Genes, Environment-Lifestyle, and Common Diseases

MATCH THE DEFINITIONS

Match the definitions on the left with the words on the right.

_____ 1. Shared by both members of a twin pair

_____ 2. Not shared by both members of a twin pair

_____ 3. Present at birth

_____ 4. Variation is caused by combined effects of multiple genes

_____ 5. Variation is caused by combined effects of environment and genes

A. Congenital

B. Polygenic

C. Discordant trait

D. Multifactorial

E. Concordant trait

CALCULATE THE RATES

Use the data provided to calculate the specified rates. You will not need all of the data, so consider which data you need before you calculate.
   All of these data apply to Fictiveville:

Number of people in Fictiveville	150,000
Number of people newly diagnosed with coronary heart disease in 2022	4050
Number of people who had coronary heart disease on January 31, 2022	16,500
Incidence rate of coronary heart disease among people who did not smoke cigarettes	1.5%
Prevalence rate of coronary heart disease among people who did not smoke cigarettes	6%
Incidence rate of coronary heart disease among people who smoked cigarettes	3.3%
Prevalence rate of coronary heart disease among people who smoked cigarettes	14%

6. What is the prevalence rate of coronary heart disease in Fictiveville? _____

7. What is the incidence rate of coronary heart disease in Fictiveville? _____

8. What is the relative risk for coronary heart disease in smokers compared with nonsmokers?

_____

Copyright © 2024 by Elsevier, Inc. All Rights Reserved.

CIRCLE THE CORRECT WORDS

Circle the correct word from the choices provided to complete these sentences.

9. According to the threshold model, multifactorial diseases that are either present or absent must exceed a (distribution, liability) threshold before the disease occurs.

10. (Similar, In contrast) to most single-gene disorders, occurrence of multifactorial disorders can change greatly from one population to another.

11. Recurrence risks for multifactorial disorders are higher if (only, more than) one family member is affected.

12. Many factors that can be measured numerically, such as blood pressure, are (multifactorial, sex-linked liability distributed).

13. Recurrence risks for multifactorial disorders are higher if the disease is (more, less) severe in the proband.

COMPLETE THE SENTENCES

Write one word in each blank to complete these sentences.

14. Traits that have a _____ distribution usually are caused by additive effects of many genetic and environmental factors.

15. Recurrence risks are calculated for single-gene disorders, but _____ risks may be calculated instead for multifactorial disorders.

16. An individual with whom a pedigree begins is called a _____.

17. Monozygotic twins also are called _____ twins.

18. Genetic variations that promote autoimmunity are associated with type _____ diabetes.

INTERPRET THE TABLE

Examine this table and answer the questions to interpret the numbers.

Concordance Rates in MZ and DZ Twins for Selected Traits and Diseases		
	CONCORDANCE RATE	
Trait or Disease	**MZ Twins**	**DZ Twins**
Bipolar disorder	0.79	0.24
Cleft lip/palate	0.38	0.08
Clubfoot	0.32	0.03
Measles	0.95	0.87
Multiple sclerosis	0.28	0.03
Myocardial infarction (males)	0.39	0.26
Myocardial infarction (females)	0.44	0.14
Schizophrenia	0.47	0.12
Spina bifida	0.72	0.33

DZ, Dizygotic; *MZ,* monozygotic.

Copyright © 2024 by Elsevier, Inc. All Rights Reserved.

19. The concordance rates for measles are similar for monozygotic and dizygotic twins. What does that indicate?

20. The concordance rates for spina bifida are very different for monozygotic and dizygotic twins. What does that indicate?

21. Compare the concordance rates for bipolar disorder for monozygotic and dizygotic twins. What does that indicate?

MATCH THE GENE VARIANTS

Match the genes on the right with the conditions on the left for which variants in these genes increase the risk.

_____ 22. Hypertension

_____ 23. Obesity

_____ 24. Coronary heart disease

_____ 25. Alzheimer's disease

_____ 26. Schizophrenia

A. Presenilin genes

B. Angiotensinogen genes

C. Leptin genes

D. Genes whose products interact with glutamate receptors

E. LDL receptor genes

TEACH PEOPLE ABOUT PATHOPHYSIOLOGY

Write your response to each situation in the space provided.

27. Mr. Medlow's daughter has phenylketonuria (PKU), an autosomal recessive disorder. "Is high blood pressure autosomal recessive?" asks Mr. Medlow. "A lot of my relatives have high blood pressure, but I exercise and diet to control my blood pressure without drugs. Is high blood pressure really genetic?"

28. "What does dizygotic mean?" asks Mrs. Hendel. "I heard the doctor say that my twin boys are dizygotic. Does that mean something bad like a birth defect?"

29. "I wish people would quit telling me to exercise and stop smoking," says Mr. van Cleeve. "That will not do me any good because my father died from a heart attack when he was only 52. I hear that the tendency to heart attack is inherited, so I am doomed to die early."

Copyright © 2024 by Elsevier, Inc. All Rights Reserved.

Chapter **5 Genes, Environment-Lifestyle, and Common Diseases**

MATCH THE DEFINITIONS

Match the word on the right with its definition on the left.

_____ 1. Protein around which DNA winds   A. Transcription

_____ 2. Process of making mRNA from a section of DNA   B. Chromatin

_____ 3. Proteins and DNA in the nucleus   C. Gene

_____ 4. Section of DNA that carries the code for a protein or noncoding RNA   D. Histone

CIRCLE THE CORRECT WORDS

Circle the correct word from the choices provided to complete these sentences.

5. Epigenetics is regulation of gene expression (caused by, not caused by) altered DNA sequence.

6. DNA methylation leads to (activation, silencing) of genes.

7. Epigenetic modifications (are, are not) maintained in successive mitotic cell divisions.

8. The process of predictable gene silencing on one copy of a chromosome but not on the other, depending on which parent transmits the chromosome, is known as (imprinting, epigenetics).

9. (miRNA, mRNA) carries the code for a protein to a ribosome, but (miRNA, mRNA) can regulate gene expression.

10. (Some, No) epigenetic modifications can be reversed.

11. Abnormal methylation of tumor-suppressor genes may be a factor in (regression, progression) of specific types of cancer.

EXPLAIN THE PICTURES

Examine the pictures and answer the questions about them.

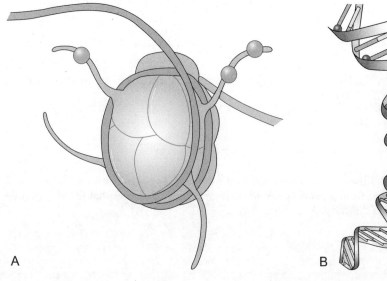

A   B

Copyright © 2024 by Elsevier, Inc. All Rights Reserved.

12. Which picture shows a nucleosome? _____

13. Acetylation of histone tails activates genes by allowing chromatin to unwind, which gives transcription factors access to the DNA. Which picture has histones in it? _____

14. Which picture shows specifically where transcription occurs? _____

15. When histone deacetylase removes the acetyl groups from a histone, what effect does that have on gene transcription? Why?

16. When excessive methylation occurs in picture B, what effect does that have on gene transcription? Why?

COMPLETE THE SENTENCES

Write one word in each blank to complete these sentences.

17. A gene that has methylation in its _____ region is less likely to be transcribed into mRNA.

18. MicroRNAs that stimulate development and progression of cancer are called _____.

19. Genes that are necessary to maintain function of all types of cells and that normally remain transcriptionally active are called _____ genes.

20. Hereditary transmission of epigenetic changes to successive generations is called epigenetic _____ inheritance.

21. Environmental chemicals, dietary factors, and alcohol intake can modify gene expression by causing _____ modifications.

TEACH PEOPLE ABOUT PATHOPHYSIOLOGY

Write your response to each situation in the space provided.

22. "I am reading a journal article about cancer development," says another nurse. "What happens when the promoter region of tumor suppressor genes is hypermethylated? Does that encourage or discourage development of cancer?"

23. "What is noncoding RNA?" asks Mr. Stevens. "When I studied biology in college, we learned about the genetic code and RNA, but I do not understand what noncoding RNA would be. Please explain."

Copyright © 2024 by Elsevier, Inc. All Rights Reserved.

24. "How is it possible for several types of cells to arise from one kind of stem cell?" asks a medical student. "I know that all cells have the same DNA, but different genes are active in different cell types. Help me understand."

CLINICAL SCENARIO

Read the clinical scenario and answer the questions to explore your understanding of genomic imprinting.

Robbie, age 4, who has Prader-Willi syndrome, has come for a well-child examination. No symptoms reported by parents or child. Moderate mental developmental delay verified by psychologist.

Physical Examination

- Vital signs normal
- Muscle tone diminished
- Height below normal for age; BMI in obesity range
- Hands and feet appear small in relation to body size
- Genitals underdeveloped for age

25. *Complete the sentence by choosing from the lists of options.*

    Robbie's assessment is consistent with _____(1)_____ syndrome, which is caused by a deletion of a portion of chromosome 15 that was inherited from his _____(2)_____.

Options for 1	Options for 2
Angelman	Father
Prader-Willi	Mother

26. In the syndrome that Robbie has, which copy of the crucial genes is imprinted?

27. Does imprinting of these genes occur normally, or is this an abnormal occurrence?

28. How is it possible for Prader-Willi syndrome and Angelman syndrome to arise from a defect in the same location of the same chromosome?

Copyright © 2024 by Elsevier, Inc. All Rights Reserved.

7 Innate Immunity: Inflammation and Wound Healing

MATCH THE DEFINITIONS

Match each word on the right with its definition on the left.

_____ 1. A signaling molecule that attracts white blood cells

_____ 2. A pattern recognition protein on innate immune cells

_____ 3. Substance released by damaged cells that activates coagulation

_____ 4. Enzyme that degrades fibrin polymers in clots

A. Toll-like receptor

B. Tissue factor

C. Plasmin

D. Chemokine

MATCH THE FUNCTIONS

Match the functions on the right with the cells on the left.

_____ 5. Eosinophils

_____ 6. Mast cells

_____ 7. Natural killer cells

_____ 8. Macrophages

_____ 9. Neutrophils

A. Eliminate virus-infected cells

B. Phagocytize microorganisms and cellular debris; secrete chemicals that promote tissue healing; activate adaptive immunity

C. Defend against parasites; degrade vasoactive substances released by mast cells

D. Phagocytize microorganisms and cellular debris soon after injury; secrete chemicals that call in longer-acting phagocytes

E. Release chemicals that initiate the inflammatory response

CIRCLE THE CORRECT WORDS

Circle the correct words from the choices provided to complete these sentences.

10. The first line of defense against microorganisms is (anatomic barriers, phagocytic cells).

11. Surfactant and other chemical defenses produced by lung epithelium are called (collectins, resistin-like molecules).

12. The microorganisms that typically colonize the body surfaces are called the normal (microbiome, bacteriocins).

13. (Kinins, Defensins) are a type of chemical barrier, but (kinins, defensins) are chemicals involved in the inflammatory response.

Copyright © 2024 by Elsevier, Inc. All Rights Reserved.

14. One innate immune cell can recognize many different types of pathogenic bacteria because it has (pattern recognition receptors, adhesion molecules).

15. A membrane attack complex, formed by the activated (complement, coagulation) cascade, causes (clot formation, cell lysis).

COMPLETE THE OVERVIEW TABLE

Complete this table by writing the correct letter in each blank in the table.

A. T and B lymphocytes, antibodies
B. Skin, mucous membranes, gastric acid, microbiome
C. Phagocytes and some nonphagocytic immune cells

Nonspecific Defense Mechanisms of Innate Immunity		Specific Defense Mechanisms
First Line of Defense: Physical and Biochemical Barriers	Second Line of Defense: Inflammation	Third Line of Defense: Adaptive (Acquired) Immunity
16. _____	17. _____	18. _____

CATEGORIZE THE IMMUNE CELLS

Write the type of immune cell beside its name. Choices: phagocytic innate, nonphagocytic innate, adaptive.

_____ 19. Mast cell

_____ 20. Lymphocyte

_____ 21. Macrophage

_____ 22. Neutrophil

ORDER THE STEPS

Sequence the events that occur during acute inflammation.

23. Write the letters here in the correct order of the steps: _____
    A. Local edema
    B. Tissue damage caused by injury
    C. Increased vascular permeability
    D. Leakage of plasma into tissues
    E. Vasodilation
    F. White blood cell margination and entry into tissues

Sequence the events that occur when a circulating neutrophil enters tissue and phagocytizes a microorganism.

24. Write the letters here in the correct order of the steps: _____
    A. Diapedesis
    B. Engulfment and formation of phagosome
    C. Margination
    D. Recognition and attachment
    E. Formation of phagolysosome
    F. Destruction of the microorganism
    G. Increased adhesion molecules
    H. Chemotaxis

 Copyright © 2024 by Elsevier, Inc. All Rights Reserved.

DESCRIBE THE DIFFERENCES

Describe the difference between each pair of terms.

25. What is the difference between a PAMP and a DAMP?

26. What is the difference between the specificity of innate and adaptive immunity?

27. What is the difference between opsonins and cytokines?

EXPLAIN THE PICTURES

Examine the pictures and answer the questions about them.

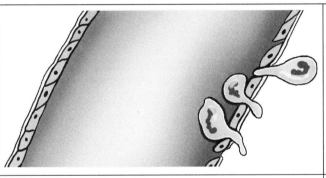

28. What one word describes what these cells are doing? _____

29. After these cells have left the blood vessel, what directs them to the site of tissue injury?

30. What does PMN mean? _____

31. Which cell is the PMN? _____

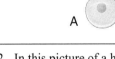

A   B

32. In this picture of a healing wound, fibroblasts are migrating into the area. Which phagocytic cells secrete chemicals to attract them? _____

_____

33. What is the function of these fibroblasts? _____

_____

34. Does wound contraction occur before or after fibroblast migration and proliferation? _____

_____

33

Copyright © 2024 by Elsevier, Inc. All Rights Reserved.

COMPLETE THE SENTENCES

Write one word in each blank to complete these sentences.

35. Physical barriers such as the skin and mucous membranes are part of _____ immunity.

36. During chronic inflammation, the body may wall off an infectious agent by forming a _____.

37. Plasma protein systems such as complement are called _____ because each component of the system activates the next component.

38. A raised scar that extends beyond the original boundaries of the wound is called a _____.

39. Wound _____ is the pulling apart of a wound at the suture line.

40. Normal neonates have increased risk for sepsis and meningitis because they are partially deficient in the blood protein cascade known as _____.

41. Age-associated changes in older adults that delay tissue healing include loss of _____ that normally bring blood to the area.

42. Activated mast cells release preformed inflammatory mediators immediately by _____ and release other inflammatory mediators more slowly after _____ them.

COMPLETE THE TABLE

Complete this table by filling in the empty boxes.
Characteristics of Immune Defenses

Aspect	Barrier Function of Innate Immunity	Inflammatory Response of Innate Immunity	Adaptive Immunity
43. How soon does this defense begin working after first contact with a pathogen?			
44. Does this defense remember the pathogen and act more rapidly upon subsequent exposure?			
45. Does each component of this defense work against many different antigens (nonspecific) or only one antigen (specific)?			

CHARACTERIZE THE EXUDATES

Match the characteristics on the right with the types of exudates on the left.

_____ 46. Fibrinous exudate   A. Watery, with few proteins or cells

_____ 47. Purulent exudate   B. Another term for purulent exudate

_____ 48. Hemorrhagic exudate   C. Thick and clotted

_____ 49. Suppurative exudate   D. Containing many red blood cells

_____ 50. Serous exudate   E. Containing many white blood cells

 Copyright © 2024 by Elsevier, Inc. All Rights Reserved.

Apply your knowledge by choosing the best answer for each question in these clinical situations.

51. Mr. Mewe lay on a concrete floor for 9 hours after a heroin overdose and developed a deep pressure injury on his sacrum. He was taken to drug rehabilitation, and his wound is healing with no complications. Which term should a nurse use when describing this mode of healing to a professional colleague?
    A. Callus formation
    B. Primary intention
    C. Remodeling
    D. Secondary intention

52. Emily, age 6, has an infected finger and has just been given an antibiotic. Her mother is very worried because the finger is red and swollen. After a nurse tells her that these signs will go away as the infection and inflammation resolve, Emily's mother asks, "Is inflammation really bad for you? It feels so bad." She needs to know that inflammation does what?
    A. Creates serious delays in wound healing.
    B. Causes pain and tissue destruction.
    C. Promotes the spread of bacteria to the other tissue.
    D. Neutralizes and destroys microorganisms.

53. A new nurse asks, "Why is fever associated with inflammation? What causes it?" Choose the best response.
    A. Inflammatory chemicals called cytokines cause fever.
    B. Mast cell degranulation causes fever.
    C. Infection, especially bacterial infection, causes fever.
    D. Macrophage chemotaxis causes fever.

54. Mrs. Tuttle had a hysterectomy 2 days ago. A nurse who is doing discharge teaching is discussing the importance of rest and nutrition when Mrs. Tuttle interrupts. "I can take pain pills if it hurts," she says. "I am a very busy person, and I do not have time to rest!" What principle should underlie the nurse's response?
    A. Débridement is a necessary component of wound healing.
    B. Wound contraction takes time, and rest and good nutrition will assist it.
    C. Reconstruction and maturation enable a healing wound to be strong.
    D. When epithelialization has occurred, tissue healing is nearly complete.

55. Mrs. Kienow has inflamed knuckles from rheumatoid arthritis. "Why do my poor inflamed finger joints feel so hot when I touch them?" she asks. Choose the best response.
    A. More warm blood comes to the inflamed area.
    B. Heat means that your small blood vessels are leaky.
    C. Infecting bacteria produce heat by fast metabolism.
    D. Invading immune cells from your blood cause the heat.

TEACH PEOPLE ABOUT PATHOPHYSIOLOGY

Write your response to each situation in the space provided.

56. "What is innate immunity?" asks Mr. Birde. "I thought you had to be vaccinated to get immunity."

57. "Why is my knee so red?" asks Jessica, age 7, who scraped her knee when she fell in the park. "I want to know why!"

Copyright © 2024 by Elsevier, Inc. All Rights Reserved.

58. "I understand why it hurts, but what makes a sprained ankle swell up like that?" asks Mrs. Kellerman.

59. "How do my white blood cells know how to get to this infected mosquito bite?" asks David, age 14. "I thought white blood cells are in the blood."

60. "That nurse said that healing this sore is only her secondary intention," says Mr. Dow, who has a deep sacral pressure injury. "That is ridiculous! This sore is the reason that I am here!"

61. "My doctor said I got this fungus because penicillin killed off my normal microbiome," says Mrs. Hunt. "What does 'normal microbiome' mean?"

62. "What does it mean that my C-reactive protein is increased?" asks Mr. Jek. "The doctor said it is an 'acute-phase reactant,' but I do not know what that is."

WORK WITH THE CLINICAL SCENARIO

Stage 1:

Mr. Moreno and his brother Miguel were on their way to work when they had an automobile accident in which they both sustained multiple cuts, but no head injuries, broken bones, or spinal cord injuries. Mr. Moreno was barely on time for his shift at the chicken processing plant, where he worked in maintenance. Other than wiping the blood off his hands while he put on his coveralls, he did not take time to wash or cover the cuts on his arm because he was afraid his supervisor would penalize him for being late. Miguel, who worked at a fast food restaurant across the street, also was barely on time for his shift. His supervisor saw the fresh wounds on his arm and told him to wash and use bandages from the first aid kit before he started taking orders.

Assess risk factors and select the best words to complete this sentence.

63. Based on the circumstances, _____(1)_____ has the greater risk of developing _____(2)_____.

Options for 1	Options for 2
Mr. Moreno	Inflammation
Miguel	Wound infection

Copyright © 2024 by Elsevier, Inc. All Rights Reserved.

Stage 2:

Several days later, Mr. Moreno and Miguel come to the neighborhood clinic where you are a nurse. Two of Mr. Moreno's cuts are very red and swollen on their edges, which are not fully approximated (the cut edges do not touch). One of the cuts is oozing a thick whitish liquid. Miguel's wounds are all slightly red and swollen on their edges, with no discharge; they are fully approximated. One wound on his forearm is an open crater; the edges of the wound do not meet because skin and underlying tissue were gouged away. This wound is light red under the bandage and is not weeping.

Interpret each assessment finding by placing an X in the appropriate square.

Assessment Finding	Normal Tissue Healing	Possible Wound Infection
64. Cuts very red and swollen on their edges, which are not fully approximated		
65. Cuts slightly red and swollen on their edges; no discharge and fully approximated		
66. Open crater; light red and not weeping		
67. Cut oozing a thick whitish liquid		

Copyright © 2024 by Elsevier, Inc. All Rights Reserved.

Chapter **7** Innate Immunity: Inflammation and Wound Healing

8 Adaptive Immunity

MATCH THE DEFINITIONS

Match the word on the right with its definition on the left.

_____ 1. Antibody-producing cell

_____ 2. Cell that suppresses immune response to self-antigens

_____ 3. Small antigen that binds to large molecules and induces an immune response

_____ 4. Portion of an antigen that is recognized and bound by an antibody or specific lymphocyte receptor

_____ 5. Molecule that activates an unusually large population of immune cells

A. Hapten

B. Superantigen

C. Epitope

D. Plasma cell

E. T-regulatory cell

COMPLETE THE OVERVIEW

Fill in the two blanks to complete the overview of immunity.

6.

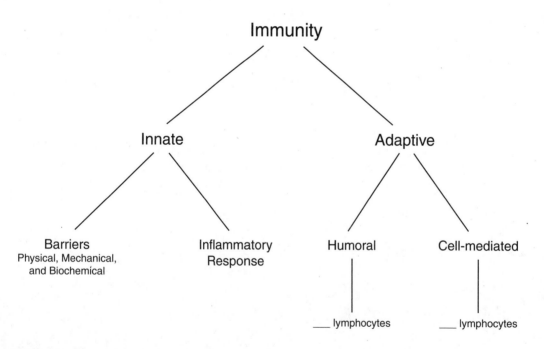

CIRCLE THE CORRECT WORDS

Circle the correct words from the choices provided to complete these sentences.

7. Human MHC molecules are known as (APC, HLA) antigens.

8. All nucleated cells have (MHC I, MHC II) molecules, whereas antigen-presenting cells have (MHC I, MHC II, both MHC I and MHC II) molecules.

Copyright © 2024 by Elsevier, Inc. All Rights Reserved.

9. (Dendritic cells, Macrophages) are the most effective in presenting antigen to naive immunocompetent Th cells.

10. In the last trimester, a fetus can produce (IgE, IgG, IgM) in response to an in utero infection.

11. Physical interactions between B lymphocytes and (Th1, Th2) cells are necessary for B lymphocytes to become activated.

12. Involution of the thymus with aging causes decreased capacity for (B lymphocyte function, T lymphocyte differentiation).

CATEGORIZE THE CLINICAL EXAMPLES

Write the type of immunity beside each clinical example. Choices: active, passive.

_____ 13. Neonate does not develop an infection because they have maternal antibodies that they received in breast milk.

_____ 14. Child does not develop an infection because they have been immunized against it.

_____ 15. Adult does not develop an infection because they were infected with that same microorganism previously and recovered.

_____ 16. Adult does not develop an infection because they were given gamma globulin after being exposed to an infected person.

ORDER THE STEPS

Sequence the events that occur during development of a mature CD4$^+$ cell.

17. Write the letters here in the correct order of the steps: _____
    A. APC presents processed antigen with MHC class II molecules to T cell.
    B. Lymphoid stem cell migrates to thymus.
    C. T cell differentiates and matures to CD4$^+$ cell.
    D. Cell divides and differentiates, developing T-cell receptors and surface markers.
    E. Immunocompetent naive T cell migrates to secondary lymphoid organ.

DESCRIBE THE DIFFERENCES

Describe the difference between each pair of terms.

18. What is the difference between central and peripheral tolerance?

19. What is the difference between the targets of antibodies and cytotoxic T cells?

20. What is the difference between the location of MHC class I molecules and MHC class II molecules?

Copyright © 2024 by Elsevier, Inc. All Rights Reserved.

EXPLAIN THE PICTURES

Examine the pictures and answer the questions about them.

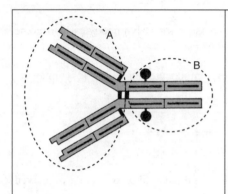

21. Which circle shows the Fab fragment of this Ig? _____

22. Why is the Fab fragment important?

23. Which circle shows the Fc fragment? _____

24. In what way is it beneficial that some innate immune cells have Fc receptors?

25. Look at the labels on the graph. Does this graph pertain to the innate immune system or the adaptive immune system?

26. Which curves rise sooner after exposure to antigen, those in section A or section B? _____

27. Why do the curves you identified rise sooner after antigen exposure?

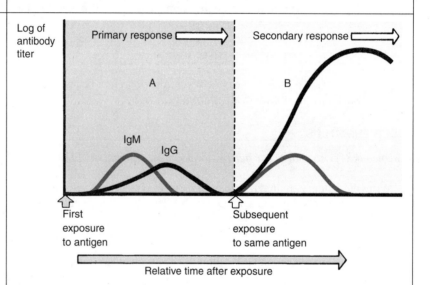

COMPLETE THE SENTENCES

Write one word in each blank to complete these sentences.

28. Another name for antigenic determinant is _____.

29. A substance included in a vaccine to stimulate immune response is called an _____.

30. CD1 antigen-presenting molecules present exogenous _____ antigens.

31. Helper T cells recognize molecules bound on MHC class _____ molecules, but cytotoxic T cells recognize molecules bound on MHC class _____ molecules.

32. The secondary immune response is produced by _____ cells.

33. Cytokines secreted by Th1 cells promote _____ immunity; cytokines secreted by Th2 cells promote _____ immunity; cytokines secreted by Th17 cells promote _____; cytokines secreted by Treg cells _____ the immune response.

Copyright © 2024 by Elsevier, Inc. All Rights Reserved.

34. The term *class switch* indicates that a B lymphocyte changes from producing _____ to producing another class of immunoglobulin.

35. Cytotoxic T cells kill their target cells by secreting _____ that make a pore in the membrane and injecting _____ through the pore, causing apoptosis.

36. Th1 cells activate macrophages by secreting _____.

CHARACTERIZE THE IMMUNOGLOBULINS (IGS)

Match the characteristics on the right with the types of immunoglobulin on the left.

_____ 37. IgE   A. Most abundant class of Igs; are transported across the placenta

_____ 38. IgM   B. Low concentration in blood; are surface receptors on developing B lymphocytes

_____ 39. IgG   C. Active against parasites; are important mediators of allergic responses

_____ 40. IgA   D. Produced during the primary response to antigen; are the largest Igs

_____ 41. IgD   E. Most abundant in body secretions

TEACH PEOPLE ABOUT PATHOPHYSIOLOGY

Write your response to each situation in the space provided.

42. Mr. Jeffers has multiple myeloma, a plasma cell cancer. "I have two questions," he says. "First, what is a plasma cell? I know mine are cancerous, but I do not know what they are. Second, my cancer doctor said I have Bence-Jones protein in my urine, as he expected. He says Bence-Jones protein is 'immunoglobulin light chains,' but I have no idea what that is. Please explain."

43. A nurse tells Jason, age 14, that he will make antibodies after his immunization. "What good are antibodies, anyway?" asks Jason.

44. "Antibodies are proteins," says Nurse Lee. "How can infants get antibodies through breast milk? I think they would be destroyed by digestion."

45. "The medical student said that NK cells are my friends when I have a virus infection," says Ms. Collins. "What are NK cells? Are they the ones that make antibodies?"

Copyright © 2024 by Elsevier, Inc. All Rights Reserved.

9 Alterations in Immunity and Inflammation

MATCH THE DEFINITIONS

Match the word on the right with its definition on the left.

_____ 1. Adaptive immune response misdirected against the body's own cells

_____ 2. Immune system of one individual produces an immunologic reaction against tissues of another individual

_____ 3. Altered adaptive immune response that causes disease or damage to the host

_____ 4. Deleterious effects of hypersensitivity to noninfectious environmental antigens

A. Allergy

B. Hypersensitivity

C. Alloimmunity

D. Autoimmunity

CIRCLE THE CORRECT WORDS

Circle the correct word from the choices provided to complete these sentences.

5. An individual is (allergic, sensitized) when an adequate amount of antibodies or T cells is available to cause a noticeable reaction on reexposure to the antigen.

6. Delayed hypersensitivity reactions involve (B, T) lymphocytes, but not (B, T) lymphocytes.

7. In antibody-dependent cell-mediated cytotoxicity, target cells often die by (phagocytosis, lysis).

8. Defective peripheral tolerance is a factor in development of (type II hypersensitivity, autoimmunity).

9. Individuals with type O blood are universal (recipients, donors) because their RBCs have (no A and B antigens, both A and B antigens).

10. Genetic predisposition to autoimmunity often involves (MHC, CD_4) alleles.

11. Graft-versus-host disease occurs in graft recipients who are (immunocompetent, immunocompromised).

12. Histamine released from mast cells causes signs and symptoms of inflammation by binding to (H1, H2) receptors.

13. Although type II hypersensitivity reactions can affect cells by several different mechanisms, they all involve antigens that are expressed in (many different, only specific) tissues.

CATEGORIZE THE CLINICAL EXAMPLES

Write the type of hypersensitivity beside each clinical example. Choices: type I (IgE-mediated), type II (tissue-specific), type III (immune complex), type IV (cell-mediated).

_____ 14. Child develops systemic anaphylaxis after eating peanut butter.

Copyright © 2024 by Elsevier, Inc. All Rights Reserved.

_____ 15. Adult develops rejection of a transplanted heart.

_____ 16. Adult develops rash on legs from poison ivy after hiking in shorts.

_____ 17. Adult develops hemolysis after mismatched blood transfusion.

_____ 18. Adolescent develops systemic anaphylaxis after being stung by a wasp.

ORDER THE STEPS

Sequence the events that occur during development of a type I hypersensitivity response.

19. Write the letters here in the correct order of the steps: _____
    A. B lymphocytes produce IgE against the allergen.
    B. IgE attaches to mast cells.
    C. Individual has initial exposure to the allergen.
    D. Mast cells degranulate.
    E. IgE circulates in blood.
    F. IgE on mast cells binds allergen.
    G. Individual has additional allergen exposure.
    H. Individual has clinical signs and symptoms of allergy.
    I. Individual has genetic predisposition to allergy.

EXPLAIN THE PICTURE

Examine the picture of immune complex–mediated hypersensitivity and answer the questions about it.

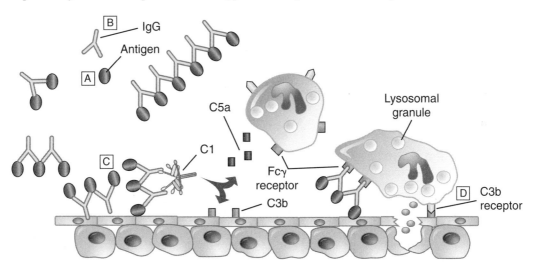

20. Which letter shows the immune complexes? _____

21. What happens to the larger and smaller immune complexes that do not bind to tissue?

22. Why do the neutrophils migrate to this area?

Copyright © 2024 by Elsevier, Inc. All Rights Reserved.

23. What causes the clinical manifestations?

COMPLETE THE SENTENCES

Write one word in each blank to complete these sentences.

24. Autoimmunity occurs when the immune system reacts against _____ to such a degree that autoantibodies or autoreactive T cells damage the person's own tissues.

25. Hypersensitivity reactions require _____ against a particular antigen that results in primary and secondary immune responses.

26. Complement deficiencies often involve recurrent infections with encapsulated bacteria because C3b is an

    _____.

27. Hypogammaglobulinemia is classified as a _____ lymphocyte deficiency.

28. Severe deficit in calories and protein impairs function of _____ lymphocytes and neutrophils.

29. DiGeorge syndrome involves deficient _____ lymphocyte immunity due to complete or partial lack of

    the _____.

30. Antibodies can _____ target cell receptors, as in Graves' disease; antibodies also can destroy or

    _____ receptors, as in myasthenia gravis.

31. Unusual or recurrent severe infections are common indicators of immune _____.

32. The technical term for hives is _____.

TEACH PEOPLE ABOUT PATHOPHYSIOLOGY

Write your response to each situation in the space provided.

33. "When immune complexes form, phagocytic cells are supposed to remove them," says a nurse. "Why does immune complex hypersensitivity occur instead?"

34. "What does the 'combined' mean in severe combined immunodeficiency disease?" asks Mrs. Quoit, whose son has SCID.

35. "My physician said my cancer drugs gave me a secondary immunodeficiency, so I get sick easily," says Mr. Erie. "I think it is important! Why did she say it is secondary?"

Copyright © 2024 by Elsevier, Inc. All Rights Reserved.

36. "Why not just look at this TB skin test in an hour or so?" asks Mr. Rush. "I am going on a business trip tomorrow and cannot come back later this week."

CLINICAL SCENARIO

Read the clinical scenario and answer the questions to explore your understanding of systemic lupus erythematosus.

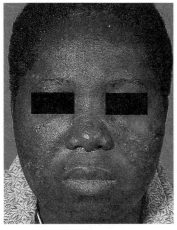

(From Forbes CD, Jackson WF: *Color atlas and text of clinical medicine*, ed 3, London, 2003, Mosby.)

Ayisha Walker, a 36-year-old woman studying medicine, has aching in her joints (arthralgia) and a new rash on her face. She states that the rash gets worse when she goes out into the sun. She also feels fatigued and gets a sharp pain in her chest when she breathes deeply. She has had "flare-ups" of these symptoms from time to time in the past, but this is the worst episode ever.

Physical Examination

- Vital signs normal

- Facial rash over her cheeks and the bridge of her nose

- Discoid scaling red rash on extremities, especially the extensor surfaces of the arms

- Finger and ankle joints with pain and stiffness on passive and active movement

- Chest examination reveals pleural friction rub heard on deep inspiration

- Cardiac, abdominal, and neurologic examinations normal

Laboratory Results

- Serum electrolytes normal

- Hematocrit and hemoglobin low; platelet count slightly low; white blood count normal

- Blood urea nitrogen (BUN) and creatinine elevated; protein present in the urine

- Chest radiograph shows a small collection of pleural fluid

- Anti-DNA antibodies positive; antinuclear antibody (ANA) positive

Copyright © 2024 by Elsevier, Inc. All Rights Reserved.

Ms. Walker's diagnosis is systemic lupus erythematosus (SLE).

37. What is the common descriptive term for Ms. Walker's facial rash?

38. Why should Ms. Walker be taught to avoid sunlight?

39. Which of Ms. Walker's laboratory results indicate renal dysfunction? Is renal dysfunction associated with SLE, or is it more likely that she also has a renal disease unrelated to SLE?

40. What other aspects of her history, physical examination, and laboratory results are manifestations of SLE?

41. What does ANA mean? Why is it important in SLE?

42. How can SLE cause such widespread tissue damage? What is the pathophysiology?

43. What is a type III hypersensitivity reaction?

Copyright © 2024 by Elsevier, Inc. All Rights Reserved.

10 Infection

MATCH THE DEFINITIONS

Match the word on the right with its definition on the left.

_____ 1. Ability to spread from one individual to others and cause disease

_____ 2. Agent that carries infectious microorganisms from an infected organism to uninfected ones

_____ 3. Capacity of an organism to cause severe disease

_____ 4. Normally not causing disease, but able to do so when an individual's immune system is suppressed

A. Virulence

B. Communicability

C. Opportunistic

D. Vector

CIRCLE THE CORRECT WORDS

Circle the correct word from the choices provided to complete these sentences.

5. Previously unknown infections are known as (emerging, pathogenic) infections.

6. A housefly is an example of a (biologic, mechanical) vector.

7. The term *horizontal transmission* refers to microorganisms spread from (mother to child, one person to another) through blood and body fluids.

8. (Endotoxins, Exotoxins) are secreted, but (endotoxins, exotoxins) are released when the bacteria die.

9. An organism's ability to adhere to host tissue is important in the process of (inflammation, colonization).

10. Bacteria that have a (capsule, nucleus) are difficult to phagocytize.

11. Antigenic variation helps a pathogen to (reproduce much more rapidly, avoid recognition by the host).

CATEGORIZE THE ORGANISMS

Write the type of organism beside its name. Choices: bacterium, virus, fungus, parasite.

_____ 12. *Aspergillus*

_____ 13. *Staphylococcus*

_____ 14. *Candida*

_____ 15. *Plasmodium*

_____ 16. *Pneumocystis*

_____ 17. *M. tuberculosis*

_____ 18. *Histoplasma*

Copyright © 2024 by Elsevier, Inc. All Rights Reserved.

_____ 19. *E. coli*

_____ 20. *Giardia*

_____ 21. *Salmonella*

_____ 22. *Clostridium*

ORDER THE STEPS

Sequence the events that occur when HIV infects a host cell.

23. Write the letters here in the correct order of the steps: _____
    A. HIV envelope fuses with host cell membrane, and viral contents enter host cell.
    B. HIV virion in body fluids encounters a susceptible host cell.
    C. New virion is assembled, buds from host cell, matures, and becomes infectious.
    D. Viral enzyme integrase inserts viral DNA into host cell DNA.
    E. Viral DNA is transcribed.
    F. Viral enzyme reverse transcriptase converts viral RNA into viral DNA.
    G. Viral envelope gp120 binds host cell CD4 and a chemokine co-receptor.
    H. mRNA for viral proteins is translated.

EXPLAIN THE PICTURES

Examine the pictures and answer the questions about them.

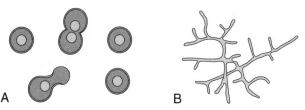

A   B

(From Goering R et al: *Mim's medical microbiology,* ed 5, London, 2013, Saunders.)

24. These pictures show fungi. Which one is the mold? _____

25. What term is used to describe the fungal form in the picture that is not mold? _____

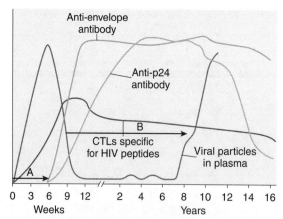

Time in this graph is the time of HIV infection.
CTL, cytotoxic T-lymphocytes

(From Kumar V, Abbas A, Fausto N: *Robbins & Cotran pathologic basis of disease,* ed 8, Philadelphia, 2010, Saunders.)

Copyright © 2024 by Elsevier, Inc. All Rights Reserved.

26. What two-word term indicates the time span denoted by the arrow marked A? _____

27. What happens in the body during this time?

28. What two-word term indicates the time span denoted by the arrow marked B? _____

29. What signs and symptoms would the individual experience during this time? _____

DESCRIBE THE DIFFERENCES

Describe the difference between each pair of terms.

30. What is the difference between endemic and epidemic?

31. What is the difference between epidemic and pandemic?

32. What is the difference between pathogenicity and immunogenicity?

33. What is the difference between biologic and mechanical vectors?

COMPLETE THE SENTENCES

Write one word in each blank to complete these sentences.

34. Some bacteria use rod-like projections called _____ to adhere to the tissues they colonize.

35. During the _____ stage of infectious disease, the individual has the first symptoms, which often include mild fatigue.

36. Gram-_____ bacteria have lipopolysaccharide in the outer membrane that is known as _____.

37. A man developed an upper respiratory infection 3 days after his sick daughter sneezed in his face. His infection had a 3-day _____ period.

38. Bacteria that grow in complex multicellular masses called _____ have some protection from host immune responses and antibiotics.

Copyright © 2024 by Elsevier, Inc. All Rights Reserved.

39. The HIV glycoprotein gp120 binds to the _____ molecule in the plasma membrane of its host cells.

40. The technical term for fungal infections is _____.

41. *Plasmodium* replication occurs in _____ and often causes _____ from lysing them.

42. Fungal infections that are localized in healthy individuals can become _____ in immunosuppressed individuals.

43. Bacteria that produce _____ are resistant to many of the penicillins.

44. An infection that transmits from an animal reservoir is called a _____ infection.

TEACH PEOPLE ABOUT PATHOPHYSIOLOGY

Write your response to each situation in the space provided.

45. Ms. Desmond says, "If viruses reproduce inside cells, why should I get a flu shot to make antibodies that are outside the cells?"

46. "The doctor said I have an opportunistic infection," says Mr. Levine, who has AIDS. "What does that mean?"

47. Billy, age 6, is scheduled for his MMR (measles, mumps, rubella) booster shot. "Why do I have to have this measles shot?" he asks. "Mommy said I had this shot when I was a baby."

48. Mrs. Hayes has been HIV positive for 1 year. Her CD4$^+$ cell count is normal. "Wonderful!" she says. "I thought HIV destroyed CD4$^+$ cells. I guess I was wrong."

49. Mr. Lee has AIDS and is hospitalized with dehydration from diarrhea. His nurse wears gloves when cleaning his perineum and emptying his bedpan. "You do not need to wear gloves," he says. "The Internet says that bowel movements do not transmit HIV." How should his nurse respond?

50. Mrs. Hedges took an HIV test after her husband died of AIDS. Her test is positive, and her CD4$^+$ cell count is normal. "Oh, no!" she exclaims. "Now I have AIDS and am going to die too!"

Copyright © 2024 by Elsevier, Inc. All Rights Reserved.

51. "Why such excitement about Kaposi sarcoma?" asks Mr. Thew, who has AIDS. "It is ugly, but it is just a skin cancer. I am more worried about dying of AIDS."

CLINICAL SCENARIO

Read the clinical scenario and answer the questions to explore your understanding of HIV infection and AIDS.

Kevin Hohner, age 37, has shortness of breath and cough. He reports weight loss of 10 pounds in the last 2 months. He states that he has had pneumonia twice in the past year. He has a prior history of unprotected anal sex with multiple partners but has been in a stable relationship for the past 6 years. His partner is HIV negative, but Mr. Hohner has not been tested for HIV.

Physical Examination

- Vital signs normal except for elevated respiratory rate

- Crackles in the lower half of lung fields, with inspiratory and expiratory rhonchi

- Reddish-brown, flat lesions on the chest and arms (see figure)

- Cardiac, abdominal, and neurologic examinations normal

- Perianal vesicular and ulcerative lesions

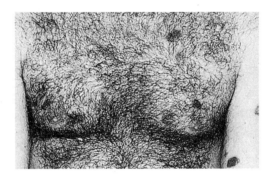

Laboratory Results

- Serum electrolytes, BUN, and creatinine normal

- Chest radiograph shows diffuse infiltrates

- CD4+ T cells 180 cells/microliter (low); CD4+/CD8+ cell ratio below normal

- Anti-HIV antibodies present; HIV viral particle load substantial

Copyright © 2024 by Elsevier, Inc. All Rights Reserved.

Mr. Hohner's diagnoses are AIDS, Pneumocystis pneumonia, Kaposi sarcoma, and perianal herpes simplex virus.

52. Why did Mr. Hohner develop Kaposi sarcoma, an unusual type of cancer?

53. Why is his CD4$^+$ T cell count so low?

54. What is the relationship between his low CD4$^+$ T cell count and Mr. Hohner's *Pneumocystis* pneumonia?

55. Given the usual course of HIV infection, for how long has Mr. Hohner most likely been HIV positive?

    _____

56. Why did he have HIV infection for so long before it was discovered?

Interpret each assessment finding by placing an X to mark the diagnosis with which it is associated.

Assessment Finding	Kaposi Sarcoma	Pneumocystis Pneumonia
57. Shortness of breath and cough		
58. Reddish-brown, flat lesions on chest and arms		
59. Elevated respiratory rate		
60. Crackles in the lower half of lung fields, with inspiratory and expiratory rhonchi		

Copyright © 2024 by Elsevier, Inc. All Rights Reserved.

11 Stress and Disease

MATCH THE DEFINITIONS

Match each word on the right with its definition on the left.

_____ 1. Chronic overactivation of adaptive regulatory physiologic systems that increases susceptibility to disease

_____ 2. The process of managing stressful challenges that impact the individual's resources

_____ 3. Dynamic physiologic regulation around a changed or changing set point

_____ 4. Physiologic regulation around a narrow set point

A. Homeostasis

B. Allostasis

C. Allostatic overload

D. Coping

IDENTIFY THE EFFECTS OF SYMPATHETIC NERVOUS SYSTEM ACTIVATION

Write "increased" or "decreased" beside each item to indicate whether activation of the sympathetic nervous system increases or decreases it from the normal value.

_____ 5. Heart rate and contractility

_____ 6. Blood pressure

_____ 7. Blood glucose

_____ 8. Skin blood flow

_____ 9. Peristalsis in gastrointestinal tract

_____ 10. Sphincter tone in gastrointestinal tract

_____ 11. Diameter of bronchioles

CIRCLE THE CORRECT WORDS

Circle the correct word from the choices provided to complete these sentences.

12. The general adaptation syndrome is a (specific, nonspecific) response to noxious physiologic stimuli, as described by (Hans Selye, Walter Cannon).

13. Posttraumatic stress disorder occurs in response to (anticipation, memory) of traumatic events, whereas a conditioned response occurs in response to (anticipation, memory) of traumatic events.

14. Research demonstrates that immune modulation by psychosocial stressors or interventions (leads directly to, does not influence) health outcomes.

15. Repetitive negative thinking was reported to be a potential risk factor for (PTSD, dementia).

16. Epinephrine (increases, decreases) blood levels of free fatty acids.

17. The cortisol effect on protein metabolism is (anabolic, catabolic) in the liver and (anabolic, catabolic) in muscle and other tissues.

18. Cortisol (decreases, increases) blood glucose and (decreases, increases) secretion of gastric acid.

53

Copyright © 2024 by Elsevier, Inc. All Rights Reserved.

19. Low socioeconomic status of the family is associated with increased (cortisol, growth hormone) during childhood.

20. Adverse life events that have a large negative impact on immunity are those that are perceived as (predictable, uncontrollable).

CATEGORIZE THE CLINICAL SITUATIONS

Write the type of stress response beside each situation. Choices: reactive, anticipatory.

_____ 21. Adult develops pounding heart, dry mouth, and shaking hands when her boss tells her she is fired from her job.

_____ 22. Student develops pounding heart, dry mouth, and shaking hands halfway through an examination.

_____ 23. Student develops pounding heart, dry mouth, and shaking hands the night before an examination while studying.

_____ 24. Adult develops pounding heart, dry mouth, and shaking hands after finding a rat in the apartment building garbage area.

_____ 25. Child develops pounding heart, dry mouth, and shaking hands when his brother tells him that a monster is under the bed.

_____ 26. Adult develops pounding heart, dry mouth, and shaking hands in the car on the way to a chemotherapy appointment.

EXPLAIN THE PICTURE

Examine the picture and answer the questions about it.

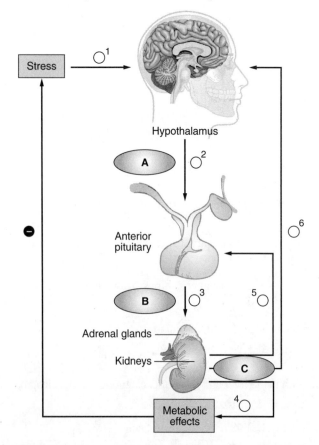

27. Write the names of the hormones represented by the letters.

    A. _____

    B. _____

    C. _____

28. In the circles labeled 1 though 6, write either + (plus) or − (minus) to indicate whether the process is activating or inhibitory.

29. What two-word physiology term is used for the inhibitory effects noted in this picture? _____
    _____

30. Which numbered circle shows the potentially deleterious actions on the body that occur with chronic stress? _____

Copyright © 2024 by Elsevier, Inc. All Rights Reserved.

IDENTIFY THE EFFECTS OF COPING STRATEGIES

Write "beneficial" or "maladaptive" by each item to indicate the general result of the coping strategy.

_____ 31. Regular exercise

_____ 32. Mindfulness

_____ 33. Cigarette smoking

_____ 34. Diet rich in sugar and fat

_____ 35. Seeking social support

COMPLETE THE SENTENCES

Write one word in each blank to complete these sentences.

36. Many researchers believe that acute inflammation is beneficial, whereas chronic low-grade _____ inflammation is associated with numerous chronic diseases.

37. When a physiologic or psychological demand exceeds an individual's coping abilities, the individual experiences _____.

38. Epinephrine and norepinephrine are called _____.

39. The hypothalamic hormone called _____-releasing hormone activates the _____ axis.

40. Catecholamines bind to _____ receptors.

41. Cortisol delays tissue healing by decreasing proliferation of _____ in connective tissue.

42. Norepinephrine in the brain promotes arousal, _____ vigilance, and _____ anxiety.

43. The cumulative effects of physiologic responses to stressors are known as _____ load.

44. The hormone _____, which has increased release during a response to stressors, promotes social attachment.

45. Estrogen tends to _____ immune responses, while androgens tend to _____ immune responses.

46. Poor wound healing occurs in people who have elevated _____ levels.

47. Regular physical activity has an _____ effect that decreases the risk of many diseases.

TEACH PEOPLE ABOUT PATHOPHYSIOLOGY

Write your response to each situation in the space provided.

48. A nurse asks, "When I bring the oximeter into the room, why do some of my patients get a sympathetic response with tachycardia and others do not?"

Copyright © 2024 by Elsevier, Inc. All Rights Reserved.

49. "How can stress affect immunity?" asks a nurse. "Immune cells are not connected to sympathetic nerves; they are moving around in the body."

50. Farley, age 11, receives outpatient chemotherapy. "Why does my heart pound when I have to come to the hospital for chemo?" he asks. "It is scary enough without my heart pounding so fast!"

51. "When I get stressed, my allergies always get worse," says Mr. Williams. "I know my allergies involve antibodies, but I would like to know how being stressed makes my allergies worse."

WORK WITH THE CLINICAL SCENARIO

Clinical Scenario:

Samir has type 2 diabetes that he manages well with medications, diet, and regular exercise. He has come to your clinic for his usual appointment to review his blood glucose logs and check his blood values. On the sidewalk in front of the clinic, he fell when he jumped out of the way of two people riding scooters while looking at their cell phones. Samir was not injured, but his hands still were shaking while these parameters were measured: body weight, blood glucose, plasma free fatty acids, heart rate, blood pressure, waist-hip ratio.

52. Highlight or underline the assessment parameters in the above scenario that you would expect to be higher than Samir's usual baseline.

53. What physiologic response was responsible for increasing all of these assessment parameters?
    A. HPA axis
    B. Sympathetic nervous system
    C. Immune system activation
    D. Low-grade systemic inflammation

Copyright © 2024 by Elsevier, Inc. All Rights Reserved.

12 Cancer Biology

NAME THE NEOPLASMS

Match the description on the right with the neoplasm name on the left.

_____ 1. Lipoma

_____ 2. Sarcoma

_____ 3. Carcinoma

_____ 4. Osteogenic sarcoma

_____ 5. Rhabdomyoma

_____ 6. Liposarcoma

_____ 7. Adenocarcinoma

_____ 8. Leiomyoma

_____ 9. Hepatocellular carcinoma

_____ 10. Rhabdomyosarcoma

A. Malignant tumor arising from connective tissue

B. Malignant tumor of glandular epithelium

C. Malignant tumor of fat cells

D. Malignant tumor of skeletal muscle

E. Benign tumor of fat cells

F. Benign tumor of smooth muscle

G. Malignant bone tumor

H. Benign tumor of skeletal muscle

I. Malignant tumor arising from epithelial tissue

J. Primary liver cancer

CIRCLE THE CORRECT WORDS

Circle the correct word from the choices provided to complete these sentences.

11. If the cancer stem cells in a tumor survive cytotoxic chemotherapy, the tumor is likely to (self-destruct, regrow).

12. Progression from a benign polyp to a malignant tumor requires (multiple, one or two) mutations.

13. The normal (oncogene, proto-oncogene) *ras* becomes the (oncogene, proto-oncogene) *ras* when a mutation makes the RAS protein active all the time.

14. Malignant tumors in the intestines most commonly metastasize to the (lungs, liver).

15. Malignant tumors are (heterogeneous, homogeneous) in their cellular composition.

16. In the presence of oxygen, normal cells metabolize glucose by (glycolysis, oxidative phosphorylation), and cancer cells metabolize it by (glycolysis, oxidative phosphorylation).

17. For a cell to become cancerous, multiple changes must occur in its (genes, enzymes).

18. (Acute, Chronic) inflammation predisposes to development of cancer.

Copyright © 2024 by Elsevier, Inc. All Rights Reserved.

MATCH THE DEFINITIONS

Match the word on the right with its definition on the left.

_____ 19. Having variable size and shape

_____ 20. The process by which a cell develops a specialized organization and function

_____ 21. Having no cellular differentiation

_____ 22. The process by which a normal cell becomes a cancer cell

_____ 23. A new growth

_____ 24. Abnormal growth caused by uncontrolled proliferation

A. Anaplastic

B. Tumor

C. Transformation

D. Neoplasm

E. Pleomorphic

F. Differentiation

CATEGORIZE THE CHANGES

Write the potential effect of the change beside its description. Choices: procancer effect, anticancer effect.

_____ 25. Point mutation inactivates one tumor suppressor gene allele; epigenetic change silences the other.

_____ 26. Chromosome translocation creates Philadelphia chromosome.

_____ 27. Point mutation inactivates proto-oncogene.

_____ 28. Decreased expression of specific noncoding RNAs causes increased expression of oncogenes.

_____ 29. Gene amplification creates multiple copies of gene for epidermal growth factor receptor.

_____ 30. DNA methylation occurs in the promoter regions of both copies of a tumor suppressor gene.

_____ 31. Epigenetic modification silences an oncogene.

_____ 32. Mutation disrupts caretaker gene.

_____ 33. Chromosome instability causes loss of both copies of tumor suppressor genes.

ORDER THE STEPS

Sequence the events that occur when a carcinoma successfully metastasizes through the blood.

34. Write the letters here in the correct order of the steps: _____
    A. Cancer cells attach to endothelium, attracted by tissue-specific characteristics and survival signals.
    B. Tumor microenvironment drives cell dedifferentiation by epithelial-to-mesenchymal transition.
    C. Cancer cells circulate, evading the immune system by associating with platelets or other mechanisms.
    D. Mutations enable self-renewal, anchorage independence, increased motility, and secretion of proteases.
    E. Cancer cells secrete chemical signals that co-opt local and circulating cells, creating a new cancerized micro-environment where they proliferate.
    F. Cancer cells intravasate, facilitated by leaky blood vessels created through angiogenesis.
    G. Cancer cells extravasate, facilitated by their motility characteristics and vascular remodeling.

Copyright © 2024 by Elsevier, Inc. All Rights Reserved.

COMPLETE THE CHART

Fill in the blank spaces within the chart to compare and contrast the characteristics of benign and malignant tumors.

Characteristic	Benign Tumors	Malignant Tumors
Appearance of the Cells	Well differentiated	
Usual Rate of Growth	Slow	
Presence of Capsule		
Vascularization	Slight	
Mode of Growth	Expansile	
Ability to Metastasize		

EXPLAIN THE PICTURE

Examine the picture and answer the questions about it.

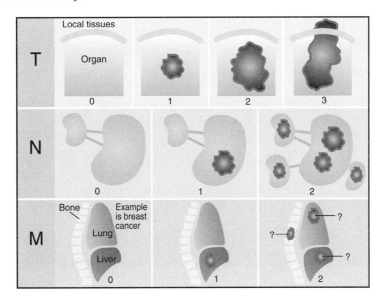

This picture shows a TNM system for breast cancer.

35. What do these letters represent?

    T = _____ ; N = _____ ; M = _____

36. Does assigning the TNM numbers grade or stage the cancer? _____

37. Write the TNM numbers for a woman with breast cancer that has metastasized to her lungs, has invaded her chest wall, and has involved several fixed lymph nodes. _____

Copyright © 2024 by Elsevier, Inc. All Rights Reserved.

Chapter **12 Cancer Biology**

DESCRIBE THE DIFFERENCES

Describe the difference between each pair of terms.

38. What is the difference between a proto-oncogene and an oncogene?

39. What is the difference between a proto-oncogene and a tumor-suppressor gene?

40. What is the difference between a driver mutation and a passenger mutation?

COMPLETE THE SENTENCES

Write one word in each blank to complete these sentences.

41. Stem cells and cancer cells are able to divide indefinitely because they make the enzyme _____.

42. Tumors stimulate formation of new blood vessels by secreting _____ factors.

43. Abnormal premalignant growths in epithelial tissues that have not crossed the basement membrane are called carci-noma _____ _____.

44. Mutations in caretaker genes contribute to _____ instability, which _____ the risk for devel-oping cancer.

45. A cancer cell that secretes growth factors that stimulate its own growth engages in _____ stimulation.

46. Characteristics of cancer cells that enable them to survive and proliferate include loss of resistance to apoptosis and development of anchorage _____.

47. Survival of malignant tumors is facilitated by tumor-associated _____ that secrete cytokines and other factors that assist cancer cell survival and proliferation.

48. Most cervical cancers are caused by infection with certain strains of _____.

TEACH PEOPLE ABOUT PATHOPHYSIOLOGY

Write your response to each situation in the space provided.

49. A nurse asks, "Why do so many of our cancer patients have hypercalcemia, even when they do not have bone metastases?"

Copyright © 2024 by Elsevier, Inc. All Rights Reserved.

50. "My uncle has liver cancer and so does my mom," says Sandi Mauntz. "But the doctor said his cancer is primary and hers is metastatic. What does that mean?"

51. Mr. Winslow has small cell carcinoma of the lung with persistent hyponatremia. "The doctor told me that my husband has 'ectopic production' of some hormone and 'paraneoplastic syndrome,' but then her beeper rang and she had to leave in a hurry," says Mrs. Winslow. "Please finish the explanation. What hormone? What do ectopic and paraneoplastic mean?"

52. "What is the Warburg effect?" asks Nurse Davidson, who is reading a journal article about cancer treatments. "What does that mean?"

53. "Now please explain the reverse Warburg effect," says Nurse Davidson. "Does that mean the cancer cells make glucose instead of burning it for energy?"

CLINICAL SCENARIOS

Read the clinical scenarios and answer the questions to explore your understanding of cancer.

Ms. Lavenia Smith, age 67, went to see a nurse practitioner because of dyspnea and a chronic cough. When asked, Ms. Smith stated that she has smoked cigarettes since she was a teenager. Pulmonary function tests show a definite blockage in her airflow, a chest radiograph shows a lesion, and bronchoscopy washings contain malignant cells. Her diagnosis is bronchogenic lung cancer. Histologically, it is a squamous cell carcinoma.

54. Why did Ms. Smith have a blockage in her airflow?

55. Did Ms. Smith's lung cancer metastasize from cancer in another location in her body, or did it arise in her lungs? What information provides this answer?

56. Why did Ms. Smith develop dyspnea?

Copyright © 2024 by Elsevier, Inc. All Rights Reserved.

57. The lining of the bronchi normally is pseudostratified columnar epithelium, not squamous cells. Why did Ms. Smith's cancer develop from squamous cells?

Ms. Smith is scheduled for surgery, followed by radiation therapy and chemotherapy. Surgery will remove the bulk of the tumor, and the radiotherapy is expected to shrink remaining lung tumor cells. The chemotherapy is aimed at metastatic liver tumors that were discovered. Ms. Smith has stopped smoking.

58. Why did Ms. Smith's oncologist order a liver scan after discovering that Ms. Smith had bronchogenic carcinoma?

59. Why had Ms. Smith's cancer metastasized before she had enough signs and symptoms to seek out a nurse practitioner?

Mrs. Gillespie died from stage 4 colon cancer. Her son Tom, age 52, was diagnosed with stage 1 colon cancer that was treated successfully with surgery and chemotherapy. Tom Gillespie has a lot of questions as he reflects on his experiences.

60. "My mother had stage 4 cancer and she died; I had stage 1 cancer and I survived," says Tom. "Obviously stage 4 is worse, but how do the doctors determine what stage a cancer is?"

61. "I remember the oncologist telling my sister and me that our mother's cancer had spread to her liver. What was that fancy meta- word that he used?" asks Tom.

62. Tom asks, "Does everybody who gets liver cancer have cancer someplace else first?"

63. "I am grateful that I survived chemotherapy," says Tom. "I knew I would lose my hair, but I was surprised when I got those painful sores in my mouth. How did the chemo cause the sores?"

64. Tom says, "I got so tired during the chemo. My doctor said I was anemic. Did the chemo kill off my red blood cells too?"

65. "My mother had a lot of pain, but the nurses managed the pain medications very well," says Tom. "What surprised me is that I did not feel any pain, except from the surgery and those mouth sores. Why didn't I have cancer pain?"

Copyright © 2024 by Elsevier, Inc. All Rights Reserved.

13 Cancer Epidemiology

MATCH THE DEFINITIONS

Match the word on the right with its definition on the left.

_____ 1. Smoke exhaled by a smoker

_____ 2. Smoke from the burning end of a cigarette, cigar, or pipe

_____ 3. Smoke from the burning end of a cigarette, cigar, or pipe plus the smoke exhaled by the smoker

A. Sidestream smoke

B. Environmental tobacco smoke

C. Mainstream smoke

CIRCLE THE CORRECT WORDS

Circle the correct word from the choices provided to complete these sentences.

4. Epigenetic changes that (silence, activate) tumor-suppressor genes by DNA (breakage, methylation) facilitate cancer initiation and progression.

5. Infiltration of (red blood, immune) cells supports the progression of a malignant tumor.

6. Potentially damaging radiofrequency radiation is emitted by (cell phones, CT scans).

7. Studies suggest that malnutrition can (increase, decrease) repair of DNA.

8. Chemicals that are not synthesized in the body but may be found in foods are called (xenobiotics, nutrigenomics).

9. Exercising muscle secretes (adipokines, myokines) with numerous effects that (increase, decrease) the risk for several types of cancer.

10. B vitamins are modulators of DNA (double strand breakage, methylation).

11. Obesity (decreases, increases) the risk for numerous types of cancer.

CATEGORIZE THE DIETARY FACTORS

Write the type of cellular effect beside each dietary factor. Choices: procancer, anticancer.

_____ 12. Lycopene from tomatoes

_____ 13. Polyphenols from tea

_____ 14. *N*-nitroso compounds from nitrites

_____ 15. Organosulfur compounds from garlic

_____ 16. Aflatoxin from moldy peanuts

Copyright © 2024 by Elsevier, Inc. All Rights Reserved.

COMPLETE THE SENTENCES

Write one word in each blank to complete these sentences.

17. Cancer-causing substances are called _____.

18. Secondhand smoke is a common term that means _____ tobacco smoke.

19. The term _____ means the study of the interactions between nutrition and an individual's genetic makeup.

20. The degree to which development of a fetus depends on its environment is called developmental _____.

21. Regular exercise decreases the risk for several types of cancer, independent of changes in body _____.

22. Adipose tissue releases _____, which influence inflammation and insulin resistance.

23. _____ radiation from sunlight causes _____ cell and squamous cell carcinomas and increases the risk for malignant _____.

24. _____ radiation from x-rays and computed tomography scans can initiate premalignant cell changes and promote preexisting ones.

25. _____ increases the risk for malignant mesothelioma and lung cancer; _____ released from rocks and soil increases the risk for lung cancer.

26. Ionizing radiation can contribute to carcinogenesis by _____ oncogenes and _____ tumor-suppressor genes.

MATCH THE MICROORGANISMS

Match the microorganisms on the right with their associated types of cancer on the left.

_____ 27. Gastric cancer

_____ 28. Cervical cancer

_____ 29. Liver cancer

_____ 30. Kaposi sarcoma

A. Hepatitis B and C viruses

B. *Helicobacter pylori*

C. Human herpesvirus type 8

D. Human papillomavirus types 16 and 18

TEACH PEOPLE ABOUT PATHOPHYSIOLOGY

Write your response to each situation in the space provided.

31. "My doctor said that I should avoid processed foods containing nitrites," says Mrs. Golt, who has a family history of colon cancer. "I know that means hot dogs, but are there others? And what do nitrites have to do with colon cancer anyway?"

Copyright © 2024 by Elsevier, Inc. All Rights Reserved.

32. "I hear that drinking too much alcohol increases the risk for cancer," says Mr. Taylor. "I do not drink hard liquor like vodka or gin. I drink beer, so I am not at risk. Right?"

33. "I have HPV, and it caused early cervical cancer. My doctors removed the cancer and said not to worry, but I am concerned that the HPV may have spread to my bones and caused cancer there. My aunt had cancer, and it went to her bones before she died. Should I get my bones checked for cancer?"

34. "I heard the radiologist talking about bystander effects," says Mr. Merino, whose cancer is being treated with radiation therapy. "Was someone standing too close to the machine when it was turned on? Or is the machine leaking radiation?"

35. "Help me understand this research about environmental carcinogens," says another nurse. "It talks about transgenerational effects and multigenerational effects. What is the difference?"

WORK WITH THE CLINICAL SCENARIO

Highlight or circle the risk factors for cancer that are part of this scenario.

36. Mr. Ortiz works in the dye department of a textile factory. He lives 3 blocks from a petrochemical plant. Several times a week, he goes to a bar with his friends after their work shift, and drinks beer until closing time. He usually eats hot dogs or sausages at the bar for dinner. He does not smoke cigarettes, but the bar is smoky from others who do smoke. Mr. Ortiz cannot afford a cell phone or a car. If he needs to ask a friend to drive him somewhere that is not within walking distance, he repays them by helping remove old siding and flooring from abandoned houses they are trying to make livable.

Copyright © 2024 by Elsevier, Inc. All Rights Reserved.

14 Cancer in Children

DESCRIBE THE CANCERS

Match the description on the right with the neoplasm name on the left.

_____ 1. Leukemia

_____ 2. Embryonal tumor

_____ 3. Wilms tumor

_____ 4. Retinoblastoma

A. Tumor that originates during fetal life and involves immature cells

B. Malignant eye tumor associated with specific genetic mutations

C. Malignant renal tumor associated with congenital abnormalities

D. Malignancy of blood-forming cells

CATEGORIZE THE CANCERS

Write the age group with the highest incidence beside each type of cancer. Choices: children/adolescents, adults.

_____ 5. Prostate cancer

_____ 6. Brain tumors

_____ 7. Neuroblastoma

_____ 8. Lung cancer

_____ 9. Wilms tumor

_____ 10. Acute leukemia

CIRCLE THE CORRECT WORDS

Circle the correct word from the choices provided to complete these sentences.

11. Children appear to be (less, more) sensitive to radiation than adults, which is a concern with CT scans.

12. Children who have Down syndrome have increased risk of developing acute (leukemia, retinoblastoma).

13. In general, childhood cancers grow (slowly, rapidly).

14. Childhood cancer has a bimodal distribution with the peaks at age (less than 5 years, 5-10 years) and age (10-15 years, 15-19 years).

15. Mutations in (oncogenes, proto-oncogenes) that convert them to (oncogenes, proto-oncogenes) drive development of cancer by causing uncontrolled cell growth.

16. The letters (oma, blast) in the name of a tumor indicate that it is an embryonal tumor.

Copyright © 2024 by Elsevier, Inc. All Rights Reserved.

MATCH THE RISKS

Match the type of cancer on the right with its potential risk on the left.

_____ 17. Adolescent uses anabolic steroids to increase muscle mass.

_____ 18. Child has Fanconi anemia.

_____ 19. Adolescent's mother received DES during pregnancy.

_____ 20. Child has MYCN oncogene.

A. Acute myelogenous leukemia

B. Vaginal adenocarcinoma

C. Neuroblastoma

D. Hepatocellular carcinoma

COMPLETE THE SENTENCES

Write one word in each blank to complete these sentences.

21. The cancers that cause the most deaths in children are brain tumors and _____.

22. Cryptorchidism (undescended testicles) is a risk factor for _____ cancer.

23. Children who have environmental exposure to insecticides and pesticides have increased incidence of _____.

24. Children who have AIDS have increased risk for developing _____ sarcoma and non-Hodgkin _____.

25. The concept that includes interaction of many factors to produce cancer is called _____ etiology.

26. Retinoblastoma and Wilms tumor are associated with disabled _____ _____ genes.

TEACH PEOPLE ABOUT PATHOPHYSIOLOGY

Write your response to each situation in the space provided.

27. Mr. Johnson's 2-year-old daughter has been diagnosed with neuroblastoma. He says, "I know that many adult cancers are linked with chemicals in the environment. Why can't the doctors tell us what chemicals are linked with her kind of cancer so that we can have our house tested for them?"

28. "The doctor said Calvin's cancer came from the mesodermal germ layer," says Mrs. Klughart, whose young son has cancer. "What does that mean? Was there an infection?"

29. Mr. Talison's son has just received a cancer diagnosis. "Oh, no! My son has cancer! Now he is going to die!" he exclaims.

Copyright © 2024 by Elsevier, Inc. All Rights Reserved.

30. Another nurse is reading a research study that links exposure to pesticides to development of leukemia. "A big percentage of the children who were exposed to pesticides did develop leukemia, but some of them did not," she says. "So how can I interpret this study?"

31. An oncology nurse who works with adults says, "I see carcinomas commonly in my adult cancer patients, but I just learned that carcinomas are uncommon in children. Why?"

Copyright © 2024 by Elsevier, Inc. All Rights Reserved.

15 Structure and Function of the Neurologic System

MATCH THE DEFINITIONS

Match each word on the right with its definition on the left.

_____ 1. A bundle of axons

_____ 2. Protective membranes surrounding the brain and spinal cord

_____ 3. Brain system that includes the amygdala, hippocampus, and thalamus

_____ 4. Composed of the midbrain, pons, and medulla oblongata

_____ 5. Insulating lipid material that surrounds axons

_____ 6. Neuron extension that carries impulses away from the cell body

_____ 7. Neuron extension that carries impulses toward the cell body

_____ 8. The structure that connects the cerebral hemispheres

_____ 9. Cranial nerve II

_____ 10. Cranial nerve X

A. Axon

B. Corpus callosum

C. Myelin

D. Tract

E. Vagus

F. Meninges

G. Optic

H. Brainstem

I. Dendrite

J. Limbic

CATEGORIZE THE PHYSIOLOGIC EFFECTS

Write the branch of the autonomic nervous system whose stimulation would cause each effect. Choices: sympathetic, parasympathetic.

_____ 11. Increased diameter of pupils

_____ 12. Dry mouth

_____ 13. Contraction of bladder detrusor muscle

_____ 14. Increased plasma free fatty acids

_____ 15. Bradycardia

_____ 16. Increased salivation

_____ 17. Cool, pale skin

_____ 18. Hyperglycemia

Copyright © 2024 by Elsevier, Inc. All Rights Reserved.

_____ 19. Dilation of bronchioles

_____ 20. Increased blood pressure

_____ 21. Increased peristalsis in intestines

EXPLAIN THE PICTURES

Examine the pictures and answer the questions about them.

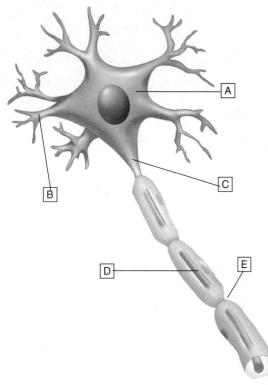

(From Patton KT, Thibodeau GA: *Anatomy & physiology,* ed 8, St Louis, 2013, Mosby.)

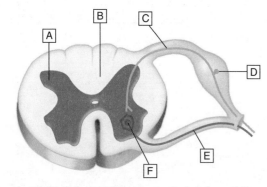

(From Patton KT, Thibodeau GA: *Anatomy & physiology,* ed 8, St Louis, 2013, Mosby.)

22. Which letter in the picture indicates an axon?

_____

23. Which letter in the picture indicates a dendrite?

_____

24. Which letter indicates the location where an action potential begins? _____

25. Name the location where an action potential begins.

_____

26. Draw an arrow on the picture to indicate which way the action potential normally travels.

27. Is this neuron unipolar, bipolar, or multipolar?

_____

28. Name the structure marked E in the picture.

_____

29. What is the benefit of having this type of structure on neurons?

30. Which letter in the picture of the spinal cord indicates the cell body of a sensory neuron? _____

31. Which letter in the picture indicates the cell body of a motor neuron? _____

32. What neural structures are marked C and E?

_____

33. Why is the area marked A darker in color than the area marked B?

Copyright © 2024 by Elsevier, Inc. All Rights Reserved.

CIRCLE THE CORRECT WORDS

Circle the correct word from the choices provided to complete these sentences.

34. Neurons (need, do not need) insulin in order to take in glucose.

35. The principle of neural (malleability, plasticity) indicates that the central nervous system is capable of change.

36. An example of (convergence, divergence) is a primary afferent neuron whose axons synapse with several spinal cord neurons at different levels of the spinal cord.

37. The epidural space is (potential, real) in the skull and (potential, real) in the spinal cord.

38. The basal ganglia are part of the (pyramidal, extrapyramidal) pathways.

39. Cell bodies of spinal lower motor neurons are located in the (white, gray) matter of the spinal cord; their axons synapse with (skeletal, vascular smooth) muscles.

40. The thoracolumbar division of the autonomic nervous system is (sympathetic, parasympathetic), and the craniosacral division is (sympathetic, parasympathetic).

41. The term *adrenergic* refers to (sympathetic, parasympathetic) nerves that are (preganglionic, postganglionic, both preganglionic and postganglionic).

ORDER THE STRUCTURES

Start with the skin and place the structures in their anatomic order, moving inward to the cerebral cortex.

42. Write the letters here in the correct order of the structures: _____
    A. Skin
    B. Pia mater
    C. Periosteum externum
    D. Subarachnoid space
    E. Dura mater
    F. Arachnoid mater
    G. Skull
    H. Subdural space
    I. Cerebral cortex
    J. Muscle

Copyright © 2024 by Elsevier, Inc. All Rights Reserved.

MATCH THE FUNCTIONS

Match the functions with the brain areas designated by letters.

_____ 43. Voluntary motor movement

_____ 44. Vision

_____ 45. Goal-oriented behavior, decision making

_____ 46. Touch and other sensations

_____ 47. Hearing

_____ 48. Motor coordination

_____ 49. Speech

DESCRIBE THE DIFFERENCES

Describe the difference between each pair (or group) of terms.

50. What is the difference between efferent nerves and afferent nerves?

51. What is the difference between the somatic nervous system and the autonomic nervous system?

52. What is the difference between a gyrus, a sulcus, and a fissure in the brain?

53. What is the difference between the anatomic routes that the cranial nerves and the spinal nerves travel to exit the central nervous system on their way to the periphery of the body?

Copyright © 2024 by Elsevier, Inc. All Rights Reserved.

54. What is the difference between an EPSP and an IPSP?

COMPLETE THE SENTENCES

Write one word in each blank to complete these sentences.

55. The peripheral nervous system consists of _____ pairs of spinal nerves and 12 pairs of _____ nerves.

56. The general term for nervous system cells that are not neurons is _____.

57. Interneurons transmit impulses from neuron to _____ within the central nervous system.

58. In the central nervous system, _____ form the myelin sheaths, but in the peripheral nervous system _____ _____ form the myelin sheaths.

59. Groups of cell bodies in the peripheral nervous system are called _____, but groups of cell bodies in the central nervous system are called _____.

60. The _____ plexuses produce cerebrospinal fluid, which returns to the blood at the _____ villi.

61. In a synapse, the space between the two neurons is called the synaptic _____.

62. The _____ body secretes melatonin.

63. Neurons with cell bodies in the substantia nigra use _____ as a neurotransmitter.

64. The technical word for motor nerves crossing contralaterally in the medulla oblongata is _____.

65. When an axon in the peripheral nervous system is severed, a process called _____ degeneration occurs, causing the axon to disappear and the _____ cells to line up in a pathway that facilitates nerve regeneration.

66. Cranial nerves III, IV, and VI are necessary for normal movement of the _____; cranial nerve XII is necessary for normal movement of the _____; cranial nerve _____ is necessary to shrug the shoulders normally against resistance.

TEACH PEOPLE ABOUT PATHOPHYSIOLOGY

Write your response to each situation in the space provided.

67. "When my father had a stroke that affected his left arm and leg, the doctor said the stroke was in the right side of my father's brain," says Mr. Yarrow. "But my cousin lost coordination of the left side of her body after injury to her cerebellum, and the doctor said the injury was on the left side, not the right side. Is one of the doctors wrong?"

Copyright © 2024 by Elsevier, Inc. All Rights Reserved.

68. Mrs. Goldblatt may have trigeminal nerve injury. What tests should be used to assess her trigeminal nerve function?

69. "All these names are so confusing!" exclaims a new nurse. "Rubrospinal tract, spinothalamic tract! How can I remember where they go so I can understand what happens if they are damaged?"

70. Mrs. Espinoza's son has a recent head injury and is in the hospital. "Why did they tell me to be sure his neck is straight and his head does not lean to the side?" she asks.

PUZZLE OUT THESE TECHNICAL TERMS

Use the clues to complete the puzzle, demonstrating your knowledge of important technical terms.

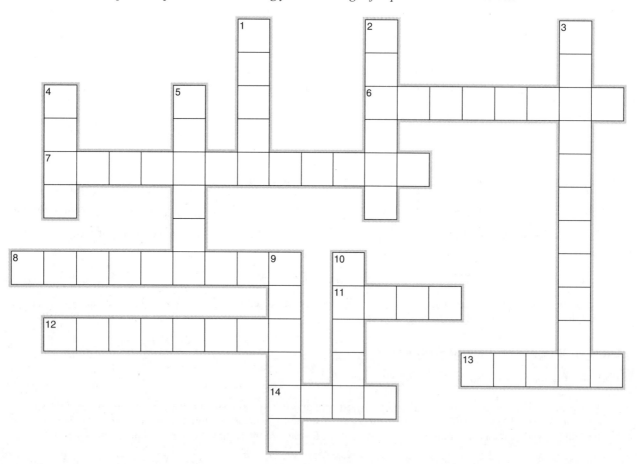

Chapter **15** **Structure and Function of the Neurologic System**   Copyright © 2024 by Elsevier, Inc. All Rights Reserved.

Across

6. Protective membranes surrounding the brain and spinal cord

7. The space that contains cerebrospinal fluid

8. Composed of the midbrain, pons, and medulla oblongata

11. Neuron extension that carries impulses away from the cell body

12. Neuron extension that carries impulses toward the cell body

13. A bundle of axons

14. The result of hyperpolarization of a postsynaptic membrane

Down

1. Cranial nerve II

2. Brain system that includes the amygdala, hippocampus, and thalamus

3. Neuron that relays impulses toward a synapse

4. The result of depolarization of a postsynaptic membrane

5. With callosum, the structure that connects the cerebral hemispheres

9. Insulating lipid material that surrounds axons

10. Cranial nerve X

Copyright © 2024 by Elsevier, Inc. All Rights Reserved.   Chapter **15 Structure and Function of the Neurologic System**

16 Pain, Temperature Regulation, Sleep, and Sensory Function

MATCH THE DEFINITIONS

Match the word on the right with its definition on the left.

_____ 1. Inflammation of the cornea

_____ 2. Inflammation of the eyelid

_____ 3. Cloudy or opaque portion of the lens of the eye

_____ 4. Sensation of spinning around

_____ 5. Lipogranuloma of oil-secreting gland of the eyelid

_____ 6. Eyelid margin turned inward against the eyeball

A. Vertigo

B. Chalazion

C. Blepharitis

D. Entropion

E. Keratitis

F. Cataract

CIRCLE THE CORRECT WORDS

Circle the correct word from the choices provided to complete these sentences.

7. A patient who lies on a cold examination table without sufficient padding will lose body heat to the table by (convection, conduction).

8. Nonshivering (chemical) thermogenesis occurs when (norepinephrine, acetylcholine) acts on (white, brown) fat.

9. Fever (inhibits, increases) many immune defenses against bacteria and viruses.

10. Children develop (lower, higher) fevers than do adults for minor infections; older adults often have (lower, higher) fevers during infection.

11. Heat stroke is characterized by a very high body temperature, (presence, absence) of sweat, and a (slow, rapid) heart rate.

12. Increased intraocular pressure is the defining characteristic of (macular degeneration, glaucoma).

13. Pain (transmission, transduction) is conversion of chemical or other stimuli into electrophysiologic activity.

14. Pain that is interpreted as coming from a foot after it had been amputated and the stump that had healed is called (phantom, imaginary) limb pain.

Copyright © 2024 by Elsevier, Inc. All Rights Reserved.

CATEGORIZE THE SLEEP DISORDERS

Write the type of sleep disorder beside its name. Choices: dyssomnia, parasomnia. Then match the examples in the right column with each disorder.

_____ 15. Insomnia

Example is _____

_____ 16. Sonnambulism

Example is _____

_____ 17. Hypersomnia

Example is _____

_____ 18. Obstructive sleep apnea syndrome

Example is _____

_____ 19. Jet-lag disorder

Example is _____

A. Obese man snores and gasps at night, frequently falls asleep at his computer at work

B. Woman awakens every night with hip pain and has difficulty falling asleep again

C. Person who flew to Poland from the U.S. has difficulty concentrating and thinking clearly during a meeting

D. Child walks while asleep several nights per month

E. Student often falls asleep while studying and sometimes while driving

ORDER THE SLEEP STAGES

Sequence the stages that occur during a sleep cycle, starting with the individual being awake.

20. Write the letters here in the correct order of the stages: _____
    A. Awake
    B. Stage N3
    C. REM sleep
    D. Stage N2
    E. Stage N1

EXPLAIN THE PICTURE

Examine the picture and answer the questions about it.

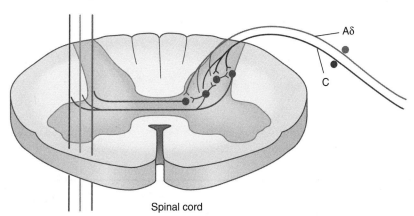

Spinal cord

Copyright © 2024 by Elsevier, Inc. All Rights Reserved.

21. This picture shows pain pathways. Which labeled fibers are unmyelinated? _____

22. What is the clinical significance of the pain pathways crossing to the other side in the spinal cord?

23. What are the names of the tracts in which axons of pain neurons ascend to the brain? _____

24. Which type of pain fiber, A-delta or C, conveys impulses that are interpreted as sharp pain that is highly localized?

_____

25. Where in the spinal cord do the primary pain afferent neurons synapse with the interneurons? _____

_____

DESCRIBE THE DIFFERENCES

Describe the difference between each pair of terms.

26. What is the difference between anosmia and ageusia?

27. What is the difference between conductive and sensorineural hearing loss?

28. What is the difference between fever and hyperthermia?

29. What is the difference between strabismus and nystagmus?

30. What is the difference between presbycusis and presbyopia?

COMPLETE THE SENTENCES

Write one word in each blank to complete these sentences.

31. The _____ is responsible for thermoregulation and modifies heat production, heat _____, or heat loss mechanisms, based on input from thermoreceptors.

78

          Copyright © 2024 by Elsevier, Inc. All Rights Reserved.

32. Growth hormone release occurs during the _____ stages of sleep.

33. The sleep stage in which dreaming occurs is _____.

34. An external hordeolum, commonly called a _____, is infection of the _____ glands of the eyelids.

35. Neonates enter _____ sleep immediately upon falling asleep.

36. Pinkeye is an acute bacterial _____.

37. Papilledema is edema of the _____ nerve where it enters the eyeball and is associated with _____ intracranial pressure.

38. A person who sees double has _____; a person whose eyelid droops has _____.

39. Pain that is felt in an area remote from its point of origin is called _____ pain.

40. Increased sensitivity of dorsal horn neurons that lowers their threshold in neuropathic pain situations is called _____ _____.

41. Visceral pain is transmitted by _____ afferent nerves.

TEACH PEOPLE ABOUT PATHOPHYSIOLOGY

Write your response to each situation in the space provided.

42. "When I started exercising at the gym, the trainer told me not to wipe off my sweat but let it stay on my skin so I would not get heat illness," says Ms. Golan. "Why should I do that? Being sweaty is not lady-like!"

43. "I understand why my patients get fevers from exogenous pyrogens when they have bacterial infections," says another nurse. "But how can a patient who does not have an infection get a mild fever after surgery?"

44. Mr. Smythe is receiving therapeutic hypothermia after a brain injury. His wife says, "I understand why his hand feels so cold, but should I worry because his skin is so pale?"

45. Mr. Nguyen was diagnosed with open-angle glaucoma during a routine eye examination. "I can see fine," he says. "And my eyes do not hurt. Why should I use those glaucoma eyedrops that were prescribed?"

Copyright © 2024 by Elsevier, Inc. All Rights Reserved.

CLINICAL SCENARIOS

Read each clinical scenario and answer the questions.

Dave Redd, age 25, was hired to do physical labor in a factory near large furnaces that melt metals before processing. After several hours of work, during which his clothes became soaked with sweat, Mr. Redd began to feel weak. He kept working because his supervisor yelled at him when he went to get water and he was afraid he would be fired. Near the end of his shift, Mr. Redd became light-headed and nauseated, and then he fainted. He was taken to the employee heath office, which has no laboratory facilities.

Physical examination

- Blood pressure low, tachycardia, no dysrhythmias, increased respiratory rate, body temperature high

- Skin warm and damp

- Reflexes normal

46. Complete the sentence by choosing from the lists of options.

    Mr. Redd is experiencing signs of _____(1)_____ and he should be positioned _____(2)_____.

Options for 1	Options for 2
Heat cramps	Prone
Heat exhaustion	With head and shoulders elevated
Heat stroke	Lying flat, supine

47. What is the reason for positioning Mr. Redd appropriately?

48. Why did Mr. Redd develop this condition?

49. Why did he faint?

50. What caused Mr. Redd's tachycardia?

51. After a short time at the employee heath office, Mr. Redd regained consciousness. What type of fluid should he be given to drink?

   Copyright © 2024 by Elsevier, Inc. All Rights Reserved.

52. What teaching should the health care provider in the employee health office do to help prevent heat exhaustion in the future?

Sandi Howell, age 23, who has type 1 diabetes, fell while skating. She came to the emergency department, stating that her left arm hurt badly and rubbing her left forearm. She denied hitting her head when she fell.

Physical examination

- Tachycardia, no dysrhythmias, blood pressure high, increased respiratory rate

- Skin cool and clammy

- Pupils dilated

- Abrasions on both knees and forearms and left hand

Laboratory results

- Blood glucose and free fatty acids elevated

- Serum electrolytes, BUN, and creatinine normal

- Radiograph of the left forearm shows transverse fracture of the ulna

53. Tissue trauma caused excitation of Ms. Howell's nociceptors when she fell. What factors are causing excitation of her nociceptors now that her broken bone has been immobilized in a cast?

54. What neurotransmitter did her primary-order pain neurons release in the dorsal horn of her spinal cord?

55. What specific physiologic mechanism caused Ms. Howell's tachycardia and increased blood pressure?

56. Which of her other physical examination or laboratory results were caused by the same physiologic mechanism?

57. What benefit might have occurred from Ms. Howell's rubbing her left forearm before the cast was applied?

Copyright © 2024 by Elsevier, Inc. All Rights Reserved.

Mr. Boult, age 61, reports "awful burning pain" in his feet and calves for the past 4 months. He was diagnosed with type 2 diabetes 24 years ago. He manages his diabetes with basal insulin and oral antidiabetic medications.

Physical examination

- Heart rate, blood pressure, and respiratory rate normal

- Cardiac and abdominal examinations normal

- Skin dry

- Lack of touch sensation in the feet and to the midpoint of the calves bilaterally

Laboratory results

- Blood glucose and free fatty acids normal

- Serum electrolytes, BUN, and creatinine normal

Mr. Boult's new diagnosis is diabetic neuropathy.

58. What type of pain does diabetic neuropathy cause? _____

59. Why does Mr. Boult not have physiologic manifestations of pain such as tachycardia and elevated blood pressure?

60. What basic physiologic mechanism causes his neuropathic pain? How is that different from nociceptive pain?

    Copyright © 2024 by Elsevier, Inc. All Rights Reserved.

17 Alterations in Cognitive Systems, Cerebral Hemodynamics, and Motor Function

MATCH THE DEFINITIONS

Match the word on the right with its definition on the left.

_____ 1. Loss of language production or comprehension

_____ 2. Involuntary rapid contractions of muscle groups in a random pattern

_____ 3. Impaired recognition of tactile, visual, or auditory stimuli

_____ 4. Involuntary rhythmic, oscillating movement of a body part

_____ 5. Shock-like, non-patterned muscle contractions causing limb movement; may occur during sleep

_____ 6. Inability to perform purposeful or skilled motor actions

_____ 7. Involuntary slow, twisting, writhing movements

_____ 8. Motor restlessness; compulsion to move lower extremities

A. Agnosia

B. Athetosis

C. Myoclonus

D. Apraxia

E. Akathisia

F. Aphasia

G. Chorea

H. Tremor

CIRCLE THE CORRECT WORDS

Circle the correct words from the choices provided to complete these sentences.

9. Damage to the cerebellum causes (resting, intention) tremor and (ataxic, shuffling) gait.

10. Cheyne-Stokes respirations include a (hypoventilatory, hyperventilatory) response to stimulation by (carbon dioxide, hypoxia).

11. Changes in the pupils are useful to evaluate (cortical, brainstem) function because the areas that control arousal are located (nearby, contralaterally).

12. When autoregulation of intracranial arterioles fails, small increases in blood volume cause intracranial pressure to rise (minimally, greatly).

13. Inflammation from brain injury causes (vasogenic, cytotoxic) cerebral edema.

14. Hypertonia is caused by damage to (upper, lower) motor neurons when the (upper, lower) motor neurons remain functional.

15. Lateral corticospinal tract damage causes (flaccidity, spasticity).

16. Amyotrophic lateral sclerosis involves degeneration of (upper, lower, both upper and lower) motor neurons.

17. Extrapyramidal motor syndromes involve (abnormal movement, paralysis).

18. Nondeclarative memory is (language, motor) memory, but declarative memory is (language, motor) memory.

Copyright © 2024 by Elsevier, Inc. All Rights Reserved.

CATEGORIZE THE DYSFUNCTIONS

Write the type of dysfunction beside each name. Choices: hyperkinesia, hypokinesia, hypertonia.

_____ 19. Loss of associated movements

_____ 20. Chorea

_____ 21. Dystonia

_____ 22. Akathisia

_____ 23. Bradykinesia

_____ 24. Tremor

_____ 25. Myoclonus

_____ 26. Spasticity

_____ 27. Athetosis

_____ 28. Muscle rigidity

ORDER THE LEVELS OF CONSCIOUSNESS

Sequence the progressive changes that occur when a fully alert individual becomes comatose.

29. Write the letters here in the correct order of decreasing consciousness: _____
    A. Light coma
    B. Disorientation
    C. Lethargy
    D. Confusion
    E. Obtundation
    F. Deep coma
    G. Stupor

Copyright © 2024 by Elsevier, Inc. All Rights Reserved.

Examine the pictures and answer the questions about them.

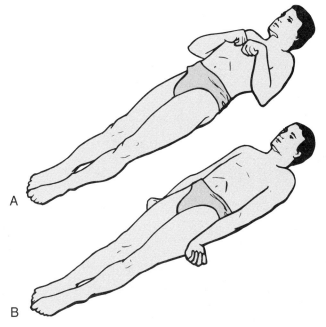

A

B

(From Rudy EB: *Advanced neurological and neurosurgical nursing,* St Louis, 1984, Mosby.)

30. In the posture shown in Figure A, the upper extremities are _____, and the lower extremities are _____.

31. Figure A shows _____ posture.

32. Interruption of inhibitory messages from what part of the brain is believed to cause this posture?

_____

33. In the posture shown in Figure B, the upper extremities are _____, and the lower extremities are _____.

34. Figure B shows _____ posture.

35. This posture is believed to occur from severe damage to the cerebrum and the _____.

DESCRIBE THE DIFFERENCES

Describe the difference between each pair of terms.

36. What is the difference between hyperkinesia and hypertonia?

37. What is the difference between arousal and awareness?

38. What is the difference between delirium and dementia?

39. What is the difference between paralysis and paresis?

Copyright © 2024 by Elsevier, Inc. All Rights Reserved.

40. What is the difference between paraplegia and hemiplegia?

COMPLETE THE SENTENCES

Write one word in each blank to complete these sentences.

41. When muscle contractions of dystonia last for longer than a few seconds, such as in torticollis, they are called dystonic _____.

42. A person who has expressive aprosody is unable to express_____ in their speech.

43. Obstruction of the flow of cerebrospinal fluid causes _____.

44. When intracranial pressure equals systolic blood pressure, cerebral blood flow _____.

45. Severely increased intracranial pressure can cause brain tissue to _____ into another cranial compartment.

46. Huntington's disease is an autosomal- _____ condition characterized by progressive loss of cognitive function, _____ motor movements, and emotional lability.

47. Lower motor neuron damage causes muscle _____, but upper motor neuron damage causes _____.

48. Supratentorial lesions are located above the tentorium _____.

49. Yawning and hiccups are motor responses integrated in the _____.

50. Executive attention cognitive functions are mediated in the _____ area of the brain.

51. A person in a persistent _____ state is unaware of self or environment and has lost all cognitive function but maintains blood pressure and breathing without support.

COMPARE THE DEMYELINATING DISORDERS

Compare and contrast multiple sclerosis and Guillain-Barré syndrome by filling in the blank spaces.

Characteristic	Multiple Sclerosis	Guillain-Barré Syndrome
Location of the Demyelinated Axons		
Pathogenesis of the Demyelination		
Signs and Symptoms		
Usual Clinical Course		
Cells that Produce Myelin during Remyelination		Schwann cells

 Copyright © 2024 by Elsevier, Inc. All Rights Reserved.

Read each clinical scenario and answer the questions.

Mrs. Czerny, age 81, was diagnosed with Alzheimer disease when she had difficulty learning the names of her new grandchildren and then got lost several times on the way to her local grocery store. Her family had noticed several years of increasing forgetfulness before her diagnosis, but had thought that was part of aging. Over the next 4 years after diagnosis, Mrs. Czerny became more in need of care because of decreased judgment and self-care ability, and her family hired a full-time caregiver. Eventually, she failed to recognize her family members when they came to visit her, which distressed them greatly. A nurse referred them to a family support group, which they found very helpful.

52. What two classic pathologic changes that contribute to neuronal death are visible in the brain tissue of a person who had Alzheimer disease? Describe each briefly.

53. How soon do clinical manifestations of Alzheimer disease arise after the pathologic changes in the brain begin?

54. Mrs. Czerny's initial symptom was forgetfulness, which is the most common initial manifestation of Alzheimer disease. What portion of her brain was most affected by the pathology at that time?

55. "First she kept forgetting, and now she has poor judgment too," says Mrs. Czerny's son. "I understand that the memory part of her brain is damaged, but now I see more problems. How is this possible?" How should a nurse respond?

Mr. Armstrong, age 73, has advanced Parkinson disease. His disease has progressed until his medications do not control all of the clinical manifestations. He fell this morning and landed on his right side. His wife called an ambulance, which took him to the emergency department. Admission assessment is as follows:

Physical Examination and Subjective Data

- Heart rate, respiratory rate, and blood pressure elevated

- Speaks very softly, with slow response

- Reports right hip pain at a level of 8 on a 0 to 10 scale (10 is worst pain), but has no facial expression of pain

- Saliva dribbling from corner of the mouth

- Bilateral pill-rolling resting tremor of the hands, more pronounced on the right

- Remainder of examination delayed until return from Radiology

Copyright © 2024 by Elsevier, Inc. All Rights Reserved.

Laboratory Results

- Radiograph: right broken femoral head

- Serum electrolytes normal, blood glucose slightly elevated

Mr. Armstrong's admission diagnoses are right hip fracture, Parkinson disease.

56. What clinical manifestations of Parkinson disease put Mr. Armstrong at risk for falling?

57. Is Parkinson disease a pyramidal or extrapyramidal disorder? What basic pathophysiology causes the motor manifestations of Parkinson disease?

58. Why is Mr. Armstrong speaking so softly?

59. A nurse says, "He says he is in pain, but his face does not show it. Maybe he does not need this pain medication." What is the appropriate response?

Mrs. Torrentia has myasthenia gravis, which was diagnosed 2 months ago. She is stabilized on anticholinesterase medications. She telephones the telephone advice line, where you work, to ask questions.

60. Mrs. Torrentia asks, "Tell me again why I started seeing double after I had been awake for several hours."

Copyright © 2024 by Elsevier, Inc. All Rights Reserved.

Mrs. Torrentia says, "I lost the paper that tells me about the two types of crisis I need to recognize early and get help. Please tell me about them again." After noting her contact information so you can send the information, you need to discuss with her the difference between a myasthenic crisis and a cholinergic crisis in myasthenia gravis.

61. Put an X to specify the type of crisis most likely associated with each assessment finding. One of these assessment findings can be associated with both conditions.

Assessment Finding	Myasthenic Crisis	Cholinergic Crisis
Muscle weakness and twitching, often starting within an hour after taking prescribed anticholinesterase medication		
Increasing muscle weakness, especially after using the muscles, with no twitching		
Diarrhea and intestinal cramping		
Increased saliva and tears		
Extreme difficulty breathing		
Severe difficulty swallowing		
Constricted pupils		
Heart beating slowly		
Heart beating fast		

Copyright © 2024 by Elsevier, Inc. All Rights Reserved.

18 Disorders of the Central and Peripheral Nervous Systems and the Neuromuscular Junction

MATCH THE DEFINITIONS

Match the word on the right with its definition on the left.

_____ 1. Forward displacement of a vertebra

_____ 2. Degeneration of vertebral structure

_____ 3. Abnormal narrowing of the spinal canal

_____ 4. Disorder of the spinal nerve root

A. Radiculopathy

B. Spinal stenosis

C. Spondylolysis

D. Spondylolisthesis

CIRCLE THE CORRECT WORDS

Circle the correct words from the choices provided to complete these sentences.

5. Trauma that causes an open head injury occurs when a break in the (skull, dura mater) exposes cranial contents to the environment.

6. A person who is hit forcefully in the back of the head with a bat can sustain a (coup, contrecoup) injury when the brain hits the front of the skull and a (coup, contrecoup) injury where the bat hit.

7. Subdural hematomas typically involve (arterial, venous) bleeding.

8. (Infection, Hyperactivity) is a significant complication of a compound skull fracture.

9. In diffuse axonal injury, the axons are damaged by (stretching and tearing, penetrating injury).

10. Vertebral injuries tend to occur at the most (rigid, mobile) portions of the vertebral column.

11. Migraine causes (unilateral, bilateral) head pain.

12. Lacunar infarcts are small (hemorrhagic, ischemic) lesions and are associated with smoking and (hypoglycemia, hypertension).

13. Blood in the subarachnoid space after hemorrhage causes (infection, inflammation) and can (impair, potentiate) circulation of cerebrospinal fluid.

14. Hyperextension and hyperflexion vertebral injuries most often occur in the (cervical, lumbar) spine.

15. Most cases of encephalitis are caused by (bacteria, viruses).

16. The most common brain tumors are (primary, metastatic) and cause both local and (focal, generalized) effects.

17. Activation of the trigeminal vascular system is an important part of the pathophysiology of (tension, migraine) headache.

Copyright © 2024 by Elsevier, Inc. All Rights Reserved.

CATEGORIZE THE NEURAL INJURIES

Write the type of injury beside each name. Choices: primary, secondary, tertiary.

_____ 18. Subdural hematoma compresses neurons

_____ 19. Increased intracranial pressure compresses neurons

_____ 20. Bullet severs tracts in spinal cord

_____ 21. Crushing blow to head compresses neurons and glia

_____ 22. Pneumonia occurs during hospitalization for spinal cord injury

_____ 23. Glutamate excitotoxicity causes neuronal death

COMPLETE THE CHART

Fill in the blank spaces within the chart to compare and contrast the functions after a spinal cord injury, during the period of spinal shock, and after the return of reflexes.

Function Below the Level of a Complete Spinal Cord Lesion	During the Period of Spinal Shock	After Return of Reflexes
Reflexes		
Motor	_____ paralysis	_____ paralysis
Sensory		
Bladder	Atonic	
Bowels	Atonic	

MATCH THE CLINICAL MANIFESTATIONS

Match the clinical manifestations on the right with the phases of a migraine with aura on the left.

_____ 24. Premonitory phase

_____ 25. Migraine aura

_____ 26. Headache phase

_____ 27. Recovery phase

A. Throbbing pain beginning on one side and spreading to entire head; fatigue, nausea, and vomiting

B. Irritability, fatigue, or depression

C. Tiredness, irritability, loss of concentration, yawning, or food craving

D. Visual, sensory, or motor symptoms that may last up to an hour

DRAW YOUR ANSWERS

Read the questions and draw your answers.

28. Draw a saccular aneurysm on this artery.

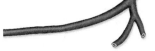

Copyright © 2024 by Elsevier, Inc. All Rights Reserved. Chapter **18** **Disorders of the Central and Peripheral Nervous Systems and the Neuromuscular Junction**

29. Draw a fusiform aneurysm on this artery.

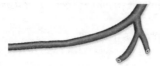

DESCRIBE THE DIFFERENCES

Describe the difference between each pair of terms.

30. What is the difference between a brain contusion and a concussion?

31. What is the difference between mass reflex and autonomic dysreflexia?

COMPLETE THE SENTENCES

Write one word in each blank to complete these sentences.

32. When continuous seizures last more than 5 minutes, the person is said to have _____ _____.

33. Bleeding between the dura mater and the skull causes an _____ hematoma.

34. A moderate traumatic brain injury is characterized by loss of _____ for more than 30 minutes and less than 6 hours, often accompanied by posttraumatic anterograde _____.

35. Release of excitatory neurotransmitters after brain injury causes secondary neural injury known as _____.

36. Neurogenic shock, also called _____ shock, is characterized by bradycardia and _____ blood pressure.

37. Any brain abnormality caused by blood vessel pathophysiology is called _____ disease.

38. The nucleus _____ is the gelatinous inner portion of an intervertebral disk that protrudes if the disk herniates.

39. Clinical manifestations of an ischemic stroke vary, depending on which _____ is obstructed.

40. A person who has a _____-type headache experiences bilateral headache with a sensation of a tight band or pressure around the head.

41. A localized collection of pus in the brain is called a brain _____.

42. Seizure activity often begins in an epileptogenic _____ where the neurons are activated easily.

 Copyright © 2024 by Elsevier, Inc. All Rights Reserved.

TEACH PEOPLE ABOUT PATHOPHYSIOLOGY

Write your response to each situation in the space provided.

43. Mr. Kanodi is upset. His son Calvin developed an acute subdural hematoma after being hit in the head by a golf ball during a tournament. "Why do they want to make a hole in his skull?" he asks. "They could damage his brain!"

44. Mr. Samuels had a thoracic spinal cord injury, and he has completed rehabilitation. His brother says, "I do not understand why he has so many muscle spasms in his legs. My friend had nerve damage in an auto accident and his leg is paralyzed too, but it just lies there flabby-like. Why are my brother's legs so spastic?"

45. Mrs. Kelso, who has multiple sclerosis, asks, "Why did it take my doctors 7 years to figure out that my symptoms were caused by multiple sclerosis?"

46. A college campus has an outbreak of meningococcal meningitis. The student health personnel are preparing fliers to post in the dormitories to inform students about signs and symptoms of this infection. What two major signs and symptoms should they list on the fliers, telling students to seek immediate medical assistance if they occur?

47. Mr. Gardner has an astrocytoma that was discovered when he had a seizure. "What does astrocytoma mean?" asks his wife. "Does that mean his brain cells that transmit messages have made a tumor?"

CLINICAL SCENARIOS

Read the clinical scenarios and answer the questions.

Mr. Tom Costa, age 71, had a stroke last year that left his right upper and lower extremities quite weak. He has smoked for 55 years and is obese. He was diagnosed with atrial fibrillation, high blood pressure and type 2 diabetes mellitus while he was hospitalized with his stroke. His father died of a heart attack at age 50; his paternal grandfather had a stroke and died a year later after a second stroke. His mother and both of her parents had type 2 diabetes.

48. What technical term should be used to describe Mr. Costa's weak right upper and lower extremities?

_____

49. The lesion that caused his motor dysfunction is located on which side of his brain? _____

50. Given his history, is it more likely that Mr. Costa had an ischemic or a hemorrhagic stroke? _____

Copyright © 2024 by Elsevier, Inc. All Rights Reserved. Chapter **18** **Disorders of the Central and Peripheral Nervous Systems and the Neuromuscular Junction**

51. What is a potential relationship between Mr. Costa's atrial fibrillation and his stroke?

52. What is a potential relationship between Mr. Costa's other risk factors and his stroke?

53. Mrs. Costa says, "Tom's grandfather had a stroke and he could not talk anymore, but he could walk. Now my husband has a stroke, and he can talk but he cannot walk. I do not understand this! Why?" Explain to Mrs. Costa.

54. "The doctor said to call her if I had a TIA," says Mr. Costa. "Why should I do that? A TIA goes away." Explain to Mr. Costa.

Mr. Goff, who had a complete T4 spinal cord transection 2 years ago, was admitted today for treatment of a sacral pressure injury. While a nurse is obtaining his admission history, Mr. Goff says that he just got a pounding headache and is getting very anxious. His upper body has become flushed.

55. What two words describe the likely reason for Mr. Goff's symptoms? _____ _____

56. What findings should be anticipated when the nurse measures Mr. Goff's blood pressure and heart rate? _____
_____

57. What pathophysiologic mechanisms account for the changes in the blood pressure and heart rate?

58. What makes this situation potentially life threatening?

59. What are common triggers for this situation?

60. Would those triggers cause this situation in a person who has a T10 injury? Why or why not?

    Copyright © 2024 by Elsevier, Inc. All Rights Reserved.

Jason Bowen, age 59, has type 2 diabetes that has not been managed well with oral medication. Recently, his physician added insulin to his medication regimen. Mr. Bowen accidentally injected too much insulin and had a tonic-clonic seizure, which his wife saw and called an ambulance. After Mr. Bowen has been stabilized in the hospital emergency department, Mrs. Bowen is crying in the hall. "I cannot bear any more!" she says. "First he gets diabetes and now he has epilepsy!"

Physical examination

- Vital signs normal

- Level of consciousness decreased: confused, disoriented to time and place, but not person

- Obese, with abdominal fat distribution

Laboratory results

- Initial blood glucose in ambulance: 46 mg/dL

- Blood glucose after treatment: 116 mg/dL

Mr. Bowen's admission diagnoses are hypoglycemic seizure and type 2 diabetes.

61. How should a nurse respond to Mrs. Bowen?

62. Did Mr. Bowen have a focal or a generalized seizure? What is the pathophysiologic difference between these two types?

63. What is the "tonic" part of the seizure?

64. What is the "clonic" part of the seizure?

65. Why did Mr. Bowen's confusion and disorientation not resolve immediately when he received intravenous glucose?

66. After he recovered that afternoon, Mr. Bowen said his leg and arm muscles were aching. What most likely caused his muscle aching?

Copyright © 2024 by Elsevier, Inc. All Rights Reserved. Chapter **18** **Disorders of the Central and Peripheral Nervous Systems and the Neuromuscular Junction**

19 Neurobiology of Schizophrenia, Mood Disorders, and Anxiety Disorders

MATCH THE DEFINITIONS

Match the word on the right with its definition on the left.

_____ 1. False belief that persists despite contradictory evidence

_____ 2. Lack of verbal or nonverbal expression of emotion

_____ 3. Lack of pleasure in activities that are normally pleasurable

_____ 4. Psychiatric disorder that involves loss of contact with reality

_____ 5. Perception that occurs in the absence of external stimuli

_____ 6. Inability to connect thoughts logically

_____ 7. Psychiatric disorder involving predominant emotions that affect ability to function in society

A. Anhedonia

B. Psychosis

C. Mood disorder

D. Hallucination

E. Affective flattening

F. Delusion

G. Disorganized thinking

CIRCLE THE CORRECT WORDS

Circle the correct words from the choices provided to complete these sentences.

8. Inherited disease alleles for schizophrenia show (complete, reduced) penetrance, which means that individuals who have the disease genes (manifest, may not manifest) schizophrenia.

9. The dorsolateral prefrontal cortex is important for function of (long-term, working) memory; in schizophrenia, this brain area appears to be (hyperactive, hypoactive).

10. Brain abnormalities in schizophrenia are believed to originate in the (prenatal, adolescent) period of brain development.

11. Major depression is a(n) (mood, anxiety) disorder.

12. Proinflammatory cytokines and cortisol levels usually are (decreased, increased) in the blood in depression.

13. Atrophy of neurons in the (hypothalamus, hippocampus) is believed to participate in the neurobiology of depression.

14. Abnormally increased sensitivity to changes in (calcium, pH) in the amygdala may underlie panic disorder.

15. Cell bodies of serotonergic neurons are located in the (locus ceruleus, raphe nuclei) in the brainstem; cell bodies of adrenergic neurons are located in the (locus ceruleus, raphe nuclei) in the brainstem.

16. Posttraumatic stress disorder is characterized by (disorganized, intrusive) thoughts after exposure to a life-threatening or traumatic event and involves (decreased, increased) neural activity in the amygdala and (decreased, increased) neural activity in the prefrontal cortex.

17. Obsessive-compulsive disorder is characterized by (disorganized, repetitive) irrational thoughts and (disorganized, ritualized) behaviors.

Copyright © 2024 by Elsevier, Inc. All Rights Reserved.

CATEGORIZE THE CLINICAL MANIFESTATIONS OF SCHIZOPHRENIA

Write the type beside each clinical manifestation of schizophrenia. Choices: positive, negative.

_____ 18. Hallucinations

_____ 19. Social withdrawal

_____ 20. Delusions

_____ 21. Blunted affect

_____ 22. Incoherent speech that uses invented words

_____ 23. Wearing aluminum foil on head to deflect radio waves

_____ 24. Failure to respond to simple questions

MATCH THE ASSESSMENTS

Match the technical term on the right with the assessment on the left that it describes.

_____ 25. Mr. J says, "I used to have a lot of fun activities, but they do not make me happy anymore."

_____ 26. Mr. G believes he is Louis XIV, King of France, although he has a history book that says Louis XIV is dead.

_____ 27. Mr. A is talking so rapidly and urgently that it is difficult to understand him.

_____ 28. Mr. S is talking to his mother, whom he insists is sitting in the corner of the room, although you are the only other person present.

_____ 29. Mr. L says he is happy and excited today, but his speech is monotone and his facial expression does not change.

A. Delusion

B. Pressured speech

C. Affective flattening

D. Anhedonia

E. Hallucination

COMPLETE THE SENTENCES

Write one word in each blank to complete these sentences.

30. One hypothesis of schizophrenia involves the neurotransmitter _____ acting on NMDA receptors.

31. The dopamine hypothesis of schizophrenia suggests that an _____ of dopamine in the mesolimbic pathway causes the _____ symptoms and a _____ of dopamine in the mesocortical pathway causes the _____ and cognitive symptoms.

32. Not spontaneously talking in response to questions or to express oneself is called _____.

33. Unipolar depression also is known as _____ depression or clinical depression.

34. Monoamine neurotransmission is hypothesized to be _____ during depression but _____ during mania.

35. People who have panic disorder may develop _____, extreme avoidance of being in a crowd or other location where it is not easy to escape.

Copyright © 2024 by Elsevier, Inc. All Rights Reserved. Chapter **19 Neurobiology of Schizophrenia, Mood Disorders, and Anxiety Disorders**

36. Mood disorders are considered to arise from the interplay between susceptible genes and _____ influences.

37. The neurotransmitter _____ binds to adrenergic receptors; the neurotransmitter _____ binds to 5-HT$_{1A}$ receptors.

38. Depression neurobiology that focuses on BDNF in the hippocampus is called the _____ hypothesis of depression.

39. In children, it may be difficult to distinguish between bipolar II disorder and _____.

TEACH PEOPLE ABOUT PATHOPHYSIOLOGY

Write your response to each situation in the space provided.

40. "That doctor may know his stuff, but I think he is rude!" exclaims Mrs. Kim, whose son David has been diagnosed with schizophrenia. "The doctor kept talking about negative symptoms. David is really sweet and stays quietly in his room most of the time. I have never heard him say a negative word to anyone. I think the doctor is the one who is negative!"

41. "What is the difference between a hallucination and a delusion?" asks Mr. Hawkins. "The doctor said my wife has both. All I know is that she is acting crazy. Please help me understand."

42. "Why does the antipsychotic medication we give Mr. Gaines have Parkinson-like side effects?" asks another nurse. "What does dopamine have to do with schizophrenia?"

43. Mr. Tennyson, who lives in his own apartment, has diabetes and schizophrenia, both of which are managed with medications. He has appointments about every 2 months in the diabetes clinic. The diabetes clinic nurses have been asked to tell a physician if they see evidence that Mr. Tennyson may have discontinued his schizophrenia medication. What assessment findings could indicate Mr. Tennyson may have stopped taking his schizophrenia medication?

44. A new telephone advice nurse asks, "What is the difference between the manifestations of a panic attack and those of mania?"

Copyright © 2024 by Elsevier, Inc. All Rights Reserved.

CLINICAL SCENARIOS

Read the clinical scenarios and answer the questions.

Mr. Trainor, age 22, is brought to the emergency department after being found wandering around his college campus at 3 AM, shouting incoherently. He believes that he is Julius Caesar and is ordering people to carry out his commands. History from his college roommate: poor social skills; increasingly unwilling to leave the dormitory; did not attend class, take showers, or change clothes in the past week; began referring to himself as "Julius" yesterday morning and was gone when his roommate returned from an evening class.

Physical examination

- Vital signs normal except for elevated heart rate and respiratory rate

- No abnormal findings with limited examination; refused to remove his shirt, calling it "my royal robe"

Laboratory results

- Serum electrolytes, BUN, and creatinine normal

- Blood alcohol negative

- Urine toxicology screen for drugs negative

After psychiatric consult, Mr. Trainor's eventual diagnosis is schizophrenia.

45. What technical term describes Mr. Trainor's belief that he is Julius Caesar? _____

46. Because the brain abnormalities in schizophrenia are believed to arise during fetal development, why does schizophrenia often become apparent during the late teens and early 20s?

47. Mr. Trainor is admitted to the psychiatric unit. His mother says, "Do you have a hand mirror I can use? I brought his driver's license that has his photograph and name, and I want to prove to him that he is Gus Trainor instead of Julius Caesar." How should his nurse respond?

48. How should Mr. Trainor's signs and symptoms be expected to change after he is stabilized on effective antipsychotic medications and supportive therapy?

49. By the time his schizophrenia was diagnosed, Mr. Trainor already showed loss of cortical gray matter in his cerebral cortex, which is characteristic of schizophrenia. How will antipsychotic medications change the progression of this loss of cortical tissue?

Copyright © 2024 by Elsevier, Inc. All Rights Reserved. Chapter **19 Neurobiology of Schizophrenia, Mood Disorders, and Anxiety Disorders**

Mr. Nelson, age 56, who has type 2 diabetes and hypertension, had a minor myocardial infarction 5 weeks ago. His wife is very concerned because he is very sad all the time, has no appetite, awakens about 3 AM every night and cannot get back to sleep, is losing weight, and says he has no energy for any activities, even refusing to talk on the telephone when his friends call. His cardiologist says Mr. Nelson's heart is functioning as well as can be expected and that he should enroll in a cardiac rehabilitation program to give himself confidence in returning to normal activities.

50. Complete the sentence by choosing from the lists of options.

    Mr. Nelson needs screening for _____(1)_____ because he is experiencing _____(2)_____, _____(3)_____, and _____(4)_____.

Options for 1	Options for 2	Options for 3	Options for 4
bipolar disorder	dysphoric mood	agitation	loss of appetite
schizophrenia	episodes of mania	insomnia	hyperactivity
major depression	disorganized thinking	pressured speech	feelings of guilt

51. Many men have a myocardial infarction without developing this disorder; what is the probable explanation for why Mr. Nelson developed this disorder after a myocardial infarction?

52. Mr. Nelson refuses to take antidepressants. What neurotransmitter abnormality is most likely present in Mr. Nelson's brain?

53. Mr. Nelson has had several upper respiratory infections since his disorder developed. What hormone alteration common to this disorder predisposes him to infection? Why?

 Copyright © 2024 by Elsevier, Inc. All Rights Reserved.

20 Alterations of Neurologic Function in Children

MATCH THE DEFINITIONS

Match the word on the right with its definition on the left.

_____ 1. Protrusion of a portion of the brain and meninges through a defect in the skull

_____ 2. Small head circumference with lack of brain growth

_____ 3. Birth defect involving failure of the vertebrae to close

_____ 4. Flattening of one side of an infant's head from prolonged lying in one position

A. Spina bifida

B. Positional plagiocephaly

C. Encephalocele

D. Microcephaly

CIRCLE THE CORRECT WORDS

Circle the correct word from the choices provided to complete these sentences.

5. Neural tube defects are associated with maternal (iodine, folate) deficiency.

6. Chiari malformations involve downward displacement of the (cerebellum, motor cortex) and are a type of (defect of neural tube closure, malformation of cortical development).

7. Cerebral palsy is a (progressive, static) encephalopathy.

8. Tethered cord syndrome involving altered (gait and bladder control, speech and cognition) may develop in children born with (spina bifida occulta, myelomeningocele) as the child grows after surgical correction.

9. Cerebral palsy is caused by injury or abnormal development in the immature (spinal cord, brain) before, during, or after birth up to (1 year, 5 years) of age.

10. Cerebral palsy always involves (motor, sensory, cognitive) defects and may involve additional problems as well.

11. A ketogenic diet may be used for a child who has (phenylketonuria, epilepsy).

12. The palmar grasp reflex normally is present at birth and should disappear by the age of (3, 6) months.

Copyright © 2024 by Elsevier, Inc. All Rights Reserved.

CHARACTERIZE THE DISORDERS

Write one letter and one number by each disorder in the left column to indicate the location of damage and the clinical manifestations.

Disorder	Choose the Location of the Damage	Choose the Clinical Manifestations
_____ 13. Dystonic cerebral palsy	A. Neurons throughout the body	1. Gait difficulties, loss of balance, often hydrocephalus with headache, nausea, vomiting, and nystagmus from increased ICP
_____ 14. Spastic cerebral palsy	B. Basal ganglia or extrapyramidal tracts	2. Purposeful movements are stiff, uncontrolled, abrupt; difficulty with fine motor coordination
_____ 15. Ataxic cerebral palsy	C. Cerebellum and often the fourth ventricle	3. Excessive startle response, loss of developmental milestones, seizures, dementia, blindness, death
_____ 16. Tay-Sachs disease	D. Cerebellum	4. Increased muscle tone, prolonged primitive reflexes, hyperreflexia, clonus, contractures
_____ 17. Medulloblastoma	E. Corticospinal pathways	5. Gait disturbances, balance difficulty, intention tremor

DESCRIBE THE DIFFERENCES

Describe the difference between each pair of terms.

18. What is the difference between a meningocele and a myelomeningocele?

19. What is the difference between pyramidal and extrapyramidal cerebral palsy?

COMPLETE THE SENTENCES

Write one word in each blank to complete these sentences.

20. Children who have congenital arteriovenous malformations are at risk for _____ stroke.

21. Stenosis of the cerebral _____ causes _____ by interfering with the circulation of _____ fluid.

22. Aseptic meningitis may be caused by a virus but not by _____.

Copyright © 2024 by Elsevier, Inc. All Rights Reserved.

23. Group _____ *Streptococcus* that causes fatal bacterial meningitis in neonates is transmitted from the mother during _____.

24. Phenylketonuria is caused by mutation of a gene for an _____ that normally converts the _____ acid phenylalanine to _____.

25. The most common intraocular congenital eye tumor of young children is _____.

26. Habitually eating non-food substances such as paint chips is called _____ and it causes children who live in old buildings to have increased risk of _____ poisoning.

27. A young child who has repeated and worsening headaches should be evaluated for _____ _____ or other cause of increased intracranial pressure.

28. Signs and symptoms of a childhood brain tumor depend on its _____ in the brain and its rate of growth.

29. Craniosynostosis is premature _____ of one or more cranial sutures in an infant.

TEACH PEOPLE ABOUT PATHOPHYSIOLOGY

Write your response to each situation in the space provided.

30. Hector, age 2, has pneumococcal meningitis. "My poor sick baby!" exclaims his mother. "Please tell me why he will not bend his neck to drink from his cup of water and why he cried so hard when I tried to straighten his little legs. I am worried that he is paralyzed like my uncle who had a stroke."

31. "When he was awake, my baby used to root around for my nipple when it touched the corner of his mouth," says Mrs. Delibes. "That was so cute! But now that he is 5 months old, he does not do that anymore. Is something wrong with him?"

32. Jeannie Quantz, age 4, developed rapidly increasing intracranial pressure during an episode of bacterial meningitis, which blocked her arachnoid villi. Her doctors tell Mrs. Quantz that Jeannie has hydrocephalus and that they need to intervene quickly. "Jeannie does not have hydrocephalus!" Mrs. Quantz says to a nurse. "Hydrocephalus is having too much fluid in the brain. My friend who worked in an orphanage overseas showed me pictures of hydrocephalus. Those babies had great big heads from too much fluid inside."

Copyright © 2024 by Elsevier, Inc. All Rights Reserved.

21 Mechanisms of Hormonal Regulation

NAME THE HORMONES

Write the name of the gland and the major hormones it secretes beside each number.

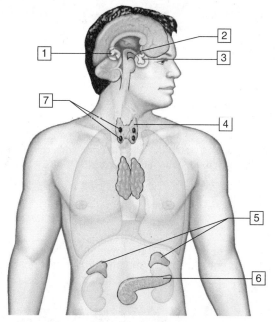

(From Patton KT, Thibodeau GA: *Anatomy & physiology,* ed 8, St Louis, 2013, Mosby.)

1. Gland: _____

   One hormone: _____

2. Gland: _____

   Six hormones: _____

3. Gland: _____

   Seven hormones from anterior: _____

   Two hormones from posterior: _____

4. Gland: _____

   Three hormones: _____

Copyright © 2024 by Elsevier, Inc. All Rights Reserved.

5. Gland: _____

   Three hormones from cortex: _____

   Two hormones from medulla: _____

6. Gland: _____

   Four hormones: _____

7. Gland: _____

   One hormone: _____

MATCH THE DEFINITIONS

Match the definitions on the right with the words on the left.

_____ 8. Up-regulation

_____ 9. Permissive effect

_____ 10. Down-regulation

_____ 11. First messenger

_____ 12. Second messenger

A. Chemical signal generated within a cell that mediates the action of a water-soluble hormone or other chemical

B. Water-soluble hormone or other chemical that binds to receptors in plasma membranes

C. Increased number or affinity of hormone receptors, often in response to low hormone concentration

D. Decreased number or affinity of hormone receptors, often in response to high hormone concentration

E. Hormone-induced changes that facilitate the maximal response or functioning of a cell

CIRCLE THE CORRECT WORDS

Circle the correct word from the choices provided to complete these sentences.

13. The hypothalamus is connected to the posterior pituitary by (portal blood vessels, a nerve tract) and to the anterior pituitary by (portal blood vessels, a nerve tract).

14. Water-soluble hormones generally have a (short, long) half-life and circulate in (bound, free) forms.

15. Low hormone concentrations usually cause cells to (down-regulate, up-regulate) receptors for that hormone, which (increases, decreases) cellular sensitivity to that hormone.

16. Water-soluble hormones bind with (cell membrane, intracellular) receptors.

17. Hormone receptors are (proteins, steroids, either proteins or steroids).

18. (GH, ACTH) is an example of a somatotropic hormone.

Copyright © 2024 by Elsevier, Inc. All Rights Reserved.

19. (Water, **Lipid**)-soluble hormones alter gene expression when the hormone-receptor complex binds to specific sites on the (RNA, **DNA**) in the (**nucleus**, ribosomes).

20. Secretion of cortisol increases when (**ACTH**, CRF) binds to receptors on cells in the adrenal (**cortex**, medulla).

21. Many of the actions of growth hormone are mediated through the effects of (**insulin-like growth factors**, incretins, ghrelins), which also are known as (somatotropins, **somatomedins**, somatostatins).

22. Catecholamines are released from the adrenal (cortex, **medulla**).

23. The action of catecholamines (**increases**, decreases) blood glucose concentration as part of the (hypothalamic/pituitary/adrenal axis, **fight or flight response**).

24. Incretins are released from the (liver, **gastrointestinal tract**) and act to (increase, **decrease**) postprandial blood glucose concentration.

25. The net effect of insulin is to (increase, **decrease**) blood glucose concentration and (**increase**, decrease) synthesis of protein and fat.

26. Cortisol acts to (**increase**, decrease) blood glucose concentration, (stimulate, **inhibit**) inflammation, and cause (only a few, **numerous**) other effects.

27. A common mechanism of hormonal regulation is (positive, **negative**) feedback.

MATCH THE FUNCTIONS

Match the altered function on the right with the hormone on the left.

A Significant Change in Secretion of this Hormone

_____ 28. Antidiuretic hormone (ADH)

_____ 29. Parathyroid hormone (PTH)

_____ 30. Insulin

_____ 31. Gonadotropin-releasing hormone (GnRH)

_____ 32. Aldosterone

Alters the Regulation of this Variable

A. Plasma calcium concentration

B. Blood glucose concentration

C. Body fluid osmolality

D. Extracellular fluid volume and plasma potassium concentration

E. Menstrual cycle regulation

Copyright © 2024 by Elsevier, Inc. All Rights Reserved.

EXPLAIN THE PICTURE

Examine the picture and answer the questions about it.

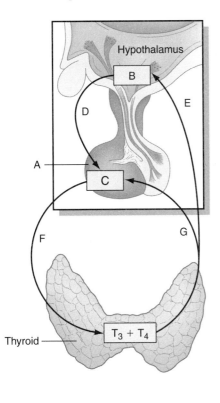

33. What gland does letter A indicate?

34. Write the hormone names and acronyms represented by the letters:

    B. _____

    C. _____

35. Look at the direction of the circular arrows and mark + or – to denote stimulation or negative feedback.

    D. _____   E. _____

    F. _____   G. _____

36. When a tumor destroys the thyroid gland, what is most likely to happen to the blood levels of hormone C? _____ of hormone B? _____ Why? _____

37. What is most likely to happen to body weight and tolerance to environmental heat or cold if a tumor destroys the thyroid gland? Why?

    _____

    _____

CATEGORIZE THE HORMONES

Write the type of hormone beside each name. Choices: peptide, steroid, amine.

_____ 38. Cortisol

_____ 39. Insulin

_____ 40. Thyroid hormones

_____ 41. Adrenocorticotropic hormone (ACTH)

_____ 42. Corticotropin-releasing hormone (CRH)

_____ 43. Aldosterone

_____ 44. Glucagon

_____ 45. Growth hormone (GH)

_____ 46. Estrogen

Copyright © 2024 by Elsevier, Inc. All Rights Reserved.

Chapter **21 Mechanisms of Hormonal Regulation**

_____ 47. Antidiuretic hormone (ADH)

_____ 48. Epinephrine

COMPLETE THE SENTENCES

Write one word in each blank to complete these sentences.

49. The neurohypophysis is the _____ pituitary, and the adenohypophysis is the _____ pituitary.

50. Steroid hormones are synthesized from _____.

51. ADH also is called arginine _____.

52. In order for a hormone to act on a cell, the cell must have _____ for that hormone.

53. Hormones that bind to receptors that activate adenylyl cyclase use _____ as a second messenger.

54. Releasing hormones are produced by the _____.

55. A person who has an iodine-deficient diet will have difficulty making enough _____ hormones.

56. In the islets of Langerhans, alpha cells produce _____ and beta cells produce insulin and _____.

57. Calcitonin is secreted by the _____ gland and helps to regulate plasma _____ concentration.

58. The term *somatopause* indicates the decrease of _____ hormone and insulin-like _____ that occurs with aging.

DESCRIBE THE DIFFERENCES

Describe the difference between each pair of terms.

59. What is the difference between a direct effect and a permissive effect of a hormone?

60. What is the difference between autocrine and paracrine action of a hormone?

61. What is the difference between negative feedback and positive feedback?

Copyright © 2024 by Elsevier, Inc. All Rights Reserved.

Write your response to each situation in the space provided.

62. A clinical research protocol includes drawing blood to measure insulin levels. "Our research subjects do not like blood draws," says a research assistant. "Can we measure urine insulin instead?"

63. "This drug information sheet says that sildenafil prolongs the action of cyclic GMP in blood vessel muscles," says Mr. Lehrner. "I asked my doctor, and he said cGMP is a second messenger. What does 'second messenger' mean? Is that an abnormal thing?"

64. Mx. Merryweather has a tumor that damaged their hypothalamus, but not their pituitary gland. Among numerous other hormone problems, they are not secreting enough antidiuretic hormone (ADH). "I do not understand this," says a nurse. "ADH comes from the pituitary and does not have a releasing hormone from the hypothalamus. How can a hypothalamic tumor cause a lack of ADH?"

65. "I understand why I need to take this antithyroid drug," says Mr. Henderson, who has newly diagnosed hyperthyroidism. "It stops my thyroid gland from making any more thyroid hormones. But why does it take several weeks to have full effects? Don't we make thyroid hormones every day?"

66. Mrs. Hillerman has breast cancer. Her cancer cells secrete uncontrolled amounts of parathyroid hormone–related peptide (PTHrP). She asks, "Why are they drawing blood again to measure calcium? Why is mine abnormal?"

67. A student is observing in an endocrine clinic. They ask, "Why do these laboratory slips have a place to request blood levels of carrier proteins for some hormones, such as thyroid, but not for others such as ADH and ACTH?"

68. "Please help me make sense of the renin-angiotensin system," says Mr. Phillipi. "If the kidney blood vessels sense low blood flow, they release renin into the blood, but how does that help fix the low blood flow? I want the details!"

Copyright © 2024 by Elsevier, Inc. All Rights Reserved.

Alterations of Hormonal Regulation

MATCH THE DEFINITIONS

Match the definitions on the right with the words on the left.

_____ 1. Ectopic hormone	A. Hormone secreted by intestinal endocrine cells
_____ 2. Hirsutism	B. Hormone secreted by nonendocrine tissues
_____ 3. Ghrelin	C. Nonpitting boggy edema caused by infiltration of mucopolysaccharides and proteins between connective tissue in the dermis
_____ 4. Incretin	D. Excessive growth of facial and body hair
_____ 5. Myxedema	E. Peptide produced in pancreatic islets and the stomach

SORT THE DISORDERS

Write the names of the endocrine disorders with their dysfunctioning organs.

Sort these seven disorders: primary hyperthyroidism, secondary hyperthyroidism, SIADH, Cushing disease, diabetes insipidus, primary hypothyroidism, secondary hypothyroidism

6. Two disorders caused by posterior pituitary dysfunction:

   _____

   _____

7. Two disorders caused by a problem within the thyroid gland:

   _____

   _____

8. Three disorders caused by a problem in the anterior pituitary gland:

   _____

   _____

   _____

CIRCLE THE CORRECT WORDS

Circle the correct word from the choices provided to complete these sentences.

9. Syndrome of inappropriate antidiuretic hormone secretion (SIADH) is characterized by (high, low) levels of ADH in the absence of normal control mechanisms.

10. An active anterior pituitary adenoma usually causes (hyposecretion, hypersecretion) of hormones from the adenoma itself and (hyposecretion, hypersecretion) of hormones from the surrounding pituitary cells.

110

Copyright © 2024 by Elsevier, Inc. All Rights Reserved.

11. Women who have gestational diabetes have (decreased, increased) risk for type 2 diabetes later in life.

12. One of the ways that obesity increases the risk of insulin resistance and type (1, 2) diabetes is increased secretion of some (adipokines, adiponectin) by the adipose tissue.

13. Metabolic syndrome increases the risk of developing type (1, 2) diabetes.

14. Untreated congenital (hypothyroidism, growth hormone deficiency) causes both decreased skeletal growth and cognitive disability.

15. In autoimmune diabetes, also called type (1, 2) diabetes, pancreatic beta cells are destroyed by autoreactive (cytotoxic T lymphocytes, natural killer cells).

16. People who have type 1 diabetes have a deficit of insulin and (glucagon, amylin) and a relative excess of (glucagon, amylin).

17. In diabetes, *microvascular disease* refers to (damage to medium-sized and large arteries, destruction of capillaries), whereas *macrovascular disease* refers to (damage to medium-sized and large arteries, destruction of capillaries).

EXPLAIN THE PICTURE

Examine the picture and answer the questions about it.

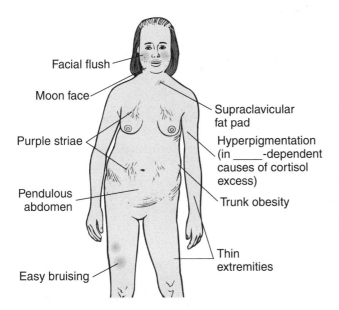

Facial flush

Moon face

Purple striae

Pendulous abdomen

Easy bruising

Supraclavicular fat pad

Hyperpigmentation (in _____-dependent causes of cortisol excess)

Trunk obesity

Thin extremities

18. The woman in this picture has _____ disease.

19. What causes her round face and truncal obesity?

20. This woman is worried that she has leukemia because she keeps bruising when she just bumps herself a little. What does she need to know about how her endocrine disorder causes this?

21. What hormone fits the blank line under the word "Hyperpigmentation"? _____
How does an excess of this hormone cause hyperpigmentation?

DESCRIBE THE DIFFERENCES

Describe the difference between each pair of terms.

22. What is the difference between a primary and a secondary endocrine disorder?

23. What is the difference between thyrotoxicosis and thyrotoxic crisis?

Copyright © 2024 by Elsevier, Inc. All Rights Reserved.

24. What is the difference between neurogenic and nephrogenic diabetes insipidus?

25. What is the difference between acromegaly and gigantism?

MATCH THE CLINICAL MANIFESTATIONS

Match the clinical manifestation on the right with the disorder on the left.

_____ 26. SIADH

_____ 27. Hypothyroidism

_____ 28. Pheochromocytoma

_____ 29. Adrenal adenoma causing hypersecretion of androgens in a woman

_____ 30. Diabetic ketoacidosis

_____ 31. Hypoglycemia

_____ 32. Primary hyperaldosteronism

_____ 33. Type 1 diabetes mellitus

_____ 34. Diabetes insipidus

_____ 35. Addison disease

A. Hypertension, tachycardia, palpitations, severe headache, diaphoresis, heat intolerance, weight loss, constipation

B. Polydipsia, nocturia, polyuria, hypernatremia, increased plasma osmolality, large volume of dilute urine

C. Polydipsia, nocturia, polyuria, increased appetite, weight loss, hyperglycemia, glycosuria

D. Weakness, fatigue, hypotension, hyperkalemia, hypoglycemia, elevated ACTH

E. Lethargy, cold intolerance, hoarseness, nonpitting boggy edema around eyes, coarse hair, decreased body temperature

F. Lethargy, hyponatremia, perhaps seizure, decreased plasma osmolality, concentrated urine

G. Tachycardia, diaphoresis, tremor, pallor, confusion, decreased level of consciousness, perhaps seizure

H. Virilization: lack of breast development, hirsutism, increased muscle bulk

I. Polyuria, decreased level of consciousness, Kussmaul breathing, acetone smell to breath, hyperglycemia, decreased blood pH, ketonuria, glycosuria

J. Hypertension, hypokalemia, increased blood pH, increased urine potassium

COMPLETE THE SENTENCES

Write one word in each blank to complete these sentences.

36. Failure of the hypothalamus to secrete its usual hormones presents clinically as _____ disease.

37. Chromaffin cell tumors of the adrenal medulla are called _____.

Copyright © 2024 by Elsevier, Inc. All Rights Reserved.

38. Increased plasma osmolality caused by inadequate response of the renal tubules to ADH is called _____ diabetes insipidus.

39. When necrosis or another problem in the anterior pituitary causes deficiency of all its hormones, the individual has

_____.

40. Prolactin-secreting tumors in the _____ pituitary are called _____; in women, they cause

_____ (milk production not associated with childbirth).

41. Chronic hyperglycemia impairs both innate and adaptive _____ responses.

42. A person who has hypothyroidism can develop a nonpitting boggy edema called _____; that same

term, when used with the word *coma,* indicates the _____ level of consciousness associated with severe hypothyroidism.

43. Enlargement of the thyroid gland is called a _____ and is a response to increased stimulation by

_____.

44. Type 1 diabetes often is diagnosed when the acute complication _____ _____ occurs.

45. People who have primary hyperparathyroidism are predisposed to form kidney _____.

46. Cushing _____ is caused by hypersecretion of ACTH from the anterior pituitary, but the term Cushing

_____ is used for any condition involving chronic exposure to excessive cortisol.

TEACH PEOPLE ABOUT PATHOPHYSIOLOGY

Write your response to each situation in the space provided.

47. A nurse says, "My type 2 diabetes patients do not get diabetic ketoacidosis as often as my type 1 diabetes patients do. Why is that?"

48. Mrs. Soderstrom has newly diagnosed acromegaly. Her husband says, "Last winter I had to buy my wife a larger pair of gloves and larger boots, even though her old ones were in good condition. Our doctor says she has too much growth hormone. Why doesn't too much growth hormone make her tall like a giant?"

49. Mr. James has a pathologic fracture and newly diagnosed hyperparathyroidism. He asks, "How can little glands in my neck make my bones weak?"

Copyright © 2024 by Elsevier, Inc. All Rights Reserved.

50. Mrs. King had thyroid surgery yesterday. She asks, "Why do the nurses keep blowing up a blood pressure cuff and looking at my hand instead of measuring my blood pressure?"

51. "Dr. Michaels said I have diabetes insipidus," says Mx. Wrey, who has an indwelling urinary catheter. "Diabetes is a sugar problem, but he said my sugar is normal. What is happening?"

52. Mrs. Santos has type 2 diabetes. She says, "Please explain to me why losing weight will help my diabetes."

53. Mr. Parks has newly diagnosed Addison disease. He asks, "Why do I get lightheaded when I stand up?"

54. Mrs. Granada says, "Please tell me why my little boy got this awful type 1 sugar diabetes!"

CLINICAL SCENARIOS

Read the clinical scenarios and answer the questions.

Mr. Cardoso, who has had type 2 diabetes for 23 years, had a myocardial infarction (MI) 2 days ago. He did not feel any chest pain with his MI. His hospital record indicates that he has gastroparesis, peripheral neuropathy, diabetic retinopathy, prior amputation of his right foot, and a previous hospitalization for hyperosmolar hyperglycemic nonketotic syndrome.

55. What are the two basic components of the pathophysiology of type 2 diabetes?

_____

Mr. Cardoso says, "I cannot eat this lunch! I still am full from breakfast."

56. *Complete the sentence by choosing from the lists of options.*

Copyright © 2024 by Elsevier, Inc. All Rights Reserved.

His statement about eating lunch indicates that Mr. Cardoso likely has _____(1)_____ caused by _____(2)_____, which is a _____(3)_____ complication of diabetes.

Options for 1	Options for 2	Options for 3
hyperglycemia	autonomic neuropathy	microvascular
gastroparesis	acute hypoglycemia	macrovascular
paresthesias	tissue ischemia	

57. Mr. Cardoso's son says, "The doctor said the diabetes is responsible for my dad's not having any pain with his heart attack. That does not make sense to me. I thought his diabetes was a sugar problem." How should a nurse respond?

58. Mr. Cardoso says, "The doctor said my diabetes contributed to my heart attack. I thought hardening of the arteries causes heart attacks! How does diabetes contribute to a heart attack?" How should a nurse respond?

59. What is the pathophysiology behind Mr. Cardoso's diabetic retinopathy?

60. What factors most likely contributed to the need to amputate Mr. Cardoso's right foot?

61. Why should Mr. Cardoso's urine be checked for microalbuminuria?

62. When Mr. Cardoso developed hyperosmolar hyperglycemic nonketotic syndrome, what signs and symptoms were likely?

Copyright © 2024 by Elsevier, Inc. All Rights Reserved.

Mrs. Jackson, age 35, is a thin, anxious woman who cannot seem to sit still. She is sweating although the room temperature is 20°C (68°F). Her eyes have a bulging, staring appearance. Her hair is fine, her skin smooth and moist. Mrs. Jackson says she is always too warm and that she does not button the top buttons on her blouses anymore because the collars are too tight. Laboratory tests confirm that Mrs. Jackson has Graves disease.

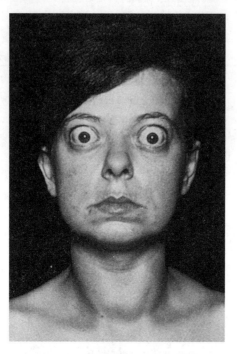

(From Stein HA, Slatt BJ, Stein RM: *The ophthalmic assistant: fundamentals and clinical practice,* ed 7, Philadelphia, 2000, Mosby.)

63. Given her diagnosis, what should be expected regarding her weight and her appetite?

64. What should assessment of her body temperature and heart rate show?

65. Why is Mrs. Jackson always too warm?

66. What is the basic pathophysiology of Graves disease?

Copyright © 2024 by Elsevier, Inc. All Rights Reserved.

67. What technical term describes Mrs. Jackson's protruding eyes? _____ Why are they protruding?

68. Why are Mrs. Jackson's collars too tight?

Walker, age 12, had not been feeling well for three days. His mother thought he had the flu and did not worry until she realized that he had consumed an entire case of soda in one day and was asking for more. When Walker became very sleepy and hard to awaken, she took him to the emergency department, where he was diagnosed with diabetic ketoacidosis. During Walker's hospitalization, type 1 diabetes was diagnosed. His mother was embarrassed that she had not recognized the symptoms because her younger sister had developed type 1 diabetes when she was four years old.

69. *Interpret Walker's assessment findings by placing an X in the appropriate column.*

Assessment Findings	Diabetic Ketoacidosis (DKA)	Type 1 Diabetes (without DKA)
Consumed an entire case of soda in one day and was asking for more		
Became very sleepy and hard to awaken		

Dasani had an autoimmune disease for which she was taking oral prednisone, a glucocorticoid drug. Although the drug controlled her signs and symptoms, she stopped looking in the mirror because she was so upset at the physical changes in her body. "I look like a fat old lady with a round face and skinny legs," she said.

70. *Complete the sentence by choosing from the lists of options.*

Dasani has _____ (1) _____ ; her round face is caused by _____

(2) _____ and her skinny legs are caused by _____ (3) _____ .

Options for 1	Options for 2	Options for 3
Cushing disease	edema	protein catabolism
Cushing syndrome	hyperglycemia	disuse atrophy
Addison disease	fat redistribution	hypoglycemia

Copyright © 2024 by Elsevier, Inc. All Rights Reserved.

Chapter **22 Alterations of Hormonal Regulation**

23 Obesity, Starvation, and Anorexia of Aging

MATCH THE DEFINITIONS

Match the word on the right with its definition on the left.

_____ 1. Cell that stores fat

_____ 2. Type of adipose tissue with adipocytes that have multiple lipid droplets and numerous mitochondria

_____ 3. Type of adipose tissue, located viscerally and subcutaneously, with adipocytes that have one lipid droplet

_____ 4. Type of adipose tissue with adipocytes that contain multiple mitochondria and are located within another type of adipose tissue

_____ 5. Type of adipose tissue located in bone marrow

_____ 6. Formation of new fat cells

_____ 7. Biologically active substance secreted by adipose tissue

_____ 8. Biologically active substance secreted by muscles, usually in response to contractile activity

A. Myokine

B. Adipokine

C. Adipocyte

D. WAT

E. BAT

F. bAT

G. MAT

H. Adipogenesis

CIRCLE THE CORRECT WORDS

Circle the correct word from the choices provided to complete these sentences.

9. When energy balance is positive, visceral white adipose tissue is more likely to store fat by (adipocyte hypertrophy, adipogenesis).

10. Visceral fat is (more, less) metabolically active than subcutaneous fat.

11. Estrogen preferentially increases deposition of (subcutaneous, visceral) white adipose tissue over (subcutaneous, visceral) white adipose tissue.

12. Hypothalamic neurons that promote appetite and decrease metabolism are called (anorexigenic, orexigenic), whereas hypothalamic neurons that suppress appetite and increase metabolism are called (anorexigenic, orexigenic).

13. High levels of leptin normally (inhibit, stimulate) food intake, whereas ghrelin (inhibits, stimulates) food intake.

14. BMI (does, does not) measure the amount and location of body fat.

15. The chronic (anti-inflammatory, proinflammatory) state of obesity increases the risk for type (1, 2) diabetes, cardiovascular disease, and numerous types of cancer.

16. In short-term starvation, energy needs are met through (glycogenolysis and gluconeogenesis, protein catabolism).

Copyright © 2024 by Elsevier, Inc. All Rights Reserved.

CATEGORIZE THE TYPES OF ADIPOSE TISSUE

Write the type of adipose tissue beside each characteristic. Choices: white, brown, beige.

_____ 17. Located within white adipose tissue

_____ 18. Major source of nonshivering thermogenesis

_____ 19. Increases with exercise and chronic exposure to cold

_____ 20. Produces minimal amounts of leptin and adiponectin

_____ 21. Located in visceral, subcutaneous, muscles, and bone marrow deposits

_____ 22. Has the highest amount of mitochondria

_____ 23. Visceral deposits produce proinflammatory cytokines and adipokines

_____ 24. Has greatly increased amounts in obesity

DESCRIBE THE DIFFERENCES

Describe the difference between each pair of terms.

25. What is the difference between adipogenesis and adipocyte hypertrophy?

26. What is the difference between orexigenic neurons and anorexigenic neurons?

27. What is the difference between anorexia nervosa and bulimia nervosa?

28. What is the difference between bulimia nervosa and binge eating disorder?

29. What is the difference between the metabolic pathways in short-term and long-term starvation?

Copyright © 2024 by Elsevier, Inc. All Rights Reserved.

COMPLETE THE SENTENCES

Write one word in each blank to complete these sentences.

30. The brown color of brown adipose tissue comes from the _____ in its many mitochondria.

31. The process of generating heat through _____ thermogenesis occurs in _____ adipose tissue.

32. Adipocytes store excess energy in the form of _____.

33. In adults, obesity is defined as BMI greater than _____ kg/m^2 and generally develops when caloric intake _____ caloric expenditure in genetically susceptible individuals.

34. Overweight is defined as BMI greater than _____ kg/m^2.

35. Neurons that regulate appetite and metabolism are located in the _____ nucleus of the _____.

36. Visceral obesity increases the risk for non-alcoholic steatohepatitis because visceral venous blood that is rich in free fatty acids drains into the _____ vein.

37. Cytokines and hormones secreted by adipose tissue are known as _____; in obesity, _____ that infiltrate adipose tissue secrete proinflammatory cytokines.

38. Rapid provision of nutrients after starvation causes _____ _____, which involves severe hypophosphatemia and other electrolyte imbalances that may be fatal.

39. Decrease in appetite or food intake in older adults may be called _____ of aging.

CHOOSE INCREASES OR DECREASES

Write "increases" or "decreases" by each item to indicate what happens to its blood level in visceral obesity compared with a lean individual.

40. Leptin _____

41. Adiponectin _____

42. Retinol-binding protein 4 _____

43. Angiotensinogen _____

44. Peptide YY _____

45. Interleukin-6 (IL-6) _____

46. Endocannabinoids _____

Copyright © 2024 by Elsevier, Inc. All Rights Reserved.

Write your response to each situation in the space provided.

47. "I learned that high leptin levels decrease food intake and increase energy expenditure," says a nurse. "However, this research article shows high leptin levels in the obese people who were studied. Am I wrong about the action of leptin?"

48. "Why do men who are obese usually have big bellies, but young women who are obese tend to have big buttocks and thighs instead?" asks Ms. Akila, who is a volunteer at a free clinic. "Is there a reason for this?"

49. "What does the word *obesogen* mean?" asks Mr. Khan. "I saw it in a health news headline on the Internet."

50. "I always overeat at Thanksgiving dinner," says Sarah Marks, age 14. "I could stop, but the food is so tasty; then I feel too full afterward. Does that mean I have an eating disorder?"

51. "This article says that tumor necrosis factor alpha is secreted by fat tissue in obesity," says Mx. Montoya. "Does that happen because there is a cancer tumor in the fat?"

Copyright © 2024 by Elsevier, Inc. All Rights Reserved.

24 Structure and Function of the Reproductive Systems

MATCH THE DEFINITIONS

Match the terms on the right with their definitions on the left.

_____ 1. Onset of sexual maturation

_____ 2. Maturation of the ovaries or testes

_____ 3. Onset of menstruation

_____ 4. Onset of breast development

_____ 5. Increased production of adrenal androgens before puberty

A. Thelarche

B. Puberty

C. Gonadarche

D. Adrenarche

E. Menarche

CIRCLE THE CORRECT WORDS

Circle the correct word from the choices provided to complete these sentences.

6. Production of ova (occurs only during fetal life, begins at puberty); production of sperm (occurs only during fetal life; begins at puberty).

7. Menopause is defined as cessation of menstrual flow for (3 months if not pregnant, 1 year).

8. The ability of the female perineum to stretch is most important during (sexual intercourse, childbirth).

9. A vaginal pH that is (low, high) protects against infection.

10. The most important estrogen is E2, also known as (estriol, estradiol).

11. Ovulation is triggered by a surge of (LH and FSH, ACTH) from the (posterior, anterior) pituitary, controlled by (GnRH, CRF) from the hypothalamus.

12. Maintaining pregnancy is an important function of the hormone (estrogen, progesterone).

13. The characteristic hormone profile of menopause is (low, high) estrogen and progesterone levels, (low, high) FSH and LH levels, and (low, high) secretion of inhibin.

ORDER THE STEPS

Sequence the events that occur during spermatogenesis.

14. Write the letters here in the correct order of the steps: _____
    A. Sperm cells migrate to the epididymis.
    B. Spermatogonia divide by mitosis.
    C. Spermatids attach to Sertoli cells and mature into sperm cells.
    D. Primary and secondary spermatocytes divide by meiosis.
    E. Sperm become motile when activated by biochemicals in semen.

122

Copyright © 2024 by Elsevier, Inc. All Rights Reserved.

EXPLAIN THE PICTURES

Examine the pictures and answer the questions about them.

UNDIFFERENTIATED

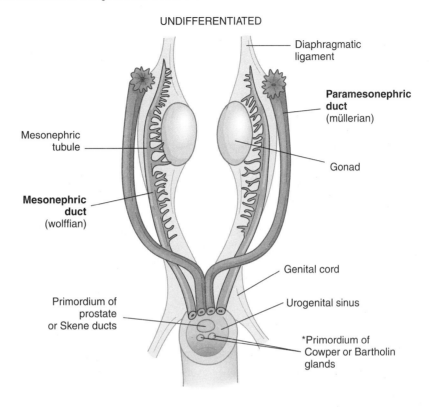

This picture shows embryonic reproductive structures that have not yet differentiated.

15. Expression of a gene on the _____ chromosome creates testes-determining factor, which stimulates the gonads to develop into _____.

16. In the absence of a Y chromosome, expression of other genes causes the gonads to develop into _____ and the regression of which of type of duct in the picture? _____

17. What happens to the remaining ducts in the presence of estrogen and absence of appreciable amounts of testosterone?

18. The primordium marked with an asterisk (*) in the picture will develop into Cowper glands in a _____ and Bartholin glands in a _____.

19. What analogous function do those glands serve in sexually mature adults?

Copyright © 2024 by Elsevier, Inc. All Rights Reserved.

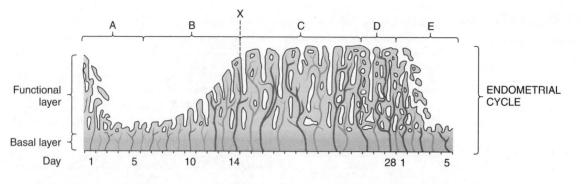

(Adapted from Lowdermilk DL et al: *Maternity nursing & women's health care,* ed 10, St Louis, 2012, Mosby.)

20. The phases of the endometrial cycle are labeled with letters. What words do the letters indicate? A = _____;
    B = _____; C = _____; D = _____; E = _____.

21. Which phase of the *endometrial* cycle occurs during the luteal phase of the *ovarian* cycle? _____

22. What hormone produced by the ovary is in greatest supply during the luteal phase of the ovarian cycle?
    _____

23. What hormone produced by the ovary is responsible for the endometrial events in phase B? _____

24. What occurs at the point marked X in the picture? _____

DESCRIBE THE DIFFERENCES

Describe the difference between each pair of terms.

25. What is the difference between puberty and adolescence?

26. What is the difference between menarche and menopause?

COMPLETE THE SENTENCES

Write one word in each blank to complete these sentences.

27. A gamete has _____ chromosomes.

28. The female structure analogous to the male penis is the _____.

29. The functional layer of the _____ sloughs off during menstruation, but the _____ layer
    remains and regenerates the functional layer.

30. The portion of the uterus located above the insertion of the fallopian tubes is called the _____.

Copyright © 2024 by Elsevier, Inc. All Rights Reserved.

31. After the release of an ovum, an ovarian follicle becomes the _____ _____ .

32. In females, LH stimulates theca cells in the primary follicle to produce _____ ; in males, LH stimulates Leydig cells to produce _____ .

33. Although menstrual (ovarian) cycles can vary in length, the _____ phase is relatively fixed at 14 days.

34. The usual site of fertilization of an ovum is in the _____ _____ .

TEACH PEOPLE ABOUT PHYSIOLOGY

Write your response to each situation in the space provided.

35. Mrs. Yarnold, age 74, says, "I never had a vaginal infection when I was young, but now that I am older, I have had two. I am keeping very good hygiene. Why would I get infections now?"

36. Ms. Francisco, age 29, is looking at a diagram of the female reproductive system. "Look at those lovely fringes on the ends of the fallopian tubes," she says. "Do they have any useful purpose?"

37. Ms. Lendler, age 36, says, "My nurse practitioner told me to wait to schedule my mammogram until right after my menstrual period. Is there a good reason for that timing?"

38. Mr. Martinelli says, "My wife and I want to have a baby. Her nurse practitioner told my wife to ask me to stay out of the hot tub until my wife gets pregnant. Why?"

39. Mr. Booker, a transgender male, has become pregnant. A nurse asks, "How is it possible for a transgender male to become pregnant?"

Copyright © 2024 by Elsevier, Inc. All Rights Reserved.

Alterations of the Female Reproductive System

MATCH THE DEFINITIONS

Match the word on the right with its definition on the left.

_____ 1. Development of the breasts in girls

_____ 2. The process of sexual maturation

_____ 3. Descent of a portion or all of the uterus into the vaginal canal

_____ 4. Abnormal hairiness

_____ 5. Pain with sexual intercourse

_____ 6. Bulging of the rectum and posterior vaginal wall into the vaginal canal

_____ 7. Descent of a portion of the posterior bladder wall and trigone into the vaginal canal

_____ 8. Herniation of the rectouterine pouch into the septum between the rectum and posterior vaginal wall

_____ 9. Benign smooth muscle tumor in the uterine muscle

A. Hirsutism

B. Cystocele

C. Enterocele

D. Puberty

E. Thelarche

F. Leiomyoma

G. Dyspareunia

H. Uterine prolapse

I. Rectocele

CIRCLE THE CORRECT WORDS

Circle the correct word from the choices provided to complete these sentences.

10. Premenstrual syndrome and premenstrual dysphoric disorder occur during the (luteal, follicular) phase of the menstrual cycle; the most prominent and distressing symptoms are (physical, emotional).

11. During the reproductive years, the (acid, alkaline) pH of the vagina protects against infection.

12. Vulvodynia is (chronic pain of, cyst formation in) the vulva; a Bartholin cyst occurs in the (duct, gland body) of the Bartholin gland.

13. Risk factors for pelvic organ prolapse include (very low body weight, obesity), familial tendency, childbirth, and (abdominal, pelvic) surgery or trauma.

14. Endometrial polyps are often related to (estrogen, progesterone) stimulation and are a common cause of (scanty, excessive) menstrual bleeding.

15. HPV-associated carcinoma in situ is most likely to develop at the (transformation, oncoprotein) zone, where the squamous epithelium meets the (ciliated, columnar) epithelium.

16. Most cervical cancers are (symptomatic, asymptomatic); the major symptom of invasive vaginal cancer is vaginal (dryness, bleeding).

Copyright © 2024 by Elsevier, Inc. All Rights Reserved.

17. The major risk factor for endometrial cancer is prolonged exposure to (estrogen, progesterone) without the presence of (estrogen, progesterone).

18. Precocious puberty occurs 2 to 2.5 (years, standard deviations) before the average age of onset of puberty.

19. Nonproliferative breast lesions generally (are, are not) associated with an increased risk for breast cancer; an example of a nonproliferative breast lesion is (ductal hyperplasia, fibrocystic disease).

20. Involuntary muscle spasm that prevents penetration during sexual intercourse is termed (dyspareunia, vaginismus).

CATEGORIZE THE DISORDERS

Write the type of disorder beside each example of sexual dysfunction. Choices: disorder of desire, disorder of orgasm, disorder of sexual pain.

_____ 21. Anorgasmia

_____ 22. Decreased libido

_____ 23. Dyspareunia

_____ 24. Vaginismus

EXPLAIN THE PICTURES

Examine the pictures and answer the questions about them.

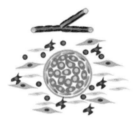 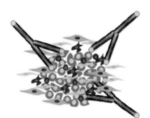

A   Ductal carcinoma in situ   B   Advanced breast cancer

25. What is the difference between the disorders in Figure A and Figure B with regard to the basement membrane?

26. Will the DCIS in Figure A invariably progress to the cancer in Figure B? _____

27. Which figure shows a lesion that might be detected clinically as a lump? _____

28. Would that lump typically be painful or painless? _____

29. The cancer in Figure B is most apt to metastasize to what location first? _____

Copyright © 2024 by Elsevier, Inc. All Rights Reserved.

30. Is it likely that the cells in the cancer in Figure B are homogeneous? Explain your answer.

CATEGORIZE THE RISK FACTORS

Write the classification beside each risk factor for breast cancer. Choices: familial, reproductive, hormonal, genetic, environmental/lifestyle.

_____ 31. *BRCA2* mutation

_____ 32. High alcohol consumption

_____ 33. Nulliparity

_____ 34. Lack of dietary fiber

_____ 35. Late menopause

_____ 36. Physical inactivity

_____ 37. Excess radiation to breasts

_____ 38. Menopausal hormone therapy

_____ 39. Breast cancer in first-degree relative

DESCRIBE THE DIFFERENCES

Describe the difference between each pair of terms.

40. What is the difference between primary and secondary dysmenorrhea?

41. What is the difference between primary and secondary amenorrhea?

42. What is the difference between endometriosis and adenomyosis?

Copyright © 2024 by Elsevier, Inc. All Rights Reserved.

COMPLETE THE SENTENCES

Write one word in each blank to complete these sentences.

43. Bacterial _____ is caused by an overgrowth of bacteria that differ from the usual vaginal bacteria.

44. Puberty is considered delayed if there are no clinical signs of puberty after age _____ in girls.

45. Central precocious puberty is driven by the hormone _____ and occurs when the hypothalamic-pituitary-gonadal axis is working normally but prematurely.

46. The most common cause of secondary dysmenorrhea is _____.

47. Primary amenorrhea can arise from failure of the _____ to synthesize GnRH, failure of the _____ pituitary to synthesize _____ and LH, failure of the ovaries to secrete _____, or anatomic defects of the uterus or vagina.

48. Inflammation of the fallopian tubes is termed _____; inflammation of the ovaries is called _____; these conditions are categorized as _____ _____ disease.

49. Ovarian cysts that may contain mature tissue such as muscle fibers or bone are called _____ cysts.

50. Oncogenic strains 16 and 18 of _____ _____ virus cause _____ cancer.

51. Inappropriate lactation is called _____; a common cause is excessive production of the hormone _____, often from a tumor in the anterior _____.

TEACH PEOPLE ABOUT PATHOPHYSIOLOGY

Write your response to each situation in the space provided.

52. "Oh no! My cousin could not get pregnant and have a baby after she had gonorrhea!" says Ms. Sokol when she learns that she has gonorrhea. After Ms. Sokol leaves, a student nurse says, "Gonorrhea is treatable with antibiotics. How could gonorrhea interfere with pregnancy?"

53. Mrs. Strider had a small lump in her breast and was worried that she had breast cancer. A biopsy of the area showed that she has fibrocystic breast disease. "I am so glad that the biopsy showed no cancer!" exclaims Mrs. Strider. "What is fibrocystic breast disease?"

54. Ms. Chavez says, "Every time I have to take antibiotics for a bladder infection, I get a vaginal yeast infection! Why is that?"

Copyright © 2024 by Elsevier, Inc. All Rights Reserved.

Chapter **25 Alterations of the Female Reproductive System**

55. A physician assistant says, "I understand the normal ovarian cycle and the formation of the dominant follicle during the ovarian cycle. But what goes wrong when a woman develops an ovarian follicular cyst?"

56. Mrs. Jacobs has endometriosis. She asks, "Why does it hurt the most when I am menstruating?"

57. Mrs. Kepler had vaginal bleeding 3 years after menopause and was diagnosed with uterine cancer. She says, "I guess I am not totally unlucky; I hear the death rate is higher with ovarian cancer. Please tell me why the ovarian cancer death rate is higher."

CLINICAL SCENARIOS

Read the clinical scenarios and answer the questions to explore your understanding of reproductive pathophysiology in people who have ovaries, uterus, fallopian tubes, and a vagina.

Jodie Nickelson, a 20-year-old college student, visits the student health center because she is experiencing pelvic pain. She reports the recent development of pain with intercourse and with defecation, as well as dysmenorrhea. Her pelvic pain increases greatly if she jumps or tries to walk briskly. Jodie states that she is sexually active but is taking oral contraceptives and is currently experiencing her normal menstrual period.

Physical Examination

- Temperature 37.8°C (100.0°F); HR, BP, and respirations within normal limits

- Tenderness on cervical movement during pelvic examination

58. *Complete the sentence by choosing from the lists of options.*

Jodie's assessment findings are consistent with _____(1)_____, caused by _____(2)_____ that usually spread from the _____(3)_____ genital tract.

Options for 1	Options for 2	Options for 3
pelvic inflammatory disease (PID)	protozoa	upper
ovarian cyst	fungi	lower
vaginitis	bacteria	

59. Why did the nurse practitioner measure Jodie's temperature?

Copyright © 2024 by Elsevier, Inc. All Rights Reserved.

60. What organs commonly are involved in this condition?

61. What is the technical term for pain with sexual intercourse? _____

62. What is the technical term for pain with defecation? _____

63. Why does pain occur with sexual intercourse and defecation in this condition?

64. During the pelvic examination, Jodie experienced pain with cervical movement. Why is this an expected finding in her situation?

65. Jodie was treated successfully with antibiotics. What potential complications of this condition might Jodie experience in the future?

Marge Orrin, age 28, visited a women's healthcare nurse practitioner because she was unable to become pregnant after trying for a year.

History

- Menses have been irregular since menarche

- Typically has five menses per year, with heavy bleeding that is heavier in the past year

- Last menstrual period 3 weeks ago

- Weight gain of 40 pounds in last 18 months

- Mother had chin hair that she shaved regularly

Physical Examination

- BP 144/90; other vital signs within normal limits

- Weight 251 pounds, BMI 35.4

- Dark hair on the chin and chest

- Moderate acne on the back

- No acanthosis nigricans

- Obese abdomen, no tenderness

- Normal external genitalia, no clitoromegaly

Copyright © 2024 by Elsevier, Inc. All Rights Reserved.

Laboratory Tests

- TSH and prolactin normal

- Testosterone elevated

- LDL elevated

- Pelvic ultrasound showed polycystic ovaries

Mrs. Orrin's diagnoses were polycystic ovary syndrome (PCOS) and hypertension.

66. What conditions characterize PCOS? Which ones did Mrs. Orrin have?

67. What are the typical blood levels of androgens in PCOS? Circle the correct answer.

Increased   Normal   Decreased

68. What are the typical blood levels of estrogens in PCOS? Circle the correct answer.

Increased   Normal   Decreased

69. Why should the nurse practitioner ask Mrs. Orrin about her fatigue level and if she feels rested after she sleeps 8 hours?

70. What is the significance of Mrs. Orrin's BMI in the context of PCOS?

Copyright © 2024 by Elsevier, Inc. All Rights Reserved.

26 Alterations of the Male Reproductive System

MATCH THE DEFINITIONS

Match the term on the right with its definition on the left.

_____ 1. Visible enlargement of breast tissue in a male

_____ 2. Foreskin of the penis

_____ 3. Narrowing of the urethra due to scarring

_____ 4. Prolonged painful penile erection

_____ 5. Inflammation of the glans penis

_____ 6. Fibrosis of the corpora cavernosa that causes penile curvature during erection

_____ 7. Undescended testicle (or both testes)

_____ 8. Inflammation of the testes

_____ 9. Inflammation of the foreskin

_____ 10. Cyst in the epididymis

_____ 11. Abnormally dilated vein within the spermatic cord

A. Peyronie disease

B. Cryptorchidism

C. Balanitis

D. Orchitis

E. Spermatocele

F. Posthitis

G. Varicocele

H. Urethral stricture

I. Prepuce

J. Priapism

K. Gynecomastia

CIRCLE THE CORRECT WORDS

Circle the correct word from the choices provided to complete these sentences.

12. Most breast cancers in men are (estrogen, androgen) positive.

13. Any factor that causes testicular temperature to (fall, rise) can impair sperm production.

14. Most penile cancer is (squamous cell carcinoma, adenocarcinoma), whereas most prostate cancer is (squamous cell carcinoma, adenocarcinoma).

15. The most common cause of orchitis in postpubertal males is (gonorrhea, mumps).

16. Testicular torsion requires immediate treatment to prevent (ischemia and necrosis, epididymitis and sterility).

17. Benign prostatic hyperplasia (BPH) begins in the (inner layers, periphery) of the prostate; most prostate cancer begins in the (inner layers, periphery) of the prostate.

18. In acute bacterial prostatitis, bacteria reach the prostate (through the blood, by ascending the urinary tract); the clinical manifestations are similar to those of (pyelonephritis, prostate cancer).

19. Arterial diseases can cause sexual dysfunction by interfering with (erection, ejaculation).

Copyright © 2024 by Elsevier, Inc. All Rights Reserved.

DESCRIBE THE DIFFERENCES

Describe the difference between each pair of terms.

20. What is the difference between phimosis and paraphimosis?

21. What is the difference between delayed puberty and precocious puberty in boys?

22. What is the difference between a varicocele and a hydrocele?

COMPLETE THE SENTENCES

Write one word in each blank to complete these sentences.

23. Priapism needs emergency treatment to prevent development of _____ _____.

24. Seminomas are a type of _____ cancer.

25. Urine reflux into the epididymis causes _____ _____.

26. The _____ hormones, such as testosterone, play important roles in development and progression of prostate cancer.

27. The prostate and other tissues can use the enzyme aromatase to convert androgens to _____.

28. Sexual dysfunction is impairment of any of these three processes (listed in the order that they normally occur): _____, _____, and _____.

29. Gynecomastia often involves imbalance of the _____ ratio.

30. The most common cause of urethritis is infection with microorganisms that were transmitted _____.

31. A man who has the *BRCA2* germline mutation has a greatly increased risk of developing _____ cancer.

TEACH PEOPLE ABOUT PATHOPHYSIOLOGY

Write your response to each situation in the space provided.

32. Mr. Montoya was diagnosed with BPH. He says, "Tell me why it takes so long for me to empty my bladder."

Copyright © 2024 by Elsevier, Inc. All Rights Reserved.

33. Mr. Hoover says, "My 90-year-old uncle has prostate cancer, but the doctor said to watch and wait rather than do surgery! Why? Isn't cancer fatal? He is healthy otherwise."

34. Mr. Ortega had burning on urination and went to see a nurse practitioner. He was diagnosed with nongonococcal urethritis. He says, "I know what urethritis means, but what about 'nongonococcal'? Do I have gonorrhea?"

35. Mr. Singh went to a clinic because he has a scrotal mass. Afterward, he says, "That doctor says I have a hydrocele and not to worry, but I am not sure he knows what he is doing! Why did he put a flashlight in back of my scrotum and look at it?"

36. Mr. Watson, age 33, noticed that his right testicle was enlarged. It did not hurt. His physician palpated Mr. Watson's testes, discovered a firm mass in the enlarged testicle, and made an appointment for Mr. Watson to have an ultrasound examination. Mr. Watson says, "I know my doctor is concerned that I might have testicular cancer, but why did he ask me if I had undescended testicles when I was an infant? And why did he feel my groin after he found the mass in my testicle?"

Copyright © 2024 by Elsevier, Inc. All Rights Reserved.

CIRCLE THE CORRECT WORDS

Circle the correct word from the choices provided to complete these sentences.

1. The risk for developing gonorrhea from vaginal or anal intercourse with an infected partner is greater for the (receptive, insertive) partner.

2. In the United States, the prevalence of syphilis is highest among (men, women) and transgender women.

3. The rash of (primary, secondary) syphilis is unusual because it appears (on the palms of the hands and soles of the feet, in lines on the backs of the hands and tops of the feet) as well as on the torso.

4. (Men, Women) who develop chancroid infection usually are asymptomatic; people who are symptomatic develop genital ulcers and abscesses of the inguinal lymph nodes called _____.

5. HPV serotypes 16 and 18 are associated with (genital warts, anogenital cancer), and HPV serotypes 6 and 11 are associated with (genital warts, anogenital cancer).

6. Trichomoniasis is caused by a (bacterium, protozoan) that (adheres to, invades) squamous epithelium.

7. A penis that is (circumcised, uncircumcised) has higher risk of *Trichomonas* infection.

8. Genital warts are (not, highly) contagious and are caused by a (bacterium, virus).

9. People who have HSV infection can transmit the virus (only when having, whether or not they have) symptoms.

CHARACTERIZE THE SEXUALLY TRANSMITTED INFECTIONS

Complete each sentence by choosing from the lists of options.

10. *Chlamydia is caused by* _____ (1) _____, *which is a(n)* _____ (2) _____.

Options for 1	Options for 2
Treponema pallidum	gram-negative intracellular bacterium
Chlamydia trachomatis	gram-negative diplococcus
Neisseria gonorrhoeae	anaerobic spirochete

11. *Gonorrhea is caused by* _____ (1) _____, *which is a(n)* _____ (2) _____.

Options for 1	Options for 2
Treponema pallidum	gram-negative intracellular bacterium
Chlamydia trachomatis	gram-negative diplococcus
Neisseria gonorrhoeae	anaerobic spirochete

Copyright © 2024 by Elsevier, Inc. All Rights Reserved.

12. Genital herpes *is caused by* _____(1)_____, *which is a(n)* _____(2)_____.

Options for 1	Options for 2
Human papillomavirus	enveloped, linear, double-stranded DNA virus that has a latent stage in neurons
Herpes simplex virus	nonenveloped, circular, double-stranded DNA virus that has numerous strains

13. *Syphilis is caused by* _____(1)_____, *which is a(n)* _____(2)_____.

Options for 1	Options for 2
Treponema pallidum	gram-negative intracellular bacterium
Chlamydia trachomatis	gram-negative diplococcus
Neisseria gonorrhoeae	anaerobic spirochete

14. Genital warts are *caused by* _____(1)_____, *which is a(n)* _____(2)_____.

Options for 1	Options for 2
Human papillomavirus	enveloped, linear, double-stranded DNA virus that has a latent stage in neurons
Herpes simplex virus	nonenveloped, circular, double-stranded DNA virus that has numerous strains

ORDER THE STEPS

Sequence the events that occur when an individual becomes infected with T. pallidum and does not receive treatment.

15. Write the letters here in the correct order of the steps: _____
    A. Signs and symptoms disappear.
    B. *T. pallidum* enters through a minor break in skin or mucous membrane.
    C. Gummas, cardiac valve damage, and/or neurologic damage may become apparent.
    D. The infection becomes systemic, causing low-grade fever, malaise, and skin or mucous membrane lesions.
    E. *T. pallidum* multiplies, and a chancre appears in that location.

EXPLAIN THE PICTURE

Examine the picture and answer the questions about it.

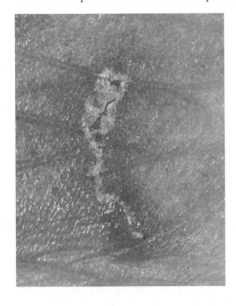

16. The picture shows the typical appearance of what condition?

    _____

17. What type of organism causes this lesion?

    _____

18. Why do the lesions have this shape?

    _____

19. What is the typical clinical manifestation at the location of these

    lesions? _____

20. In addition to transmission during sexual contact, what other ways

    can this condition be transmitted? _____

    _____

Copyright © 2024 by Elsevier, Inc. All Rights Reserved.

DESCRIBE THE DIFFERENCES

Describe the difference between each pair of terms.

21. What is the difference between a chancre and a bubo?

22. What is the difference between condylomata acuminata and condylomata lata?

23. What is the difference between "crabs" and scabies?

COMPLETE THE SENTENCES

Write one word in each blank to complete these sentences.

24. The bacteria that cause gonorrhea attach to host _____ cells of mucous membranes at the site of initial infection.

25. Untreated genital gonococcal infection that spreads can cause _____ in men and _____ _____ _____ in women, both of which can lead to sterility.

26. Gonorrhea transmitted by an infected mother before or during birth typically manifests as an _____ infection in the neonate and develops 1 to 12 _____ after birth.

27. Excessive scratching of pruritic lesions such as from scabies or pubic lice can lead to _____ infection.

28. Granuloma inguinale, also known as _____, is a chronic, progressive, destructive bacterial infection of genitals.

29. The chronic STI lymphogranuloma venereum begins as an infection of the genital _____ and then spreads to the _____ tissue.

30. The major routes of transmission of hepatitis _____ are sexual contact and nonsexual exposure to infected blood and other body fluids.

31. Typical lesions of genital herpes begin as painful _____ that break open and then crust over before they heal.

32. Recurrent episodes of genital herpes typically are _____ severe and have _____ duration than the primary episode.

Copyright © 2024 by Elsevier, Inc. All Rights Reserved.

Write your response to each situation in the space provided.

33. "Our son says he got gonorrhea from his girlfriend, but she did not have any symptoms," says Mrs. Alvid. "Is that really possible?"

34. Katrina, age 16, asks, "Why should I get that HPV shot? I am not afraid of a few warts!"

35. Jesse, age 24, developed molluscum contagiosum. "What is a fomite? Is it a type of insect?" he asks. "The Internet said that this infection can be spread by fomites at a public swimming pool."

36. Mrs. Escudero has bacterial vaginosis. "My nurse practitioner said something about having the wrong bacteria in my vagina," she says. "Please explain that."

37. Mr. Bowers has a large syphilitic chancre on his penis and will receive penicillin today. He asks, "Is that sore going to make a scar?"

38. Ms. Bagai developed genital herpes and took valacyclovir as prescribed. Four months later, she has another outbreak. She says, "I took all my medicine the first time, just as the nurse practitioner told me to do, and I have not had sex since then. Why do I have herpes again?"

Copyright © 2024 by Elsevier, Inc. All Rights Reserved.

Read the clinical scenario and answer the questions to explore your understanding of Chlamydia infection.

Ms. Ward, age 21, came to a nurse practitioner for her yearly check-up. The nurse practitioner noticed abnormal redness of Ms. Ward's cervix and took a swab to test for gonorrhea and *Chlamydia*. The test was negative for gonorrhea and positive for *Chlamydia*.

39. Why did the nurse practitioner test for both gonorrhea and *Chlamydia*?

40. Ms. Ward says, "I do not have any symptoms, so why should I take this antibiotic?" How should the nurse practitioner respond?

41. Why should the nurse practitioner ask Ms. Ward if she feels burning when she urinates?

42. How does *Chlamydia* reproduce?

43. Ms. Ward says, "I hear that PID causes infertility. Is that true?" How should the nurse practitioner respond?

44. "How common is *Chlamydia* infection? Is it unusual?" asks Ms. Ward after agreeing to start taking the prescribed antibiotic.

45. If a woman who has *Chlamydia* infection becomes pregnant, what are the most common manifestations in the infant if the mother transmits the infection during birth?

   Copyright © 2024 by Elsevier, Inc. All Rights Reserved.

28 Structure and Function of the Hematologic System

MATCH THE DEFINITIONS

Match each definition on the right with its word on the left.

_____ 1. Hemoglobin

_____ 2. Hepcidin

_____ 3. Thrombopoietin

_____ 4. Tissue thromboplastin

_____ 5. Plasmin

_____ 6. Myoglobin

A. Chemical released by damaged cells that activates coagulation

B. Enzyme that dissolves clots

C. Oxygen-binding molecule in muscle cells

D. Oxygen-binding molecule in erythrocytes

E. Hormone growth factor that regulates platelet formation

F. Hormone that regulates iron homeostasis

CLASSIFY THE CELLS

Write the type of cell beside each name. Choices: granulocyte, agranulocyte.

_____ 7. Macrophage

_____ 8. Natural killer cell

_____ 9. Lymphocyte

_____ 10. Neutrophil

_____ 11. Monocyte

_____ 12. Basophil

_____ 13. Eosinophil

Copyright © 2024 by Elsevier, Inc. All Rights Reserved.

MATCH THE FUNCTIONS

Match the cell on the right with its function on the left.

_____ 14. Do active phagocytosis as part of the mononuclear phagocyte system; process and present antigens; participate in wound healing

A. Eosinophils

B. Neutrophils

_____ 15. Process antigens and present them to lymphocytes

C. Macrophages

_____ 16. Produce antibodies against specific antigens

D. B lymphocytes (plasma cells)

_____ 17. Kill tumor cells and virus-infected cells

E. Natural killer cells

_____ 18. Precursor cells for macrophages

F. Dendritic cells

_____ 19. Do phagocytosis early in inflammation; kill bacteria

G. Monocytes

_____ 20. Defend against parasites

CIRCLE THE CORRECT WORDS

Circle the correct word from the choices provided to complete these sentences.

21. Mature erythrocytes (have, do not have) a nucleus; mature neutrophils have a (round, multilobed) nucleus.

22. Neutrophils, basophils, and eosinophils are (immunocytes, granulocytes); immature neutrophils are called (segmented, bands).

23. The term *hematopoiesis* refers to production of (erythrocytes, blood cells) and occurs primarily in the (bone marrow, spleen) after birth.

24. In the bones, hematopoiesis occurs in the (yellow, red) marrow; the (yellow, red) marrow is inactive.

25. Each hemoglobin A molecule consists of (two, four) globin chains and (two, four) hemes; in order to bind oxygen, the iron portion of heme must be (ferrous Fe^{2+}, ferric Fe^{3+}).

26. The hormone (ferroportin, hepcidin) regulates absorption of dietary iron; after absorption, iron circulates attached to (ferritin, transferrin) and is stored inside cells attached to (ferritin, transferrin); large amounts of this intracellular iron complex gather as (ferroportin, hemosiderin).

27. Nitric oxide and prostacyclin (trigger, inhibit) platelet adhesion and aggregation; thromboxane A_2, epinephrine, thrombin, and collagen (trigger, inhibit) platelet adhesion and aggregation.

CATEGORIZE THE LYMPHOID ORGANS

Write the type of lymphoid organ beside each name. Choices: primary, secondary.

_____ 28. Spleen

_____ 29. Thymus

_____ 30. Lymph nodes

_____ 31. Peyer patches (gut-associated lymphoid tissue)

Copyright © 2024 by Elsevier, Inc. All Rights Reserved.

_____ 32. Tonsils

_____ 33. Bone marrow

ORDER THE STEPS

Sequence the cells that lead to a fully differentiated blood cell in the myeloid lineage.

34. Write the letters here in the correct order: _____
    A. Common myeloid progenitor cell
    B. Fully differentiated blood cell
    C. Hematopoietic stem cell
    D. Blast cell
    E. Progenitor cell
    F. Multipotent stem cell

EXPLAIN THE PICTURES

Examine the pictures and answer the questions about them.

35. What happens when platelets are exposed to subendothelial collagen?

36. The platelets on the left have smooth edges, but the platelets on the right have jagged, spiky edges. What does this change in shape indicate? _____

37. After the events in the picture, the platelets will aggregate and form a platelet plug. What stabilizes the platelet plug? _____ What is the source of that stabilizing substance?

38. How do the platelets expel the serum from the platelet plug, thus increasing its strength?

Copyright © 2024 by Elsevier, Inc. All Rights Reserved.

Chapter **28** **Structure and Function of the Hematologic System**

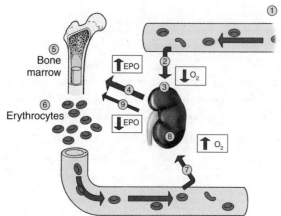

39. What does the acronym EPO mean? _____

40. In the picture, EPO is released by the _____ and acts on the _____ _____.

41. What does EPO stimulate the bone marrow to do? _____

42. What causes increased release of EPO? _____

43. Where does negative feedback occur in the picture? _____
    _____

DESCRIBE THE DIFFERENCES

Describe the difference between each pair of terms.

44. What is the difference between a leukocyte and a lymphocyte?

45. What is the difference between plasma and serum?

46. What is the difference between a multipotent stem cell and a hematopoietic stem cell?

47. What is the difference between a reticulocyte and an erythrocyte?

Copyright © 2024 by Elsevier, Inc. All Rights Reserved.

48. What is the difference between ferritin and apoferritin?

NAME THE PROGENITORS

Write the type of progenitor cell beside each mature cell or cell fragment. Choices: lymphoid, myeloid.

_____ 49. Erythrocyte

_____ 50. Natural killer cell

_____ 51. Eosinophil

_____ 52. Monocyte

_____ 53. T cell

_____ 54. Neutrophil

_____ 55. Basophil

_____ 56. Plasma cell (mature B cell)

_____ 57. Platelet

COMPLETE THE SENTENCES

Write one word in each blank to complete these sentences.

58. Fibrinogen is the most plentiful _____ factor that circulates in the blood.

59. The most abundant plasma protein is _____; the most abundant leukocytes are the _____.

60. The capacity to be _____ deformed is important for erythrocytes because it enables them to squeeze through the sinusoids of the _____ and through the smallest capillaries.

61. Platelets, also called _____, are cytoplasmic fragments of large cells called _____ that are located in the _____ _____.

62. Erythropoietin stimulates bone marrow to produce more _____; thrombopoietin stimulates bone marrow to produce more _____.

63. Tissue factor also is called tissue _____; this substance triggers the _____ pathway of clotting.

64. Plasmin is an enzyme that degrades _____ polymers; its inactive precursor is _____, which is produced by the _____.

65. Lymphocytes tend to have decreased function in _____ adults.

Copyright © 2024 by Elsevier, Inc. All Rights Reserved.

CATEGORIZE THE SUBSTANCES

Write the function of each substance with regard to blood clotting. Choices: promotes clotting, antithrombotic.

_____ 66. Plasminogen activators

_____ 67. Tissue thromboplastin

_____ 68. Thrombomodulin, protein C, and protein S

_____ 69. Tissue factor pathway inhibitor

_____ 70. Exposure of blood to collagen

_____ 71. Thrombin

_____ 72. Prostacyclin

_____ 73. Antithrombin III

_____ 74. Nitric oxide

TEACH PEOPLE ABOUT PATHOPHYSIOLOGY

Write your response to each situation in the space provided.

75. "I had a blood transfusion a few years ago," says Mx. Wilder. "Every once in a while I still think about that stranger's red cells moving around my body."

76. Mrs. Abbott received an erythropoietin injection to treat her severe anemia. "My physician said my reticulocyte count is increased, which is good," she says. "But I understand that reticulocytes are immature red blood cells. Why is that good?"

77. "My nurse practitioner told me I need more iron in my diet to help make red blood cells," says Mrs. Saleem. "What does iron have to do with red blood cells?"

78. "My brother's spleen was removed after an automobile accident," says Mr. Norton. "I just learned that the spleen normally removes worn-out red cells from the blood. Because he no longer has a spleen, how does his body get rid of old red blood cells?"

Copyright © 2024 by Elsevier, Inc. All Rights Reserved.

79. "I am reading a mystery story in which the important clue was high bilirubin in a man's blood when a poison caused a lot of his red blood cells to die," says Mrs. Verde. "What do red blood cells have to do with bilirubin?"

80. A nurse says, "I hear that platelets release various chemicals, including some proteins like clotting and growth factors, when they are activated. But protein synthesis takes time, and platelet activation occurs very fast. Please explain this!"

81. Mr. Patel has signs of deep venous thrombosis, and a blood sample was drawn to measure D-dimer. He asks, "What is D-dimer? How will measuring it help to decide whether or not I have a blood clot in my leg?"

82. Mr. Jeterman was injured in a knife fight. His partner says, "I know that his scabs eventually will fall off. What happens to clots in blood vessels inside the body? Do they fall off into the blood when the blood vessel heals? I think that would cause a problem."

Copyright © 2024 by Elsevier, Inc. All Rights Reserved.

29 Alterations of Erythrocyte, Platelet, and Hemostatic Function

MATCH THE DEFINITIONS

Match the word on the right with its definition on the left.

_____	1. Increased blood level of immature erythrocytes	A. Anemia
_____	2. Increased number or volume of circulating erythrocytes	B. Anisocytosis
_____	3. Decreased number or volume of circulating erythrocytes	C. Poikilocytosis
_____	4. Premature death of damaged erythrocytes	D. Pancytopenia
_____	5. Having erythrocytes of different shapes	E. Reticulocytosis
_____	6. Having erythrocytes of different sizes	F. Eryptosis
_____	7. Decreased number of circulating erythrocytes, leukocytes, and platelets	G. Polycythcmia

MATCH MORE DEFINITIONS

Match the word on the right with its definition on the left.

_____	8. Enlarged lymph nodes	A. Granulocytopenia
_____	9. Lower-than-normal neutrophil count in the blood	B. Leukopenia
_____	10. Lower-than-normal blood counts of white blood cells, red blood cells, and platelets	C. Lymphadenopathy
_____	11. Higher-than-normal white blood cell count	D. Granulocytosis
_____	12. Lower-than-normal white blood cell count	E. Agranulocytosis
_____	13. Higher-than-normal blood counts of neutrophils, eosinophils, and basophils	F. Leukocytosis
_____	14. Lower-than-normal blood counts of neutrophils, eosinophils, and basophils	G. Pancytopenia
_____	15. Complete absence of neutrophils, eosinophils, and basophils in the blood	H. Neutropenia

CIRCLE THE CORRECT WORDS

Circle the correct word from the choices provided to complete these sentences.

16. When plasma volume increases to compensate for anemia, the blood viscosity (increases, decreases), which causes blood flow to be (sluggish, turbulent).

17. Defective DNA synthesis in bone marrow precursors usually creates erythrocytes that are (microcytic, macrocytic) and normochromic.

Copyright © 2024 by Elsevier, Inc. All Rights Reserved.

18. Folate deficiency anemia is associated with chronic malnourishment and (cocaine, **alcohol**) use disorder.

19. The term *megaloblastic anemia* indicates that the erythrocytes are (**macrocytic**, macrochromic).

20. The incidence of iron deficiency anemia is (lowest, **highest**) in women during their reproductive years and (increases, **decreases**) after menopause.

21. Numerous cytokines released by during chronic inflammation alter (**iron metabolism**, hemoglobin function), thus contributing to (iron-deficiency anemia, **anemia of chronic disease**).

22. A major contributor to anemia in people who have chronic kidney disease is (**deficiency**, excess) of erythropoietin.

23. People who are dehydrated after extensive diarrhea have (absolute, **relative**) polycythemia; people who have hypercapneic chronic obstructive pulmonary disease have (**secondary absolute**, relative) polycythemia.

24. Hemolysis from a mismatched blood transfusion is an example of (autoimmune, **alloimmune**) hemolytic anemia that occurs (**intravascularly**, extravascularly).

25. Individuals who have congenital hemolytic disorders typically have a (small, **large**) spleen.

26. People who have thrombocythemia have a higher increased risk for (bleeding, **clotting**), although the other event also may occur.

27. The most common causes of eosinophilia are (bacterial infection, **parasite invasion**) and (autoimmune, **hypersensitivity**) reactions.

28. Monocytosis occurs during the (early, **late**) phase of inflammation, whereas neutrophilia occurs during the (**early**, late) phase of inflammation.

29. All types of leukemia are characterized by uncontrolled (**production**, destruction) of white blood cells in the (blood, **bone marrow**) that thereby (**decreases**, increases) the amount and function of erythrocytes and platelets.

30. Although (leukopenia, **leukocytosis**) may occur pathologically or normally in response to physiologic stressors, (**leukopenia**, leukocytosis) occurs only pathologically.

31. (**Localized**, Generalized) lymphadenopathy indicates drainage from areas of inflammation, but (localized, **generalized**) lymphadenopathy usually indicates a malignant or non-malignant disease.

32. In a leukemia or lymphoma that has the term *lymphoblastic* in its name, the malignant cells are (**immature**, well differentiated).

CATEGORIZE ANEMIAS BY THE APPEARANCE OF THE ERYTHROCYTES

Write the appearance of the erythrocytes beside each type of anemia. Choices: normocytic-normochromic, macrocytic-normochromic, microcytic-hypochromic.

_____ 33. Iron deficiency anemia

_____ 34. Aplastic anemia

_____ 35. Pernicious anemia

_____ 36. Posthemorrhagic anemia

_____ 37. Folate deficiency anemia

_____ 38. Anemia of chronic disease

Copyright © 2024 by Elsevier, Inc. All Rights Reserved.

CATEGORIZE ANEMIAS BY THEIR GENERAL CAUSES

Write the general cause of the anemia beside its name. Choices: impaired erythrocyte production, increased erythrocyte destruction.

_____ 39. Hereditary spherocytosis

_____ 40. Anemia of chronic disease

_____ 41. Iron deficiency anemia

_____ 42. Sickle cell anemia

_____ 43. G6PD deficiency

_____ 44. Pernicious anemia

_____ 45. Aplastic anemia

_____ 46. Folate deficiency anemia

DESCRIBE THE DIFFERENCES

Describe the difference between each pair of terms.

47. What is the difference between leukemias and lymphomas?

48. What is the difference between a lymphocytic leukemia and a myelogenous leukemia?

49. What is the difference between splenomegaly and hypersplenism?

EXPLAIN THE PICTURES

Examine the pictures and answer the questions about them.

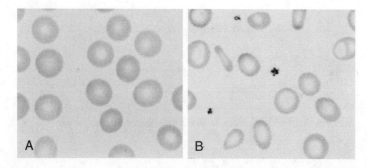

Copyright © 2024 by Elsevier, Inc. All Rights Reserved.

50. Picture A shows normal erythrocytes. What technical term indicates that they have normal size?_____

51. What technical term indicates that the erythrocytes in picture A have normal color, and thus a normal amount of hemoglobin? _____

52. What technical term describes the color (and thus the amount of hemoglobin) of the erythrocytes in picture B?

_____

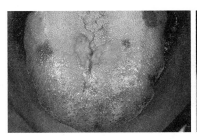 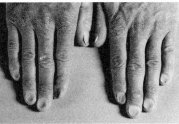

53. These pictures show the tongue and the fingernails from a person whose erythrocytes look like those in picture B. The tongue has lost papillae and looks fissured. What technical term describes it? _____

54. What technical term applies to the concave, brittle fingernails? _____

55. These pictures are characteristic of what type of anemia? _____

56. Would you expect this person to develop pallor or jaundice? Why?

57. Write a common scenario in which this type of anemia occurs.

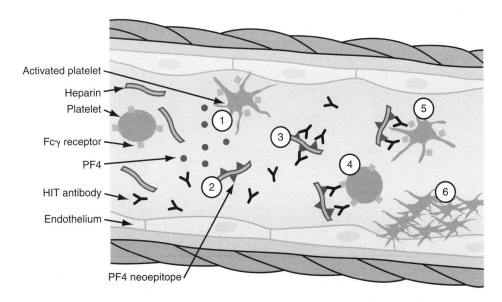

58. The picture shows activation of HIT antibodies. What does HIT mean? _____

Copyright © 2024 by Elsevier, Inc. All Rights Reserved.

Chapter **29** Alterations of Erythrocyte, Platelet, and Hemostatic Function

59. What is the activated platelet numbered 1 releasing? _____

60. What does this substance bind? _____

61. When a person develops HIT antibodies, they react specifically against what? _____

62. By what mechanism do more platelets become activated, causing more clotting?

63. Where do clots usually form in HIT?

MATCH THE ABNORMALITIES

Match the names of the abnormal items on the right with the descriptions on the left.

_____ 64. Abnormal antibody or fragment released by malignant plasma cells in multiple myeloma

_____ 65. Mutant tyrosine kinase that drives cell proliferation and survival in some types of leukemia

_____ 66. Genetic translocation between chromosomes 9 and 22 that creates a mutant protein found in many people with CML

A. Philadelphia chromosome

B. M protein

C. BCR-ABL1 variant oncoprotein

COMPLETE THE SENTENCES

Write one word in each blank to complete these sentences.

67. When describing the appearance of erythrocytes, terms that end with _____ refer to the hemoglobin content and terms that end with _____ refer to cell size.

68. Hereditary hemochromatosis is an autosomal- _____ disorder that causes increased absorption of dietary _____.

69. Serum ferritin levels are used to evaluate _____ status when diagnosing anemia.

70. Polycythemia _____ is a slow growing cancer in which the bone marrow produces too many _____.

71. Idiopathic (primary acquired) aplastic anemia involves damage by T _____ to the hematopoietic stem cells in the _____ _____; secondary aplastic anemia occurs when those cells are destroyed by _____, drugs, or ionizing _____.

72. Release of _____ during chronic inflammation contributes to the anemia of chronic disease by decreasing the availability of _____ and inhibiting erythroid progenitors.

73. Congenital hemolytic anemias are caused by _____ defects in erythrocytes, but acquired hemolytic anemias usually are caused by the _____ system.

Copyright © 2024 by Elsevier, Inc. All Rights Reserved.

74. Hemolysis in most inherited hemolytic anemias occurs in the _____ by the action of _____.

75. Drug-induced hemolytic anemia from antibiotics usually begins when the antibiotic or other drug serves as a _____ and binds to erythrocyte proteins.

76. Hemolysis that occurs slowly will not cause anemia because bone marrow can increase erythrocyte production up to _____ times its normal rate; jaundice occurs from hemolysis only when heme destruction exceeds the liver's ability to process and excrete _____.

77. Infectious mononucleosis is an acute infection of _____ lymphocytes commonly caused by Epstein-Barr _____; typical clinical manifestations are pharyngitis, fever, and cervical _____.

78. In Africa, _____ lymphoma, a rapidly growing _____ lymphocyte tumor in the _____ and facial bones of children, is associated with Epstein-Barr _____.

79. AML stands for _____ _____ _____; CLL stands for _____ _____ _____.

80. Leukopenia creates increased risk for _____.

81. Hypercalcemia and bone lesions are characteristic of _____ _____ because the malignant cells reside in the bone marrow and not in the circulating blood.

82. The bone marrow depression of acute leukemia causes _____ due to lack of erythrocytes, fever from _____ due to lack of leukocytes, and _____ due to lack of platelets.

83. Splenomegaly secondary to infection in the body increases the risk for spleen _____ from blunt trauma.

84. Reed-Sternberg cells are the classic abnormal cells in _____ _____.

LOCATE THE DEFECT

Write the location of the erythrocyte defect beside each type of hemolytic anemia. Choices: membrane defect, enzyme pathway defect, hemoglobin synthesis defect.

_____ 85. Thalassemia

_____ 86. Hereditary spherocytosis

_____ 87. Sickle cell anemia

_____ 88. G6PD deficiency anemia

TEACH PEOPLE ABOUT PATHOPHYSIOLOGY

Write your response to each situation in the space provided.

89. "I thought red blood cells came from bone marrow," says Mrs. Weiner. "How can chronic kidney disease give me anemia?"

Copyright © 2024 by Elsevier, Inc. All Rights Reserved.

90. Mrs. Agee, who has polycythemia vera, says, "I thought red blood cells carry oxygen, not cause clotting. Why did I get a blood clot in my arm vein?"

91. Mrs. Montoya asks, "Why does anemia make me so tired?"

92. Mrs. Ferric was diagnosed recently with hereditary hemochromatosis. She says, "Tell me again how removing some of my blood regularly will help protect my liver."

93. Mr. Abbotts developed aplastic anemia from chronic benzene exposure at work. "I know that I got tired from low red cells, got infections from low white cells, and bled more from low platelets," he says. "But I had several infections and a lot of little bleeding spots on my skin before I became so tired and saw the doctor. Why did it take longer for me to get tired?"

94. Mr. Cook developed posthemorrhagic anemia after accidentally cutting his wrist on a table saw and losing 1400 mL of blood. His wife says, "I know that anemia makes a person pale and tired. But how could it make him lightheaded as he was at first?"

95. "I had penicillin with no problem," says Mrs. Capthon. "But my daughter got what they call hemolytic anemia from penicillin. I understand that means her red blood cells were destroyed. What happened?"

96. A nurse asks, "What is the difference between the composition of arterial thrombi and venous thrombi?"

97. Mr. Finn developed DIC while he was in a critical care unit with sepsis. Mrs. Finn asks, "How can he be bleeding when he is making so many bad clots?"

Copyright © 2024 by Elsevier, Inc. All Rights Reserved.

98. Mr. Ekewe bruises easily and bleeds excessively. "The doctors checked my platelets, and they are fine," he says. "Now they want to do more tests. What else could it be?"

99. Mrs. Nguyen says, "They told me I have ITP. I was so scared that I do not remember anything else. What is ITP? How does it make those red dots and purple blotches on my skin? Is it contagious?"

100. Mr. Vander Waal has thrombocytopenia from cancer chemotherapy. His son has immune-mediated thrombocytopenia. "We have similar symptoms but different treatment," Mr. Vander Waal says, "Why?"

101. Mr. Drayson was admitted to the hospital with pneumonia. A nurse says, "He has Von Willebrand disease also. What should I assess to see if it gets out of control?"

102. "The doctor said they found Bence Jones proteins in my urine," says Mx. Thea. "What are Bence Jones proteins and why are they important?"

103. "I have multiple myeloma, which my oncologist says is malignant plasma cells," says Mr. Amon. "What are plasma cells? Do they have a normal function? What happens to that function when plasma cells become malignant?"

104. "Why is Knut so tired?" asks his partner. "He has ALL, but I thought leukemia is a problem with white blood cells. Knut is tired even when he does not have an infection."

105. "The doctor said my father is anemic," says Mrs. Fields, whose father has AML. "I think she should give him some iron tablets like the ones they gave me when I was anemic."

Copyright © 2024 by Elsevier, Inc. All Rights Reserved.   Chapter **29** **Alterations of Erythrocyte, Platelet, and Hemostatic Function**

106. Mr. Squil has Hodgkin lymphoma. "When I get a sore throat, my neck nodes swell just a little and get tender," he says. "But with this Hodgkin lymphoma they swelled up a lot and were not tender at all. How can my lymph nodes swell so much but not be painful?"

107. "That medical student said my white cells are well differentiated," says Mr. Mihaly, who has CML. "What does that mean?"

CLINICAL SCENARIOS

Read the clinical scenarios and answer the questions to explore your understanding of alterations of hematologic function.

Mrs. Swenson, age 64, was taken to an urgent care center after she fell while getting off a bus. While her abrasions were being bandaged, she said, "My feet are numb and tingly, and I cannot always tell where they are." In answer to questions, she reported an 8-pound weight loss in the past 3 months, poor appetite, indigestion, sore tongue, and constant fatigue. Pallor was noted.

Laboratory Results

- Blood glucose, serum electrolytes, BUN, and creatinine normal

- Hemoglobin 8.0 g/dL (low) and hematocrit 32% (low)

- Macrocytic normochromic RBCs

Mrs. Swenson was directed to see a nurse practitioner, who diagnosed pernicious anemia after additional testing.

108. What is the normal process of absorption of dietary vitamin B_{12}?

109. What caused Mrs. Swenson's pernicious anemia?

110. How are Mrs. Swenson's numbness and tingling related to pernicious anemia?

111. Mrs. Swenson is being treated with cobalamin (vitamin B_{12}) injections. After her blood vitamin B_{12} level is brought back to normal, can her cobalamin be discontinued? Why or why not?

Copyright © 2024 by Elsevier, Inc. All Rights Reserved.

Marcia Day, age 41, is admitted to the hospital with multiple traumas from a motor vehicle accident. She has been stabilized surgically and has been in the intensive care unit for 4 days when she begins to bleed from her intravenous catheter sites and has blood in her stool. She also has poor peripheral circulation as evidenced by poor capillary refill in her extremities.

112. Ms. Day has DIC. What words are signified by the acronym DIC?

_____

113. Because the pathophysiology of DIC involves widespread clotting, why does it simultaneously involve hemorrhage?

114. What is the role of tissue factor in the pathophysiology of DIC?

115. DIC involves insufficient activity of activated protein C. What is the normal function of this protein, and how does lack of that function contribute to DIC?

116. Why is Ms. Day at high risk for multiple organ dysfunction?

Colin Bank, age 42, has bilateral swelling in his neck that has gradually increased in size over the past 2 months, causing him to purchase new dress shirts with a larger neck size. Previously he has been healthy and takes no medications.

117. Physical examination reveals significant enlargement of his cervical lymph nodes. What assessment questions should Colin be asked?

118. Colin reports an 8-pound unintentional weight loss, night sweats, and fatigue. If he has Hodgkin lymphoma, would his swollen lymph nodes be painful? Why or why not?

119. The biopsy report on Colin's cervical nodes has returned and indicates Hodgkin lymphoma. What type of cell is characteristic of Hodgkin lymphoma? _____

Copyright © 2024 by Elsevier, Inc. All Rights Reserved.

120. Given his diagnosis, would Colin's blood tests show large numbers of circulating malignant cells? Why or why not?

121. Colin was treated successfully. What other lymphomas might have caused enlarged cervical lymph nodes?

Copyright © 2024 by Elsevier, Inc. All Rights Reserved.

30 Alterations of Hematologic Function in Children

MATCH THE DEFINITIONS

Match the word on the right with its definition on the left.

_____ 1. Abnormally precipitated oxidized hemoglobin within an erythrocyte

_____ 2. An endogenous inhibitor of coagulation

_____ 3. Presence of immature nucleated red blood cells in the blood

_____ 4. Normal enzyme that protects erythrocytes from oxidative damage

_____ 5. Breakdown of red blood cells

_____ 6. Formation of red blood cells

A. Erythroblastosis

B. Erythropoiesis

C. G6PD

D. Hemolysis

E. Heinz body

F. Protein S

DRAW YOUR ANSWERS

Read the questions and draw your answers.

7. In this drawing of a young child's femur, shade in the portion where erythropoiesis normally occurs.

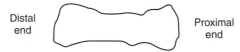

8. In this drawing of a young child's femur, shade in the portion where erythropoiesis would occur in a child with alpha thalassemia minor.

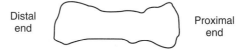

9. In this drawing of an adult femur, shade in the portion where erythropoiesis normally occurs.

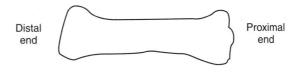

CIRCLE THE CORRECT WORDS

Circle the correct word from the choices provided to complete these sentences.

10. Variations in hemoglobin levels between the sexes arise during (infancy, adolescence) and show (lower, higher) levels in healthy males.

11. Iron deficiency anemia in children is highest before age (2, 14) due to an imbalance between dietary iron intake, the need for iron for normal (growth, G6PD function), and any occult blood loss.

Copyright © 2024 by Elsevier, Inc. All Rights Reserved.

12. A child who has a G6PD deficiency must not be given (aspirin, yogurt) because it could trigger a (hemorrhagic, hemolytic) episode.

13. Sickle cell disease is an autosomal- (dominant, recessive) condition that is expressed in the (homozygous, heterozygous) form as sickle cell trait and in the (homozygous, heterozygous) form as sickle cell disease.

14. Sickle cell anemia often is detected at (birth, 6 to 12 months of age) because fetal hemoglobin (is, is not) affected by the genetic mutation.

15. Von Willebrand disease is a genetic (thrombotic, hemorrhagic) condition.

ORDER THE STEPS

Sequence the events that occur during a sickle cell vaso-occlusive crisis.

16. Write the letters here in the correct order of the steps: _____
    A. Low temperature, hypoxemia, acidemia, or dehydration occurs
    B. Erythrocytes attach to the endothelium in microcirculation
    C. Deoxygenated hemoglobin S polymerizes inside erythrocytes in the microcirculation
    D. Erythropoiesis creates erythrocytes containing hemoglobin S
    E. Erythrocytes become sickled
    F. Microcirculation clogging by erythrocytes reduces blood flow
    G. Prolonged tissue ischemia causes pain and infarction of the local tissue
    H. Increased local hypoxemia and acidosis increase sickling and vasospasm that stop blood flow

DESCRIBE THE DIFFERENCES

Describe the difference between each pair of terms.

17. What is the difference between the hemoglobin chains of the most common form of adult hemoglobin and embryonic and fetal hemoglobins?

18. What is the difference between the frequency of hemolysis in children who have hereditary spherocytosis and children who have G6PD deficiency?

19. What is the difference between the chemical structures of hemoglobin A_1 and hemoglobin S?

20. What is the genetic difference between sickle cell anemia and sickle cell trait?

Copyright © 2024 by Elsevier, Inc. All Rights Reserved.

Examine this table and answer the questions to interpret the numbers.

Age Variations in Hematologic Values

Age	Hemoglobin (g/dL) Mean	Hematocrit (%) Mean	Reticulocytes (%) Mean	Leukocytes (WBC/mm³) Mean	Neutrophils (%) Mean
Cord blood	16.8	55	5	18,000	61
2 wk	16.5	50	1	12,000	40
3 mo	12	36	1	12,000	30
6 mo to 6 yr	12	37	1	10,000	45
7 to 12 yr	13	38	1	8000	55
Adult female	14	42	1.6	7500	55

21. What causes the hemoglobin and hematocrit to be so different between birth and 3 months?

22. What are reticulocytes? Why does cord blood have high reticulocyte levels?

23. What is the difference between the normal WBC count in an infant and a school-aged child? Why is it important for a healthcare provider to know this?

COMPLETE THE SENTENCES

Write one word in each blank to complete these sentences.

24. Before the bone marrow is functional in a fetus, production of erythrocytes takes place primarily in the _____ and to a lesser extent in the spleen and lymph nodes.

25. A child who has sickle cell anemia and develops a parvovirus infection may develop _____ crisis.

26. Acute chest syndrome in sickle cell anemia occurs when sickled erythrocytes cause vaso-occlusion in the _____.

27. Young children with sickle cell anemia may develop _____ crisis when large amounts of blood pool in the spleen and liver, potentially causing death from _____ _____.

Copyright © 2024 by Elsevier, Inc. All Rights Reserved.

28. Beta-thalassemia major also is called _____ anemia; the erythrocytes are unstable and prone to hemolysis because they have too many free hemoglobin _____ chains.

29. Children with hemophilia experience recurrent episodes of _____ and may develop limited mobility due to damage to _____ from some of these episodes.

30. The most common leukemia in children is acute _____ leukemia, which causes bone marrow _____ with pallor, fatigue, purpura, bleeding, and fever.

31. Fever in acute leukemia is caused by _____ because of decreased neutrophils and by _____ from rapid growth of leukemic cells.

32. Children who have inherited deficiencies of antithrombin III or proteins C or S have increased risk for _____.

33. Hodgkin lymphoma is characterized by _____ enlargement of supraclavicular or cervical lymph nodes and has some association with Epstein-Barr _____.

34. Childhood non-Hodgkin lymphoma can arise from any _____ tissue and therefore has signs and symptoms that are specific to its location.

MATCH THE HEMOPHILIAS

Match the types of hemophilias on the right with the descriptions on the left.

_____ 35. Autosomal-recessive factor XI deficiency

_____ 36. X-linked recessive factor VIII deficiency

_____ 37. X-linked recessive factor IX deficiency

A. Hemophilia A

B. Hemophilia B

C. Hemophilia C

TEACH PEOPLE ABOUT PATHOPHYSIOLOGY

Write your response to each situation in the space provided.

38. "What actually makes the red blood cells go into a sickle shape?" asks Mrs. Han, a chemical engineer whose son has sickle cell anemia. "Give me the details!"

39. "Why did my nephew get yellow when he had a hemolytic crisis?" asks Mr. Tage. "I thought he would get pale from not having enough red blood cells."

Copyright © 2024 by Elsevier, Inc. All Rights Reserved.

40. Archer, age 2, has hereditary spherocytosis and developed gallstones. His mother says, "The pediatrician told me that Archer's spherocytosis caused his gallstones. She explained about the gallbladder, bile, and gallstones, but I am missing a piece of the puzzle. How do abnormal red cells cause gallstones?"

CLINICAL SCENARIOS

Read the clinical scenarios and answer the questions to explore your understanding of altered hematologic function in children.

Mrs. Scott received no prenatal care during her first pregnancy because of lack of money and transportation. Her neighbor helped her during childbirth, as she had helped many women in the area. The baby, Jacob, was healthy. Although Mrs. Scott has not been tested, she is Rh negative. Mr. Scott and young Jacob are both Rh positive. Mrs. Scott now is pregnant again.

43. Why is Mrs. Scott's fetus at risk for hemolytic disease of the newborn?

42. Why did Jacob, the first baby, not develop hemolytic disease of the newborn?

43. Ashley, Mrs. Scott's second baby, did develop hemolytic disease of the newborn. When Baby Ashley was born, she was pale, and her liver and spleen were somewhat enlarged. Why were these particular organs enlarged?

44. Baby Ashley was not jaundiced when she was born, but jaundice developed soon afterward. What caused her jaundice?

45. Why was Baby Ashley not jaundiced when she was born?

Copyright © 2024 by Elsevier, Inc. All Rights Reserved.

Chapter **30** Alterations of Hematologic Function in Children

46. What is kernicterus, and why is it important in this situation?

Jim, age 10, developed unexplained multiple bruises on his torso. He did not tell anyone about them because he was afraid he would be in trouble. A few days later, his gym teacher noticed them when Jim's shirt flapped up during exercise. She reported a concern about child abuse to the authorities. After vigorous denial of abuse by Jim and his family and a visit to a physician, Jim was diagnosed with primary immune (idiopathic) thrombocytopenic purpura. His condition improved after 3 months of corticosteroid therapy.

47. The diagnostic blood work showed a low platelet count. What caused Jim's platelet count to be low?

48. Given the pathophysiology, what should the erythrocyte count have been? Why?

49. Why did Jim have multiple bruises?

  Copyright © 2024 by Elsevier, Inc. All Rights Reserved.

31 Structure and Function of the Cardiovascular and Lymphatic Systems

MATCH THE DEFINITIONS

Match each word on the right with its definition on the left.

_____ 1. Causing decreased myocardial contractility

_____ 2. Causing a decreased heart rate

_____ 3. Ability to generate action potentials in a regular pattern

_____ 4. Ability to generate spontaneous depolarization to threshold potential

_____ 5. Resistance to ejection during systole

_____ 6. Ability of the heart muscle to shorten, generating force; change in developed tension at a given resting fiber length

_____ 7. The pressure generated at the end of diastole

_____ 8. Volume of blood flowing into the systemic (or pulmonary) circuit in 1 minute

A. Automaticity

B. Afterload

C. Negative inotropic effect

D. Contractility

E. Preload

F. Negative chronotropic effect

G. Cardiac output

H. Rhythmicity

CIRCLE THE CORRECT WORDS

Circle the correct word from the choices provided to complete these sentences.

9. The right atrioventricular valve has (two, three) cusps and is called the (tricuspid, mitral) valve; the left atrioventricular valve has (two, three) cusps and is called the (tricuspid, mitral) valve.

10. Compared with skeletal muscle, cardiac muscle has (fewer, more) mitochondria and (fewer, more) T tubules.

11. Norepinephrine action on α_1-adrenergic receptors causes (vasoconstriction, vasodilation).

12. The myocardium normally extracts about (40%, 70%) of the oxygen from the coronary arteries; therefore it has a (small, large) oxygen reserve if myocardial oxygen demand increases.

13. Binding of ATP to (myosin, actin) is necessary for myocardial contraction; excitation–contraction coupling requires (calcium, magnesium).

14. At resting membrane potential, the inside of a myocardial cell is (less, more) negatively charged than the outside; when the myocardial cell depolarizes, the inside of the cell becomes (less, more) negatively charged.

15. Veins have (thinner, thicker) walls than arteries and are (less, more) compliant; valves are located in (both arteries and veins, veins only).

165

Copyright © 2024 by Elsevier, Inc. All Rights Reserved.

16. The tunica (media, intima) is the middle layer of blood vessels; it is composed of (endothelium and connective tissue, smooth muscle and elastic fibers).

17. Resistance to blood flow through an artery increases when the artery (dilates, constricts).

18. Age-related changes in the cardiovascular system include (dilation, stiffening) of myocardium and arterial walls.

MATCH THE FUNCTIONS

Name the structures with their location in the picture and then match their functions. The first one is completed as an example. Hint: Identify the structure first and then consider its function.

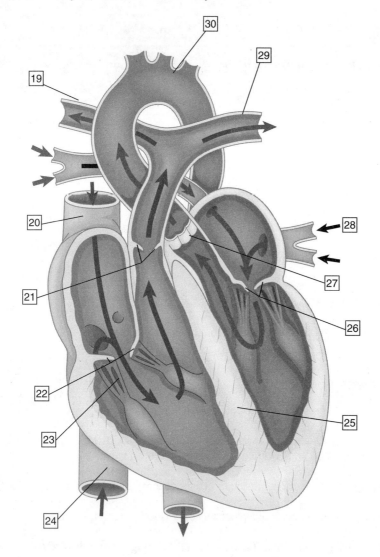

Chapter **31 Structure and Function of the Cardiovascular and Lymphatic Systems**

Copyright © 2024 by Elsevier, Inc. All Rights Reserved.

Name and Function of the Structure	Functions to Be Matched
19. Name: ___Right pulmonary artery___ Function: ___B___	A. Provides one-way flow of blood from the left ventricle into the aorta
20. Name: _____ Function: _____	B. Transports deoxygenated blood from the right ventricle to the right lung
21. Name: _____ Function: _____	C. Transports oxygenated blood from the left ventricle to the systemic circulation
22. Name: _____ Function: _____	D. Conveys deoxygenated blood from the head and upper extremities to the right atrium
23. Name: _____ Function: _____	E. Provides one-way flow of blood from the right ventricle into the pulmonary artery
24. Name: _____ Function: _____	F. Transports deoxygenated blood from the right ventricle to the left lung
25. Name: _____ Function: _____	G. Anchors the valve cusps to the papillary muscles to prevent valve prolapse
26. Name: _____ Function: _____	H. Conveys deoxygenated blood from the trunk and lower extremities to the right atrium
27. Name: _____ Function: _____	I. Transports oxygenated blood from the left lung to the left atrium
28. Name: _____ Function: _____	J. Provides one-way flow of blood from the left atrium into the left ventricle
29. Name: _____ Function: _____	K. Provides one-way flow of blood from the right atrium into the right ventricle
30. Name: _____ Function: _____	L. Separates the right and left ventricles

SELECT THE FASTER ONES

Consider the pairs and select the one that is faster.

31. Which has a faster spontaneous depolarization rate: SA node or AV node?

32. Which has a faster spontaneous depolarization rate: AV node or Purkinje fibers?

33. Which causes a faster heart rate: sympathetic nerve firing or parasympathetic nerve firing?

34. Which causes a faster heart rate: stimulation of cardiac β_1 receptors or cardiac β_3 receptors?

Copyright © 2024 by Elsevier, Inc. All Rights Reserved. Chapter **31 Structure and Function of the Cardiovascular and Lymphatic Systems**

35. Which has a faster physiologic effect on heart rate: changes in autonomic nerve activity or changes in the levels of circulating factors?

36. Which is faster: blood flow in a capillary or blood flow in an arteriole?

CATEGORIZE THE EFFECTS

Write the type of initial effect beside each stimulus, assuming that no other factors also change. Choices for arterioles: vasoconstriction, vasodilation. Choices for cardiac output or heart rate: increase, decrease.

_____ 37. Norepinephrine effect on systemic arterioles

_____ 38. Epinephrine effect on systemic arterioles

_____ 39. Increased afterload effect on cardiac output

_____ 40. Physiologically increased preload effect on cardiac output

_____ 41. Large parasympathetic stimulation effect on cardiac output

_____ 42. Falling BP causing baroreceptor reflex effect on heart rate

_____ 43. Thyroid hormone effect on cardiac output

_____ 44. Increasing core temperature causing thermoregulatory effect on cutaneous arterioles

_____ 45. Nitric oxide local effect on arterioles

_____ 46. Endothelin local effect on arterioles

_____ 47. Angiotensin II local effect on arterioles

ORDER THE STEPS

Sequence the events that occur during the cardiac cycle.

48. Write the letters here in the correct order of the steps: _____
    A. Atrial pressure rises above ventricular pressure; mitral and tricuspid valves open; ventricles fill passively; pulmonary and aortic valves remain closed
    B. Ventricular systole begins, and increasing intraventricular pressure closes the mitral and tricuspid valves; pulmonary and aortic valves remain closed
    C. Ventricles relax and have little volume; pulmonary and aortic valves close; mitral and tricuspid valves remain closed; atria begin filling
    D. Pulmonary and aortic valves are closed; mitral and tricuspid valves open; atria contract; ventricles are relaxed and they fill
    E. Ventricular pressures exceed pulmonary artery and aortic pressures; pulmonary and aortic valves open; ventricular ejection occurs; mitral and tricuspid valves remain closed

Copyright © 2024 by Elsevier, Inc. All Rights Reserved.

EXPLAIN THE PICTURE

Examine the electrocardiogram (ECG) and answer the questions about it.

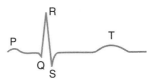

49. What electrical event occurs in the myocardium that generates the portion of the ECG marked P?

_____

50. What do the atria do in response to this event?

_____

51. Electrical signals are conducted through what parts of the heart during the PR interval?

_____

52. What are the ventricles doing during the portion of the ECG that is labeled R through the end of the T wave?

_____

53. The mitral valve closes at approximately what location on the ECG? _____

54. Why is it important for the mitral and tricuspid valves to close at that time?

DESCRIBE THE DIFFERENCES

Describe the difference between each pair of terms.

55. What is the difference between the endocardium and the epicardium?

56. What is the difference between systole and diastole?

57. What is the difference between angiogenesis and arteriogenesis?

Copyright © 2024 by Elsevier, Inc. All Rights Reserved.

58. What is the difference between laminar flow and turbulent flow?

COMPLETE THE SENTENCES

Write one word in each blank to complete these sentences.

59. The aortic and pulmonary valves are the _____ valves, and they each have _____ cusps.

60. The _____ side of the heart is a high-pressure system, and the _____ side of the heart is a low-pressure system.

61. In areas where it is attached to the heart, the visceral pericardium is called the _____.

62. The _____ arteries bring oxygenated blood to the myocardium; venous blood from the myocardium empties into the _____ atrium.

63. Two important branches of the left coronary artery are the left _____ _____ artery and the _____ artery.

64. Parasympathetic nerves to the heart release the neurotransmitter _____, which binds to _____ receptors; sympathetic nerves to the heart release the neurotransmitter _____, which binds to _____ receptors.

65. As an action potential is transmitted through the T tubules, it triggers release of _____ from the sarcoplasmic reticulum.

66. An _____ disk is a thickened portion of the cardiac sarcolemma that enables rapid spread of depolarization between myofibrils.

67. The process of _____ enables an organ to regulate its blood flow by altering the resistance in its arterioles.

68. The right lymphatic duct and the _____ duct drain lymph into the _____ veins.

69. Small blood vessels that bring blood to the walls of large arteries are called vasa _____.

70. Echocardiography uses _____ beams to evaluate the heart; SPECT uses a radiotracer that is administered _____; MRI uses a _____ field; and coronary angiography uses a catheter and a contrast _____.

CALCULATE THE ANSWERS

Use the relevant portions of the information provided to calculate your answers.

Mrs. Ghent's blood pressure is 140/80 mmHg, heart rate is 78 beats/min, stroke volume is 45 mL/beat, left ventricular end-diastolic volume is 75 mL/m^2, and respiratory rate is 18 breaths/min.

71. Her pulse pressure is _____.

72. Her mean arterial pressure is _____.

Copyright © 2024 by Elsevier, Inc. All Rights Reserved.

73. Her cardiac output is _____.

74. Her ejection fraction is _____.

SORT THE LAWS

Write the name of these laws beside their descriptions: Laplace's law, Frank-Starling law of the heart, Poiseuille's law.

_____ 75. Within limits, a greater end-diastolic volume will produce a greater contractile force during systole.

_____ 76. The amount of tension generated in a cardiac chamber or vessel to produce a given internal pressure varies directly with the radius and inversely with the wall thickness.

_____ 77. Blood flow is inversely related to resistance; resistance to blood flow is directly related to vessel length and blood viscosity and inversely related to the vessel radius to the fourth power.

TEACH PEOPLE ABOUT PHYSIOLOGY

Write your response to each situation in the space provided.

78. Kevin, age 17, says, "I am learning about the heart in high school. Why is the left ventricle muscle normally thicker than the right ventricle muscle? Why aren't they the same?"

79. A nurse who is new to the cardiac unit says, "I hear the cardiologists talking about blockage of the LAD. What are they discussing?"

80. An emergency department nurse says, "We always measure blood troponin levels in our suspected MI [myocardial infarction; heart attack] patients. I know that troponin normally is inside the myocardial cells, not in the blood. But what is the normal function of troponin?"

81. Mr. Pannopoulos asks, "When they transplant a heart, I know they cut the nerves. Do they have to put in a pacemaker to make the new heart beat after it is transplanted?"

Copyright © 2024 by Elsevier, Inc. All Rights Reserved. Chapter **31** Structure and Function of the Cardiovascular and Lymphatic Systems

32 Alterations of Cardiovascular Function

MATCH THE DEFINITIONS

Match the word on the right with its definition on the left.

_____ 1. Distended and tortuous superficial veins in which blood has pooled because of damaged valves

_____ 2. Sustained inadequate venous return due to valvular damage

_____ 3. Ischemic pain in the lower extremities that occurs while walking but disappears when resting

_____ 4. Inflammatory disease of peripheral arteries that usually is associated with smoking

_____ 5. Vasospastic disease of peripheral arteries in which episodes of ischemia and pallor are followed by rubor and paresthesias

_____ 6. Inflammation of the membranous sac that surrounds the heart

_____ 7. Compression of the heart by pericardial fluid

A. Intermittent claudication

B. Thromboangiitis obliterans

C. Raynaud phenomenon

D. Chronic venous insufficiency

E. Pericarditis

F. Tamponade

G. Varicose veins

CIRCLE THE CORRECT WORDS

Circle the correct word from the choices provided to complete these sentences.

8. Postthrombotic syndrome is characterized by chronic persistent pain and (pallor and atrophy, edema and ulceration) of a limb that had deep venous thrombosis.

9. A major danger of deep venous thrombosis is development of (cerebral, pulmonary) thromboembolism; a danger of an arterial thrombus is development of (systemic, pulmonary) thromboembolism.

10. Superior vena cava syndrome occurs when a tumor or other mass (ruptures, compresses) the superior vena cava, causing (severe hypertension, venous distention) in the upper extremities and head.

11. Factors that cause primary hypertension increase peripheral vascular (responsiveness, resistance) and/or cause sustained (increase, decrease) in blood volume.

12. In hypertension, the pressure–natriuresis relationship shifts so that the hypertensive individual excretes (more, less) sodium in the urine.

13. People who have uncomplicated hypertension usually have (no, many) signs and symptoms in addition to their elevated blood pressure; treatment usually begins with (antihypertensive medications, lifestyle modifications).

14. The term *dissecting aneurysm* means that blood enters an artery wall and (runs between the layers of the wall, bursts through the wall and causes hemorrhage).

15. Risk for myocardial infarction increases with low blood levels of (LDL, HDL) and with high blood levels of (LDL, HDL).

Copyright © 2024 by Elsevier, Inc. All Rights Reserved.

16. Cardiac valve damage in rheumatic fever is caused by (group A β-hemolytic streptococci, an abnormal immune response); cardiac valve damage in infective endocarditis is caused by (streptococci or other organisms, an abnormal immune response).

17. Constrictive pericarditis is (an acute, a chronic) condition that can (compress, dilate) the heart.

IDENTIFY THE ACRONYMS

Use the clues to identify the acronyms and then write the words that each acronym represents.

Clues	Acronyms	Words Represented by the Acronyms
18. Clot formation in a large vein, usually in lower extremities		
19. Type of lipoprotein that migrates into arterial wall in atherosclerosis		
20. Heart attack that shows ST-segment elevation on ECG		
21. Atherosclerosis in the coronary arteries		
22. Heart disease caused by atherosclerosis in the coronary arteries		
23. Atherosclerosis in arteries that supply the extremities		
24. Mitral valve cusps billow backward into valve opening when valve should be closed		

EXPLAIN THE PICTURES

Examine the pictures and answer the questions about them.

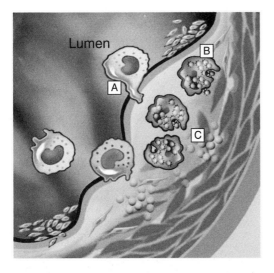
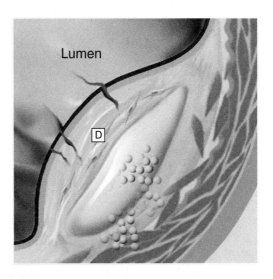

25. These pictures of artery walls show part of the disease process of _____

26. What is the monocyte labeled A doing? _____

27. What layer of the artery wall is the monocyte labeled A entering? _____

Copyright © 2024 by Elsevier, Inc. All Rights Reserved.

28. What are the abnormal globules that have accumulated in this layer of the artery wall?

_____

29. What is the cell labeled B called? _____

30. What did the cell labeled B phagocytize that gave it its characteristic appearance?

_____

31. The cell labeled C is a smooth muscle cell. What is it doing that is abnormal?

_____

32. The cells labeled D are fibroblasts. What have they created? _____

33. Which picture illustrates a fibrous plaque? _____

34. What does the other picture illustrate? _____

CATEGORIZE THE CLINICAL MANIFESTATIONS

Write the type of heart failure that typically causes each sign or symptom. Choices: left heart failure, right heart failure.

_____ 35. Orthopnea

_____ 36. Ankle edema

_____ 37. Jugular venous distention

_____ 38. Dyspnea

_____ 39. Decreased urine output

_____ 40. Coughing pink, frothy sputum

_____ 41. Crackles upon auscultation

_____ 42. Hepatomegaly

DESCRIBE THE DIFFERENCES

Describe the difference between each pair of terms.

43. What is the difference between a thrombus and an embolus?

44. What is the difference between primary and secondary hypertension?

Copyright © 2024 by Elsevier, Inc. All Rights Reserved.

45. What is the difference between myocardial hibernation and myocardial stunning?

46. What is the difference between dilated and restrictive cardiomyopathy?

47. What is the difference between valvular stenosis and valvular regurgitation?

NAME THE RISK FACTORS

Use the clues to complete the list of risk factors for hypertension.

48.   H   ___ ___ ___ ___ ___ ___

49.   ___ ___ ___ Y ___ ___ ___ ___ ___

50.   P   ___ ___ ___ ___ ___ ___ ___ ___

51.   ___ ___ E

52.   R   ___ ___ ___ ___

53.   ___ ___ ___ ___ ___ T   ___

54.   ___ ___ ___ ___ E   ___ ___ ___ ___

55.   ___ N   ___

56.   S   ___ ___ ___ ___ ___

57.   ___ **I**   ___ ___ ___ ___ ___ ___ ___

58.   ___ ___ ___ **O**   ___ ___ ___

59.   ___ **N**   ___ ___ ___ ___ ___ ___ ___ ___ ___

Clues:

48. If this is positive in the family, risk increases.

49. Genetic character of hypertension.

50. Low dietary intake of this electrolyte is a risk factor.

51. As this increases, the risk increases.

52. Substance released by the kidneys that contributes to some cases of hypertension.

53. Modifiable risk factor estimated with BMI.

Copyright © 2024 by Elsevier, Inc. All Rights Reserved.

54. Low dietary intake of this electrolyte also is a risk factor.

55. Increased firing of this portion of the autonomic nervous system is a risk factor.

56. High dietary intake of this electrolyte is a risk factor.

57. Habitual use of these is a risk factor.

58. High intake of this recreational beverage is a risk factor.

59. With the word *glucose*, a major risk factor.

COMPLETE THE SENTENCES

Write one word in each blank to complete these sentences.

60. A clot in a blood vessel that breaks loose and circulates is called a _____.

61. Sluggish circulation from chronic venous insufficiency may cause a venous _____ ulcer.

62. Sustained hypertension causes left ventricular _____ and coronary atherosclerosis, thus increasing the risk for _____ _____.

63. Rapidly progressive hypertension with a diastolic pressure above 140 mmHg is called _____ hypertension and can damage the _____.

64. Postural hypotension, also called _____ hypotension, is a systolic blood pressure decrease of at least _____ mmHg or a diastolic blood pressure decrease of at least _____ mmHg within 3 minutes of standing and is a significant risk factor for _____.

65. People who have subacute infective endocarditis are at risk for _____ embolism, whereas people who have trauma to long bones are at risk for _____ embolism.

66. The risk factors for peripheral arterial disease are the same as the risk factors for _____; the risk factors for coronary artery disease are the same as the risk factors for _____.

67. Clot formation at the site of rupture of an atherosclerotic plaque causes tissue _____, which leads to _____ if blood flow is not restored.

68. People who are obese have decreased levels of _____, an antiatherogenic adipokine.

69. Risk for myocardial infarction increases with factors that increase myocardial oxygen _____ or reduce myocardial oxygen _____.

70. Tissue healing after a myocardial infarction creates a noncontractile _____.

71. The ischemic injury from a sudden blockage of a coronary artery can be exacerbated by _____ injury when blood flow is restored.

72. Acute rheumatic fever is characterized by carditis, acute migratory _____, chorea, and _____ marginatum, which occur 1 to 5 weeks after streptococcal infection of the _____.

Copyright © 2024 by Elsevier, Inc. All Rights Reserved.

73. Heart failure in which the cardiac output is increased but still insufficient to meet the body's oxygen and nutrient needs is called _____ heart failure.

74. Vasospastic angina, also called _____ angina, is caused by unpredictable _____ of a coronary artery.

75. Angina caused by a clot temporarily occluding a coronary artery that resolves before necrosis occurs is called _____ angina.

MATCH THE CONSEQUENCES

Match the consequences on the right with the valve disorders on the left.

_____ 76. Aortic stenosis

_____ 77. Mitral regurgitation

_____ 78. Mitral stenosis

_____ 79. Tricuspid regurgitation

A. Right atrial and right ventricular dilation and hypertrophy

B. Left atrial hypertrophy and dilation

C. Left ventricular hypertrophy and dilation

D. Left atrial and left ventricular dilation and hypertrophy

TEACH PEOPLE ABOUT PATHOPHYSIOLOGY

Write your response to each situation in the space provided.

80. "Stress is all in your head!" exclaims Mr. Weiss. "I do not want to take that stress management class! How can stress affect blood pressure?"

81. Mx. Evers has a newly diagnosed aortic aneurysm. "What is an aneurysm?" asks their partner. "And why do they want to operate to fix it? My partner feels fine!"

82. Mrs. Gao developed a deep venous thrombosis during a long car ride. "Tell me again those three big causes of leg clots," she says. "I want to avoid all of them in the future!"

83. "My uncle had a heart attack, and my father had a stroke," says Mr. Carradine. "My doctor said they were caused by the same thing, but I do not see how. Can you explain?"

Copyright © 2024 by Elsevier, Inc. All Rights Reserved.

Chapter **32** **Alterations of Cardiovascular Function**

84. "Why do I get so tired and faint when I try to exercise?" asks Mr. Azul, who has mild aortic stenosis. "I am fine when I am not exercising."

85. "I heard the doctor tell the medical student that heart failure with reduced ejection fraction and heart failure with preserved ejection fraction are two kinds of heart failure," says Mr. Moon. "My doctor said I have heart failure with reduced ejection fraction, but I do not know what that means. Please explain."

86. Mr. Santos has left ventricular hypertrophy from hypertension. "How does that increase my risk of heart attack?" he asks. "I think big, strong muscles are a good thing!"

87. "My husband is in the emergency department, and they said he has acute coronary syndrome!" exclaims Mrs. Gato. "Is that a heart attack?"

88. Mrs. Fewe was diagnosed with atrial fibrillation. "Oh, no! Grandma is dying! Call 911!" says Kendra, age 11, when she hears the diagnosis. "Fibrillation is an emergency!"

CLINICAL SCENARIOS

Read the clinical scenarios and answer the questions to explore your understanding of cardiac pathophysiology.

Mr. Kent, a 57-year-old nurse, developed crushing substernal chest pain with dyspnea, dizziness, and nausea while trying to lift a patient from a bed to a chair. In the emergency department, he states that his symptoms resolved as soon as he sat down to rest. Mr. Kent indicates that he has had similar episodes in the past, particularly when trying to do strenuous yard work. After an ECG and other tests, his diagnosis is stable angina.

89. What assessment questions should you ask Mr. Kent about his risk factors for coronary heart disease?

90. Why is it important to examine the appearance of Mr. Kent's lower extremities and palpate his pedal pulses?

Copyright © 2024 by Elsevier, Inc. All Rights Reserved.

91. Now that Mr. Kent's chest pain is completely resolved, what might his electrocardiogram show?

92. "I work pediatrics, not with adults," says Mr. Kent. "Remind me what stable angina is. It has been a long time since nursing school."

93. Mr. Kent says, "I seem to remember that some people have angina pain that is not in the chest. Is that correct?"

94. "This is my wake-up call," says Mr. Kent. "I see that I need to take better care of myself. Tell me how eating less saturated fat will help. Maybe that will motivate me."

Mr. Williamson, age 81, had been feeling tired for several weeks. When he developed extreme shortness of breath, his wife took him to the emergency department. The emergency department personnel listened to his lungs, took a radiograph, and gave him an intravenous diuretic. He was admitted to the hospital with pulmonary edema from acute biventricular heart failure. After a few days, he was discharged from the hospital with various medications, including antihypertensives, and instructions to eat a low-sodium diet and weigh himself every morning.

95. What fluid imbalance did Mr. Williamson have when he was taken to the emergency department? What parts of the case scenario provide the evidence for your answer?

96. What did the emergency department personnel hear when they listened to Mr. Williamson's lungs?

97. When Mr. Williamson was admitted to the hospital, what did assessment of his ankles most likely reveal? Why?

98. When Mr. Williamson was admitted to the hospital, what was the most likely character of his pulse?

Copyright © 2024 by Elsevier, Inc. All Rights Reserved.

99. Why was Mr. Williamson instructed to weigh himself every morning?

100. Why was a low-sodium diet prescribed for Mr. Williamson?

PUZZLE OUT THE TECHNICAL TERMS

Use the clues to complete the puzzle, demonstrating your knowledge of important technical terms.

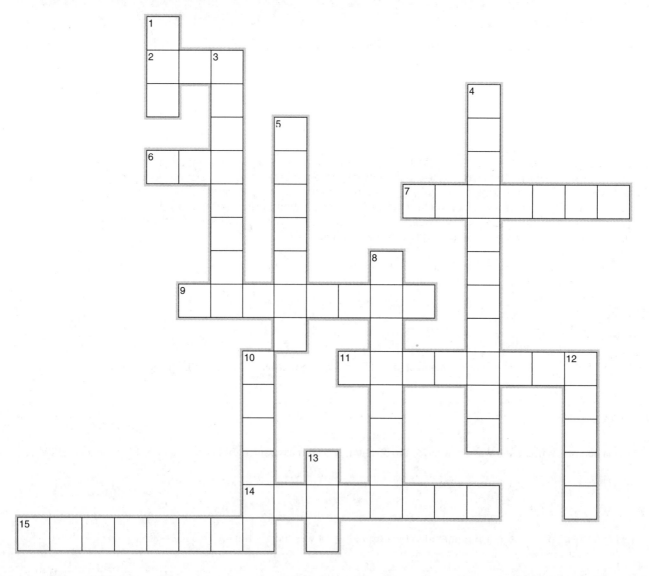

Chapter **32 Alterations of Cardiovascular Function**

Copyright © 2024 by Elsevier, Inc. All Rights Reserved.

Across

2. Acronym for clot formation in a large vein, usually in lower extremities
6. Nonspecific marker of inflammation measured to assess cardiac risk
7. Another term for Prinzmetal angina
9. Localized outpouching or dilation of a vessel wall or cardiac chamber
11. Blood clot that is attached to the endothelium in a blood vessel or cardiac chamber
14. Type of angina caused by a clot temporarily occluding a coronary artery and resolving before necrosis occurs
15. Valve cusps billow backward into valve opening when valve should be closed

Down

1. Acronym for type of lipoprotein that migrates into arterial walls in atherosclerosis
3. Cardiac biomarker measured in blood to detect myocardial infarction
4. Disturbance of cardiac rhythm
5. A bolus of matter circulating in the blood
8. Lack of oxygen in tissue due to lack of blood supply
10. The lesion of atherosclerosis
12. Acronym for a myocardial infarction that shows ST-segment elevation on ECG
13. Acronym for elevated systolic blood pressure accompanied by normal diastolic blood pressure

Copyright © 2024 by Elsevier, Inc. All Rights Reserved.

33 Alterations of Cardiovascular Function in Children

IDENTIFY THE ACRONYMS

Use the clues to identify the acronyms and then write the words that each acronym represents.

Clues	Acronyms	Words Represented by the Acronyms
1. Congenital defect involving a hole in the septum between the two top cardiac chambers		
2. Congenital defect involving failure of the fetal blood vessel between the pulmonary artery and the aorta to close		
3. Congenital defect involving a hole in the septum between the two lower cardiac chambers		

CIRCLE THE CORRECT WORDS

Circle the correct word from the choices provided to complete these sentences.

4. Abnormal movement of blood from one side of the heart to the other is called a (transposition, shunt).

5. The major determinant of the direction of blood flow through a ventricular septal defect is the (difference between, sum of) pulmonary vascular resistance and (systemic, aortic) vascular resistance.

6. Tetralogy of Fallot is the most common (acyanotic, cyanotic) heart defect.

7. A heart defect that increases pulmonary blood flow from (right-to-left, left-to-right) shunting can cause heart failure in an infant.

8. Bluish coloration of mucous membranes and nail beds caused by the presence of deoxygenated hemoglobin is called (hypoxemia, cyanosis).

9. Heart failure in children is (rarely, commonly) manifested by peripheral edema and neck vein distention.

10. If an atrial septal defect is not large, it is likely to (close spontaneously, enlarge throughout childhood).

Copyright © 2024 by Elsevier, Inc. All Rights Reserved.

CHARACTERIZE THE CONGENITAL HEART DEFECTS

Write one letter and one number beside each picture of a congenital heart defect in the left column to indicate its name and the direction of blood shunt.

Picture of Congenital Heart Defect	Name of the Defect	Direction of the Blood Shunt (Use each answer more than once)

Picture of Congenital Heart Defect

Name of the Defect

A. Ventricular septal defect

B. Tricuspid atresia

C. Coarctation of the aorta

D. Atrial septal defect

E. Tetralogy of Fallot

F. Pulmonic stenosis

G. Patent ductus arteriosus

H. Aortic stenosis

**Direction of the Blood Shunt
(Use each answer more than once)**

1. Left to right

2. Right to left

3. No shunt

_____ 11.

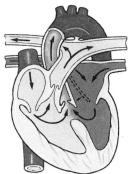

_____ 12.

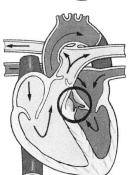

_____ 13.

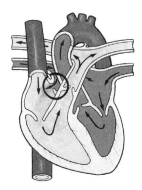

_____ 14.

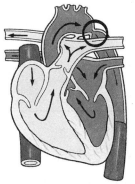

Copyright © 2024 by Elsevier, Inc. All Rights Reserved.

Chapter **33 Alterations of Cardiovascular Function in Children**

_____15.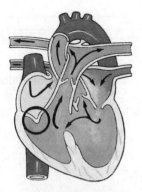

_____16.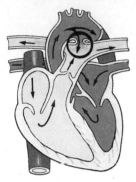

_____17.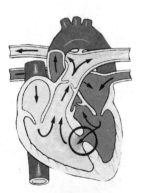

_____18.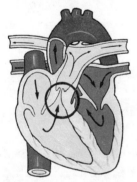

Copyright © 2024 by Elsevier, Inc. All Rights Reserved.

DESCRIBE AND EXPLAIN THE DIFFERENCES

Describe the difference between each pair of terms and then explain why the difference occurs.

19. What is the difference between the direction of blood flow through the ductus arteriosus in fetal life and the direction after birth if the ductus arteriosus does not close? Explain why the difference occurs.

20. What is the difference between the clinical manifestations of a congenital heart defect that causes a moderate right-to-left blood shunt and one that causes a moderate left-to-right blood shunt? Explain why the difference occurs.

COMPLETE THE SENTENCES

Write one word in each blank to complete these sentences.

21. Blood pressure in an infant should be measured at least _____ minutes after feeding.

22. Abnormal flow of blood in a congenital heart defect is heard as a _____, whose character and location assist with diagnosis.

23. Failure of the endocardial cushions to fuse during fetal life causes an _____ canal defect and frequently occurs in children who have _____ syndrome.

24. Underdevelopment of the left heart is termed _____ left heart syndrome.

25. With transposition of the great arteries, the aorta arises from the _____ ventricle, and the pulmonary artery arises from the _____ ventricle; unless additional defects are present, this defect is incompatible with _____ life.

26. The condition in which the pulmonary artery and the aorta are a single blood vessel is called _____ _____.

27. Young children who develop _____ disease have vasculitis of unknown cause and often develop aneurysms of their _____ arteries that may regress as the condition resolves.

28. Secondary hypertension in children often is associated with underlying _____ disease.

29. Pediatric primary hypertension causes subclinical organ damage to the heart and _____.

30. Childhood obesity is a risk factor for _____.

31. Blood flow through an abnormal cardiac opening always moves from an area of _____ pressure to an area of _____ pressure.

32. A congenital heart defect with a right-to-left shunt is characterized as a _____ defect.

Copyright © 2024 by Elsevier, Inc. All Rights Reserved.

Chapter **33** Alterations of Cardiovascular Function in Children

Write your response to each situation in the space provided.

33. Mrs. Yu says, "The doctor said my baby has coarctation of his aorta. What is that? It sounds awful! And please tell me why the nurses keep taking blood pressure in my baby's leg. Is there something wrong with his leg too?"

34. Mrs. Quaid says, "The doctor said my baby has tetralogy of Fallot and she drew me a picture of the four defects. But why does my baby's little face turn that blue color when she cries? And why won't she nurse very long? Maybe she does not like me!"

35. Mr. Voll says, "The doctor said my baby has a patent ductus arteriosus. What is that? Isn't that ductus a normal thing? I remember that from going to the 'developing baby' class with my wife."

36. Mrs. Ortiz says, "The doctor said my baby has atrial septal defect. What is that? And then he said that my baby has a heart murmur! Does my baby have two heart defects?"

WORK WITH THE CLINICAL SCENARIO

You work in a neonatal ICU. Many of the patients have congenital heart defects.

37. *Interpret the assessment findings in neonates with congenital heart defects by placing an X in the column that they are most likely to indicate. One assessment pertains to both columns.*

Assessment Findings	Cyanotic Congenital Heart Defect	Acyanotic Congenital Heart Defect
Poor feeding, diaphoresis with feeding, but no change in color of nailbeds or mucous membranes		
Episodes of bluish nailbeds and mucus membranes with crying		
Cardiac murmur		
Extremely low blood pH on the first day of life		

Copyright © 2024 by Elsevier, Inc. All Rights Reserved.

38. *Complete the sentence by choosing from the lists of options.*

You should monitor a neonate who has _____(1)_____ very carefully for changes in _____(2)_____, because it may worsen when the _____(3)_____ closes.

Options for 1	Options for 2	Options for 3
atrial septal defect	respiratory rate	foramen ovale
patent ductus arteriosus	lower extremity perfusion	ductus arteriosus
coarctation of the aorta	muscle tone	stenotic valve

Copyright © 2024 by Elsevier, Inc. All Rights Reserved.

34 Structure and Function of the Pulmonary System

MATCH THE DEFINITIONS

Match each word on the right with its definition on the left.

_____ 1. Space between the lungs that contains the heart, great vessels, and esophagus

_____ 2. Substance secreted by type II alveolar cells that helps keep alveoli from collapsing

_____ 3. What goblet cells in the bronchi secrete

_____ 4. A measure of distensibility

_____ 5. The structures that participate in gas exchange

_____ 6. Membrane attached to the external side of the lungs

_____ 7. Where the bronchi and pulmonary vessels enter the lungs

_____ 8. Fibers that give lung tissue its elasticity

_____ 9. Where the trachea divides into the two main bronchi

A. Surfactant

B. Hila

C. Elastin

D. Carina

E. Compliance

F. Acinus

G. Pleura

H. Mucus

I. Mediastinum

ORDER THE STEPS

Beginning with the nose, sequence the structures through which air moves during inhalation.

10. Write the letters here in the correct order of the steps: _____
    A. Bronchioles
    B. Trachea
    C. Nasopharynx
    D. Bronchi
    E. Nose
    F. Respiratory bronchioles
    G. Larynx
    H. Alveoli
    I. Alveolar ducts

Copyright © 2024 by Elsevier, Inc. All Rights Reserved.

MATCH THE FUNCTIONS

Match the word on the right with its function on the left.

_____ 11. Prevent airway collapse

_____ 12. Filter and humidify inspired air

_____ 13. Prevent lung collapse at end-exhalation

_____ 14. Allow pressure to equalize between adjacent alveoli

A. Surfactant

B. Cartilage rings

C. Pores of Kohn

D. Nasopharynx

CIRCLE THE CORRECT WORDS

Circle the correct word from the choices provided to complete these sentences.

15. The left lobe of the lung has (two, three) lobes; the right lobe of the lung has (two, three) lobes.

16. Stimulation of the carina often causes (inhalation, coughing).

17. The pulmonary circulation has (lower, higher) pressure and resistance than the systemic circulation.

18. Pulmonary (arteries, veins) are spaced randomly throughout the lungs, but the pulmonary (arteries, veins) run beside the branches of the airways.

19. A terminal bronchiole (has, does not have) accompanying lymphatic capillaries.

20. Pulmonary veins carry (oxygenated, deoxygenated) blood and are attached to the (right, left) atrium.

21. The most effective way to measure the adequacy of alveolar ventilation is to measure (ventilatory rate and pattern, $PaCO_2$).

22. The neurons that control respiration are located in the (basal ganglia, brainstem).

23. Parasympathetic stimulation causes airways to (dilate, constrict); sympathetic stimulation causes airways to (dilate, constrict).

24. The (internal, external) intercostal muscles are active during vigorous inspiration.

25. In a person at sea level breathing through the nose, the gas that reaches the lungs is (partially, fully) saturated with water vapor; the PaO_2 in that case is calculated by ($[(760 \times 0.209) - 47]$, $[(760 - 47) \times 0.209]$).

26. The alveolar gas equation enables a healthcare provider to estimate the (physiologic dead space, PaO_2).

27. The shift in the oxyhemoglobin dissociation curve caused by alterations in pH and $PaCO_2$ is called the (Haldane, Bohr) effect.

28. Spirometry is used to measure (Sao_2, FEV_1); oximetry is used to measure (Sao_2, FEV_1).

29. Changes in the normal (microbiota, alveolar density) in the lung are associated with tobacco smoking, corticosteroids, antibiotics, and many respiratory diseases.

Copyright © 2024 by Elsevier, Inc. All Rights Reserved.

Examine the picture and answer the questions about it.

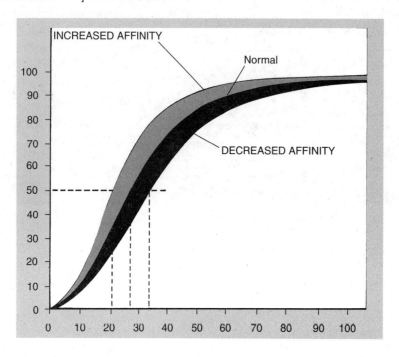

30. This picture shows an oxyhemoglobin dissociation curve. What parameter is measured on the horizontal axis?

_____

31. What parameter is measured on the vertical axis? _____

32. Which chemoreceptors, central or peripheral, will respond if the parameter measured on the horizontal axis falls to

    55 mmHg? _____

33. Which side (left or right) of the curve represents the situation of blood in the lungs? _____ In what way

    is that beneficial? _____

34. Which side (left or right) of the curve represents the situation of blood in the tissues? _____ In what way

    is that beneficial? _____

35. List three factors that cause this shift to occur in the tissues. _____

36. Which way does the curve shift when a patient is hypothermic? _____

37. In what way does the curve shift in hypothermia affect tissue oxygenation? _____

    _____

Copyright © 2024 by Elsevier, Inc. All Rights Reserved.

DESCRIBE THE DIFFERENCES

Describe the difference between each pair of terms.

38. What is the difference between a terminal bronchiole and a respiratory bronchiole?

39. What is the difference between type I and type II alveolar cells?

40. What is the difference between the visceral pleura and the parietal pleura?

41. What is the difference between PaO_2 and P_AO_2?

42. What is the difference between ventilation and respiration?

COMPLETE THE SENTENCES

Write one word in each blank to complete these sentences.

43. The nasopharynx and oropharynx are the _____ airway.

44. The mononuclear phagocytic cells in the lungs are called alveolar _____.

45. The structures that comprise the acinus are the _____ bronchioles, the _____ ducts, and the _____.

46. Gas exchange occurs across the _____ membrane.

47. A person with a respiratory rate of 12 breaths/minute and a minute volume of 6.0 L/minute has a tidal volume of _____ mL.

48. Receptors in the conducting airways that initiate the cough reflex in response to inhaled dust are called _____ receptors.

49. During inspiration, the diaphragm moves _____, which _____ the volume of the thoracic cavity, creating _____ pressure that draws air into the lungs.

50. Normal lung tissue returns to its resting state after inspiration because it has _____ recoil.

Copyright © 2024 by Elsevier, Inc. All Rights Reserved.

Chapter **34 Structure and Function of the Pulmonary System**

51. Lungs that are fibrotic and stiff have _____ compliance, which _____ the work of breathing, thus _____ oxygen demand.

52. The V/Q ratio of a normal upright lung is _____, which indicates that ventilation is _____ than perfusion.

53. Blood gas analysis in a healthy older adult is most likely to show a decrease in _____.

MATCH THE ZONES

Match the lung zones of an upright lung on the right with the descriptions on the left.

_____ 54. Perfusion is greater than ventilation because pulmonary arterial and venous pressures are greater than alveolar pressure.

_____ 55. Perfusion is happening but is not maximum because pulmonary arterial and venous pressures are opposed by alveolar pressure.

_____ 56. No perfusion occurs because alveolar pressure is greater than pulmonary arterial and venous pressures.

A. Zone I

B. Zone II

C. Zone III

TEACH PEOPLE ABOUT PHYSIOLOGY

Write your response to each situation in the space provided.

57. Mr. van Bibber brought his 4-year-old daughter Devon to the emergency department when she aspirated a peanut. "I am so glad we were close by and Devon got fast treatment!" he exclaims. "The nurse said the peanut was in the air tubes that go to her right lung. Then she said that foreign objects almost always go in the right side. Why on the right?"

58. "I read that smoking makes the cilia in airways not work well," says Mr. Lewis. "What do those cilia do when they ARE working?"

59. "Please explain why the blood in the left side of the heart in a healthy adult is not quite 100% oxygenated," says a nurse. "After blood goes through the lungs, it should be fully oxygenated."

60. "I learned that pulmonary arterioles constrict when alveolar partial pressure of oxygen is low in a portion of a lung," says a physiology student. "In what way is that beneficial?"

61. A healthcare professional says, "I need to calculate the oxygen content of Mrs. Mullen's blood. What variables do I need?"

Copyright © 2024 by Elsevier, Inc. All Rights Reserved.

62. "My respiratory patient has hypoxemia, but his $PaCO_2$ is normal," says a nurse. "How is that possible?"

PUZZLE OUT THE TECHNICAL TERMS

Use the clues to complete the puzzle, demonstrating your knowledge of important technical terms.

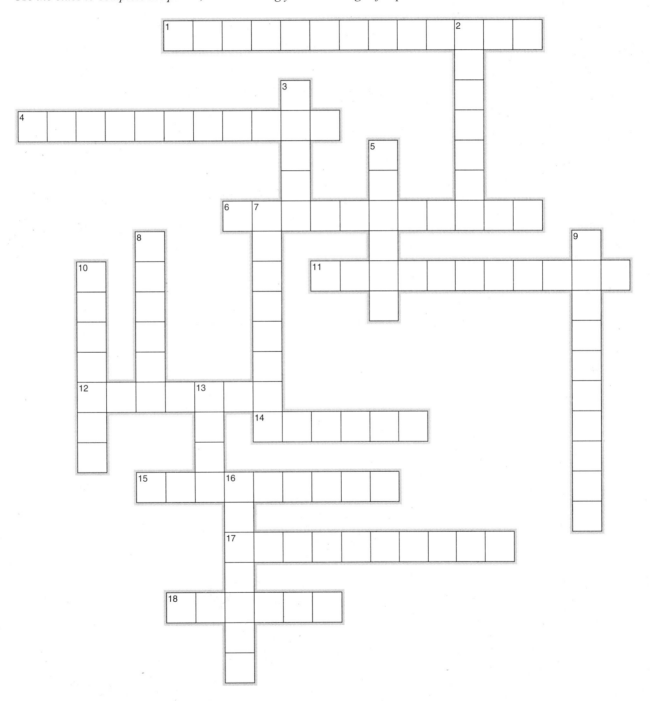

Copyright © 2024 by Elsevier, Inc. All Rights Reserved.

Chapter **34 Structure and Function of the Pulmonary System**

Across

1. Hemoglobin molecules that have bound oxygen
4. Space between the lungs that contains the heart, great vessels, and esophagus
6. Exchange of oxygen and carbon dioxide during cellular metabolism
11. Movement of air into and out of the lungs
12. Structure that connects the larynx to the bronchi
14. Structure that connects the upper and lower airways
15. Dome-shaped major muscle of inspiration
17. Substance secreted by type II alveolar cells that helps keep alveoli from collapsing
18. The structures that participate in gas exchange

Down

2. The conducting airways of the lungs
3. What goblet cells in the bronchi secrete
5. Where the trachea divides into the two main bronchi
7. Intercostal muscles used for vigorous inspiration
8. Membrane attached to the external side of the lungs
9. A measure of distensibility
10. Fibers that give lung tissue its elasticity
13. Where the bronchi and pulmonary vessels enter the lungs
16. Description of normal expiration with regard to muscle effort

Copyright © 2024 by Elsevier, Inc. All Rights Reserved.

35 Alterations of Pulmonary Function

MATCH THE DEFINITIONS

Match the word on the right with its definition on the left.

_____ 1. Presence of pus in the pleural cavity

_____ 2. Collapse of alveoli

_____ 3. Bluish discoloration of the skin caused by desaturation of hemoglobin

_____ 4. PaO$_2$ below normal

_____ 5. Coughing up bloody mucus

_____ 6. Passage of fluid and/or solid particles into the lungs

A. Cyanosis

B. Hypoxemia

C. Hemoptysis

D. Empyema

E. Atelectasis

F. Aspiration

CIRCLE THE CORRECT WORDS

Circle the correct word from the choices provided to complete these sentences.

7. Hyperventilation decreases the (PaCO$_2$, PaO$_2$).

8. Presence of fluid in the pleural space is called pleural (edema, effusion).

9. Severe kyphoscoliosis causes (increased, decreased) chest wall compliance.

10. Persons who have difficulty (coughing, swallowing) have increased risk for aspiration; aspiration of gastric acid is most likely to cause (bronchiolitis, pneumonitis).

11. A person who has pulmonary edema will have (resonance, dullness) to percussion over the lung bases, inspiratory (wheezing, crackles), and with severe pulmonary edema, (foul-smelling, pink frothy) sputum.

12. Processes that increase capillary permeability can cause (exudative, transudative) pleural effusion, but processes that increase capillary hydrostatic pressure can cause (exudative, transudative) pleural effusion.

13. Clinical manifestations of bronchiolitis include tachypnea, (productive, nonproductive) cough, use of accessory muscles, (low-grade, high) fever, and hypoxemia.

14. Silicosis is a(n) (obstructive, restrictive) respiratory disease; asthma is a(n) (obstructive, restrictive) respiratory disease.

15. People who have obstructive respiratory disorders have the most difficulty with (inspiration, expiration).

16. Clubbing of the fingers is a response to (acute, chronic) hypoxemia.

17. The most common cause of lung cancer is (poor nutrition, cigarette smoking); early lung cancer has (vague, obvious) signs and symptoms.

18. Severe asthma that is not controlled by bronchodilators and maintenance medications may be managed with (mucolytics, biologics).

195

Copyright © 2024 by Elsevier, Inc. All Rights Reserved.

CATEGORIZE THE CAUSES

Write the ventilation problem beside each cause. Choices: hypoventilation, hyperventilation.

_____ 19. Acute head injury

_____ 20. Airway obstruction

_____ 21. Reduced firing of neurons to respiratory muscles

_____ 22. Anxiety

_____ 23. Respiratory muscle weakness

_____ 24. Response to severe hypoxemia

_____ 25. Reduced compliance of chest wall

ORDER THE STEPS

Sequence the histologic events that occur during the development of acute respiratory distress syndrome.

26. Write the letters here in the correct order of the steps: _____
    A. Neutrophils release inflammatory mediators and activate complement.
    B. Proinflammatory cytokines are released.
    C. Pulmonary edema occurs from exudation.
    D. Neutrophils, macrophages, and platelets accumulate in the lungs.
    E. Pneumonia or other condition causes acute lung injury.
    F. Fibrosis destroys alveoli and bronchioles.
    G. Cell damage disrupts alveolocapillary membrane.
    H. Fibroblasts and other lung cells proliferate and form membranes.

Copyright © 2024 by Elsevier, Inc. All Rights Reserved.

EXPLAIN THE PICTURE

Examine the picture and answer the questions about it.

27. This picture shows a portion of the pathophysiology of an acute episode of _____.

28. From the information in the picture, was this the first time the individual was exposed to the antigen? Explain your answer.

29. What is the source of the IgE that binds to mast cells?

30. Which end of IgE binds to receptors in the mast cell plasma membrane?

31. What happens when antigen binds to the IgE located on the mast cells? Why is that important?

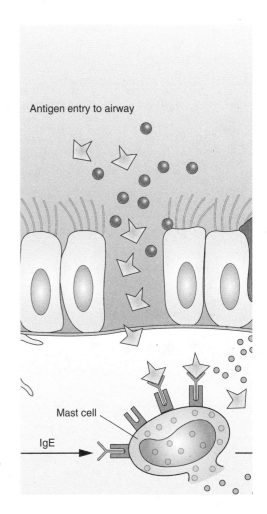

Antigen entry to airway

Mast cell

IgE

DESCRIBE THE DIFFERENCES

Describe the difference between each pair of terms.

32. What is the difference between dyspnea and orthopnea?

33. What is the difference between chylothorax and hemothorax?

34. What is the difference between absorption atelectasis and compression atelectasis?

Copyright © 2024 by Elsevier, Inc. All Rights Reserved.

35. What is the difference between communicating pneumothorax and tension pneumothorax?

MATCH THE BREATHING PATTERNS

Match the breathing patterns on the right with the descriptions on the left.

_____ 36. Alternating periods of deep and shallow breathing with apnea episodes

_____ 37. Increased ventilatory rate, small tidal volume

_____ 38. Rhythmic and effortless with normal tidal volume

_____ 39. Irregular, quick inspirations with an expiratory pause

_____ 40. Increased ventilatory rate, small tidal volume, increased effort, prolonged expiration, wheezing

_____ 41. Increased ventilatory rate, very large tidal volume, no expiratory pause

A. Kussmaul

B. Gasping

C. Cheyne-Stokes

D. Eupnea

E. Restricted

F. Obstructed

COMPLETE THE SENTENCES

Write one word in each blank to complete these sentences.

42. Waking up suddenly with dyspnea during the night and needing to sit upright or stand to breathe is called

_____ _____ _____.

43. Rib fractures that disrupt the mechanics of breathing can cause a portion of the chest wall to collapse _____ during inspiration, an acute condition known as _____ chest.

44. A person who has pneumothorax has _____ in the pleural space.

45. A person who has _____ has persistent abnormal dilations of the bronchi and a chronic cough that produces large amounts of purulent _____.

46. Pulmonary fibrosis is an excessive amount of _____ tissue in the lungs and causes _____ lung compliance.

47. In asthma, long-term airway damage that is irreversible is known as airway _____.

48. During an acute asthma episode, inflammatory mediators cause inflammation, hypersecretion of _____, and bronchial smooth muscle _____.

49. An asthma episode that does not resolve with usual treatment is called _____ _____.

50. Genetic deficiency of _____ _____ causes early-onset emphysema because this enzyme normally inhibits the action of _____ _____ that can destroy lung tissue.

51. The two disorders known as COPD are emphysema and _____ _____; this latter condition is characterized by persistent hypersecretion of _____ and chronic _____ cough.

198

Copyright © 2024 by Elsevier, Inc. All Rights Reserved.

52. Clinical manifestations of emphysema include _____ chest and _____ on exertion and eventually at rest.

53. Cor pulmonale is _____ ventricular enlargement caused by chronic pulmonary _____.

54. Laryngeal cancer is characterized by progressive _____.

55. Primary lung cancer arising from cells that line the airways is called _____ _____; small cell carcinoma in the lung often produces ectopic _____.

TEACH PEOPLE ABOUT PATHOPHYSIOLOGY

Write your response to each situation in the space provided.

56. "Why does Grandpa have to breathe so hard?" asks Ben, age 14, whose grandfather has emphysema.

57. "My uncle has ARDS," says Simon, age 10. "What does ARDS mean and what is wrong with him?"

58. "My cousin's arm tested positive for tuberculosis, but he does not feel sick and his x-ray is good," says Marsh, age 11. "When will he start coughing up blood like in the movies?"

59. "How did working in the coal mine make Grandpa have trouble breathing?" asks Jonah, age 8, whose grandfather has pulmonary fibrosis.

60. Mr. Rudofski says, "My grandfather was a sand blaster and got pulmonary fibrosis from years of exposure to silica. My uncle was a rare book librarian and got pulmonary fibrosis from years of exposure to book mold. They both had pulmonary fibrosis, with similar symptoms, but the doctors called one condition a 'pneumoconiosis' and the other a 'hypersensitivity pneumonitis.' Please explain why."

61. "My husband had difficulty breathing; at the emergency department they said he had water in his lungs because the left side of his heart was not working properly," says Mrs. Hoody. "How can a problem with the heart cause water in the lungs?"

Copyright © 2024 by Elsevier, Inc. All Rights Reserved.

62. A nurse on a respiratory unit asks, "Why do so many of our chronic bronchitis patients have polycythemia?"

CLINICAL SCENARIOS

Read the clinical scenarios and answer the questions to explore your understanding of respiratory disorders.

Mrs. Beeson, age 64, who has a long history of smoking, developed pleuritic chest pain in her right chest. She also has a high fever, dyspnea, and a cough. On examination, she has absent breath sounds on the left and a pleural friction rub.

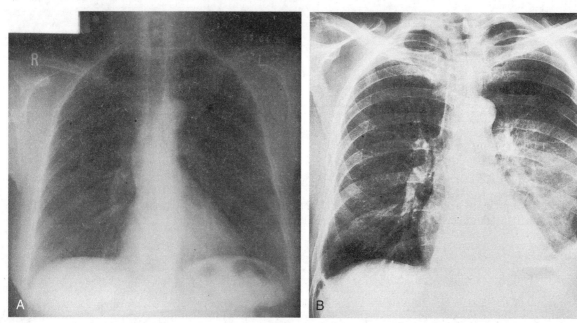

| Normal radiograph (x-ray) | Mrs. Beeson's radiograph |

A, Davies A, Moores C: *The respiratory system,* ed 2, Philadelphia, 2010, Churchill Livingstone. B, Hansell DM, et al: *Imaging of disease of the chest,* ed 5, Philadelphia, 2010, Mosby.

Mrs. Beeson's radiograph shows a dense white collection of fluid at the base of the left lung, where it obscures the left diaphragm and much of the lower left lung. Thoracentesis reveals numerous white blood cells and bacteria in her pleural fluid.

63. *Complete the sentence by choosing from the lists of options.*

   Mrs. Beeson has _____(1)_____, which is pus in the _____(2)_____.

Options for 1	Options for 2
empyema	alveoli
chronic bronchitis	pleural space
pneumonia	bronchioles

Copyright © 2024 by Elsevier, Inc. All Rights Reserved.

64. Where does the abnormal fluid usually originate?

65. Why does Mrs. Beeson experience dyspnea?

Mrs. Goh, age 46, emigrated from Southeast Asia 25 years ago. She is admitted to the hospital with low-grade fever, shortness of breath, and a cough producing discolored sputum. Further evaluation reveals that she has had an unintentional weight loss of 15 pounds in the past 4 months. Examination of her sputum is positive for *Mycobacterium tuberculosis*. Her diagnosis is active tuberculosis (TB) disease.

66. In the Mrs. Goh clinical scenario above, highlight the signs and symptoms of active TB disease.

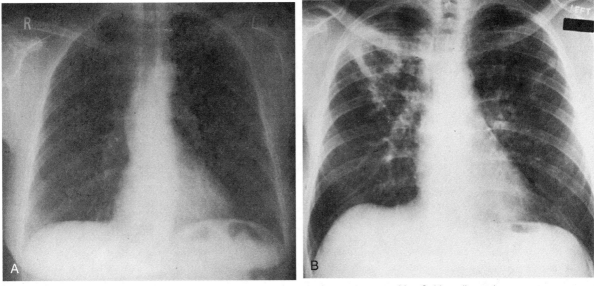

| Normal radiograph (x-ray) | Mrs. Goh's radiograph |

A, Davies A, Moores C: *The respiratory system,* ed 2, Philadelphia 2010, Churchill Livingstone. **B,** Mason RJ, Broaddus VC, Murray JF: *Murray and Nadel's textbook of respiratory medicine,* ed 4, Philadelphia, 2010, Saunders.

Mrs. Goh's radiograph shows cavitary disease in the right lung. Mrs. Goh was infected with the TB bacillus when she lived in Southeast Asia. Until several months ago, the TB bacilli were sequestered in a tubercle.

67. How is tuberculosis transmitted?

Copyright © 2024 by Elsevier, Inc. All Rights Reserved.

68. What is a tubercle?

69. When the TB bacilli were sequestered in the tubercle, did Mrs. Goh have a positive tuberculin skin test? Explain your answer.

70. Mrs. Goh's TB infection reactivated. Why might this have occurred after at least 25 years?

Mrs. Yarborough, age 47, who smokes a pack of cigarettes per day, develops fever, chills, dyspnea, and a cough productive of yellow-green sputum. Her body temperature is 38.5°C (101.3°F). She has tachypnea, tachycardia, and inspiratory crackles auscultated over her right upper and lower lung. Sputum stain reveals numerous white blood cells and bacteria.

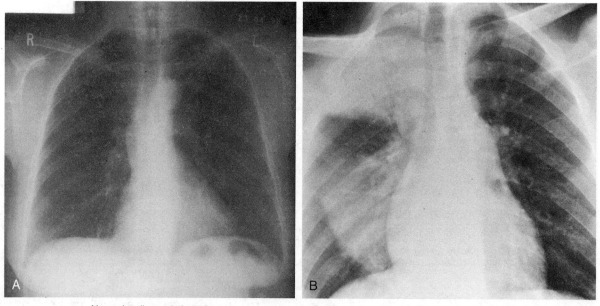

Normal radiograph (x-ray)   Mrs. Yarborough's radiograph

A, Davies A, Moores C: *The respiratory system,* ed 2, Philadelphia, 2010, Churchill Livingstone. **B,** Laufleur Brooks M: *Exploring medical language,* ed 7, St. Louis, 2009, Mosby.

71. Does Mrs. Yarborough have bacterial or viral pneumonia? Explain your answer.

Copyright © 2024 by Elsevier, Inc. All Rights Reserved.

72. What is the pathophysiology of Mrs. Yarborough's illness?

73. What will clear the consolidated exudate from her alveoli as she recovers?

74. Why is smoking cessation important for Mrs. Yarborough to help prevent another episode of pneumonia?

Ms. Kelly Silber, age 24, was admitted 2 days ago for a femur fracture from a skiing accident. She develops sudden dyspnea and pain in her left chest that is worse with breathing. Assessment reveals tachypnea, tachycardia, and some slight crackles in the lower left lung. Ms. Silber's serum D-dimer is elevated. Spiral CT arteriography confirmed her diagnosis of pulmonary embolism.

75. How did Ms. Silber develop a pulmonary embolism?

76. How does a large pulmonary embolism cause V/Q mismatch?

77. Ms. Silber asks, "What is the connection between my broken leg and this breathing problem?" Respond as if speaking directly to Ms. Silber.

Copyright © 2024 by Elsevier, Inc. All Rights Reserved.

36 Alterations of Pulmonary Function in Children

MATCH THE DEFINITIONS

Match the word on the right with its definition on the left.

_____ 1. Infection and inflammation in the terminal airways and alveoli

_____ 2. Runny nose

_____ 3. Harsh vibratory sound caused by turbulent airflow through a partially obstructed upper airway

_____ 4. Localized swelling involving the deep subcutaneous tissue

_____ 5. Acute laryngotracheitis seen in young children

_____ 6. Viral lower respiratory tract infection seen in infants and young toddlers

A. Stridor

B. Angioedema

C. Rhinorrhea

D. Pneumonia

E. Bronchiolitis

F. Croup

CIRCLE THE CORRECT WORDS

Circle the correct word from the choices provided to complete these sentences.

7. Premature infants are likely to develop (ischemia, atelectasis) due to underdeveloped alveoli and lack of (surfactant, capillaries).

8. A neonate's chest wall tends to (collapse inward, bulge outward) with increased respiratory effort because it is highly (calcified, compliant).

9. The cough associated with croup is a (productive, barking) cough.

10. Acute epiglottitis classically is a (viral, bacterial) infection that most commonly occurs in children aged (2 to 6, 6 to 12) years who have not been vaccinated against *H. influenzae* type B.

11. A child who has laryngomalacia will have partial airway obstruction during (inspiration, expiration).

12. Peritonsillar abscess usually is (unilateral, bilateral) and is a complication of (tonsillitis, infectious mononucleosis).

13. Pneumonia in young children usually is a (viral, bacterial) infection.

14. Pneumonia caused by *Mycoplasma* is known as (bacterial, atypical) pneumonia and usually is (not, very) severe.

15. PARDS (precedes, follows) a direct lung injury and is characterized by (progressive, recurrent) respiratory distress and severe (hypercapnia, hypoxemia) that is poorly responsive to supplemental oxygen.

16. MIS-C arises (during, days or weeks after) an acute SARS-COV-2 infection and involves dysfunction of (multiple organs, the lower respiratory tract).

Copyright © 2024 by Elsevier, Inc. All Rights Reserved.

CATEGORIZE THE RESPIRATORY DISORDERS

Write the type of disorder beside each name. Choices: upper airway infection, upper airway congenital malformation, lower airway infection.

_____ 17. Tonsillitis

_____ 18. Bronchiolitis

_____ 19. Bacterial tracheitis

_____ 20. Pneumonia

_____ 21. Subglottic stenosis

_____ 22. Retropharyngeal abscess

_____ 23. Croup

_____ 24. Peritonsillar abscess

EXPLAIN THE PICTURE

Examine the picture and answer the questions about it.

25. This picture shows areas associated with specific clinical manifestations in a child with upper airway obstruction. Which letter on the picture denotes the area where an obstruction will cause a weak cry or hoarse voice? _____

26. Which letter denotes the area where an obstruction will cause snoring? _____

27. What is the significance of the area marked E? _____

28. What sound is associated with obstruction in areas B and C? _____

29. Because obstruction in area B or C produces the same sound, why are they marked as different areas? _____

30. Obstructive sleep apnea is associated with sounds made in which area? _____

Copyright © 2024 by Elsevier, Inc. All Rights Reserved.

COMPLETE THE SENTENCES

Write one word in each blank to complete these sentences.

31. The acronym PARDS stands for pediatric acute _____ _____ _____.

32. Acute laryngotracheobronchitis, commonly called _____, usually is caused by a _____ that causes _____ edema.

33. The predisposing factors for childhood obstructive sleep apnea include obesity and _____ hypertrophy.

34. Respiratory distress syndrome of the newborn is caused by _____ deficiency; fibrin deposits in the alveoli create the appearance of _____ membranes.

35. Chronic lung disease of prematurity, also called _____ _____, is associated with arrested lung _____.

36. Bronchiolitis most commonly is caused by _____ _____ _____ infection; symptoms include initial _____, cough, and _____ respiratory rate.

37. Meconium aspiration causes aspiration _____.

38. Obesity is lined to both allergic and non-allergic childhood _____.

TEACH PEOPLE ABOUT PATHOPHYSIOLOGY

Write your response to each situation in the space provided.

39. Mrs. Abebe's baby has bronchiolitis. She is very worried. "If only I understood better what makes him breathe so fast! The doctor said he has a virus, but his big sister got a virus and did not breathe so fast. She just had a runny nose."

40. "Why is my baby breathing so funny?" asks Mrs. Santosa. Her little chest goes *inward* when she inhales, instead of outward as mine does. Is something wrong with her?"

41. "What is croup?" asks Sandi, age 9. "My little brother had croup, and it was scary! Will I get it?"

42. A physician assistant says, "Explain to me why a little bit of airway edema causes such severe airway obstruction in infants. I know their airways are smaller, but the severity of the obstruction puzzles me."

Copyright © 2024 by Elsevier, Inc. All Rights Reserved.

43. Mrs. Jones took her son Jason, age 9, to a nurse practitioner because his teacher reported that Jason keeps falling asleep in school and that his grades are poor. "The nurse practitioner asked if Jason snores," Mrs. Jones said. "Why did she ask that?"

44. Neonate Marks has respiratory distress syndrome of the newborn. Mr. Marks, the baby's father, says, "I read about RDS on the Internet last night. I learned about surfactant, and I think I understand that part. But why is RDS more common when a woman has an elective C-section as my wife did?"

45. "My cousin's baby died of SIDS," says Mrs. Bush, whose son Howie is 18 months old. "Now I set my alarm every 2 hours during the night to be sure that Howie is breathing."

46. Kevin, age 14, aspirated a chunk of hot dog during a hot dog eating contest. He choked and wheezed at the time, but he soon recovered and kept gobbling hot dogs until the contest concluded. Several days later, he began wheezing again, and his mother took him to a physician assistant, who discovered the aspirated item. "I am fine!" exclaims Kevin. "Why do you have to put that tube down my throat to remove that piece of hot dog? Won't it eventually dissolve anyway?"

47. Molly, age 6, developed acute cough, wheeze, and dyspnea after playing with her cousin's dog. "Why did she get asthma from the dog?" asks her brother, age 10. "Was it dog germs? I play with the dog all the time, but I do not get asthma."

CLINICAL SCENARIOS

Read the clinical scenarios and answer the questions to explore your understanding of acute epiglottitis and cystic fibrosis.

Darrell, age 4, had difficulty breathing and was drooling. His mother rushed him to the emergency department. Based on the following assessment, the admitting nurse immediately called an anesthesiologist, who intubated Darrell.

Objective Findings

- Tripod posture
- Drooling
- Voice muffled
- Inspiratory stridor
- Obvious use of accessory muscles during inspiration
- Temperature 38.9°C (102°F) (tympanic)

Copyright © 2024 by Elsevier, Inc. All Rights Reserved.

Subjective Findings

- Child reports sore throat

- Mother reports sudden onset

Darrell's diagnosis is acute epiglottitis. On follow-up, it was determined that Darrell had not received any immunizations.

48. The admitting nurse did not examine Darrell's throat. Was this an error on her part?

49. *Complete the sentence by choosing from the lists of options.*

Darrell was drooling because his swollen _____(1)_____ was _____(2)_____.

Options for 1	Options for 2
pharynx	preventing him from swallowing
epiglottis	causing production of more saliva

50. What caused Darrell's stridor?

51. Explain to Darrell's mother what the epiglottis is and what epiglottitis means.

52. Why was Darrell given intravenous antibiotics instead of the oral ones?

53. What is the usual clinical course of acute epiglottitis that is treated with intubation and antibiotics?

   Copyright © 2024 by Elsevier, Inc. All Rights Reserved.

Wilson, age 15, has cystic fibrosis that was diagnosed when he was an infant. He is thin, small for his age, and has recurrent respiratory infections.

54. Wilson asks, "If I inherited CF from my parents, why don't they have CF?"

55. What is CFTCR, and why is it important in CF?

56. Why does Wilson have recurrent respiratory infections?

57. What is the role of neutrophils in CF?

58. In what way is biofilm formation important in CF?

59. Examination of Wilson's hands is likely to reveal what findings?

60. How does the pathophysiology of CF contribute to Wilson being thin and small for his age?

Copyright © 2024 by Elsevier, Inc. All Rights Reserved.

37 Structure and Function of the Renal and Urologic Systems

MATCH THE DEFINITIONS

Match the word on the right with its definition on the left.

_____ 1. The process of urination

_____ 2. Red blood cells in the urine

_____ 3. The bladder wall muscle

_____ 4. Accumulations of precipitated material in the urine that have a cylindrical shape like a mold of a section of tubule

_____ 5. Precipitated material in the urine that increases as urine cools

_____ 6. The area of the bladder between the openings of the ureters and the urethra

_____ 7. White blood cells in the urine

_____ 8. The area of the kidney where the ureter exits and blood vessels enter and exit

_____ 9. Cone-shaped sections of the renal medulla that contain loops of Henle and collecting ducts

_____ 10. Chambers of the kidney through which urine passes into the renal pelvis

A. Detrusor

B. Trigone

C. Micturition

D. Hematuria

E. Pyuria

F. Casts

G. Crystal

H. Pyramids

I. Hilum

J. Calyces

CIRCLE THE CORRECT WORDS

Circle the correct word from the choices provided to complete these sentences.

11. All of the glomeruli are located in the renal (medulla, cortex).

12. Small openings in the glomerular endothelium, called (pores, lacunae), are maintained by the vascular epithelial growth factor secreted by the (podocytes, epithelium).

13. The (internal, external) urethral sphincter is under voluntary control and is innervated by the (pudendal, phrenic) somatic motor nerve.

14. Urea is a product of (carbohydrate, protein) breakdown; recycling of urea within the renal medulla is necessary to (concentrate, filter) urine.

15. Elimination of a substance in the urine is called (secretion, excretion).

16. The amount of plasma filtered per unit time is the (glomerular filtration rate, filtration fraction).

17. Natriuretic peptides (increase, decrease) renal excretion of sodium and water; ADH (increases, decreases) renal excretion of water, which (increases, decreases) urine specific gravity.

210

Copyright © 2024 by Elsevier, Inc. All Rights Reserved.

18. Blood entering the peritubular capillaries has (low, high) hydrostatic pressure and (low, high) oncotic pressure, which facilitates (secretion, reabsorption) of fluid from the proximal convoluted tubules.

19. Tamm-Horsfall protein, also known as (nephrin, uromodulin), is produced in the (proximal, distal) nephron segments and protects against (infection, dehydration).

20. The concentration gradient of the renal interstitium (decreases, increases) from the cortex to the tip of the medulla; this gradient is necessary in order to (dilute, concentrate) the urine.

21. The countercurrent exchange system operates because fluid flows in opposite directions through the two segments of the (loop of Henle, vasa recta), and the gradient is maintained by the (loop of Henle, vasa recta).

22. The kidneys (activate, inactivate) vitamin D, a process that is stimulated by (calcitonin, parathyroid hormone).

23. Creatinine clearance and/or blood levels of cystatin C are used to estimate (renal blood flow, glomerular filtration rate); para-aminohippurate clearance is used to estimate (effective renal plasma flow, glomerular filtration rate).

LOCATE THE STRUCTURES

Write the anatomic location in the kidney beside each structure. Choices: renal cortex, renal medulla.

_____ 24. Glomeruli

_____ 25. Collecting ducts

_____ 26. Most of the proximal tubules

_____ 27. Glomerular capillaries

_____ 28. Most of the distal tubules

_____ 29. Pyramids

_____ 30. Most of the vasa recta

_____ 31. Renal corpuscles

_____ 32. Interlobular arteries

_____ 33. Afferent arterioles

ORDER THE STEPS

Sequence the structures through which fluid flows starting in the glomerulus and ending as urine in the bladder.

34. Write the letters here in the correct order of the steps: _____
    A. Glomerular capillaries
    B. Proximal convoluted tubule
    C. Bladder
    D. Renal pelvis
    E. Filtration slits
    F. Loop of Henle
    G. Bowman capsule
    H. Distal convoluted tubule
    I. Ureter
    J. Collecting duct

Copyright © 2024 by Elsevier, Inc. All Rights Reserved.

MATCH THE FUNCTIONS

Match the portion of the nephron on the right with its function on the left.

_____ 35. Reabsorption of large amounts of sodium, water, glucose, amino acids; net reabsorption of bicarbonate; secretion of H^+, organic acids, and many medications

_____ 36. Reabsorption of sodium, chloride, and potassium but not much water

_____ 37. Secretion of potassium, ammonia, and H^+; site of action of aldosterone and ADH

_____ 38. Filtration

_____ 39. Reabsorption of water

A. Glomerulus

B. Distal tubule and collecting duct

C. Proximal tubule

D. Descending limb of loop of Henle

E. Thick ascending limb of loop of Henle

EXPLAIN THE PICTURE

Examine the picture and answer the questions about it.

40. The first cell pictured below the Bowman capsule is in what portion of the nephron?

_____

41. What is the significance of the large number of mitochondria in this cell?

42. What is the significance of the microvilli on the luminal surface of this cell?

43. Compare the cells pictured on the descending limb of the loop of Henle and the thick ascending limb. Which cell has larger mitochondria and thus is more suited for active transport of solutes?

_____

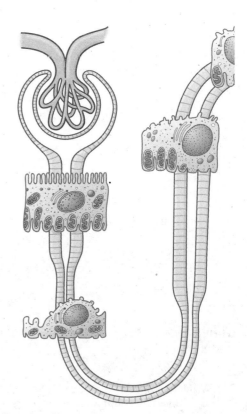

Copyright © 2024 by Elsevier, Inc. All Rights Reserved.

MATCH THE MECHANISMS

Match the mechanism on the right with its description on the left.

_____ 44. A process that regulates sodium and water balance by reabsorption of a constant fraction of the sodium load filtered at the glomerulus.

_____ 45. A process that regulates renal blood flow and glomerular filtration rate to keep them constant by altering the amount of vasoconstriction of afferent arterioles in response to changes in their circumference.

_____ 46. A process that regulates glomerular filtration rate to keep it constant by altering the amount of vasoconstriction of afferent arterioles in response to changes in the concentration of filtered sodium.

A. Tubuloglomerular feedback

B. Glomerulotubular balance

C. Myogenic mechanism

DESCRIBE THE DIFFERENCES

Describe the difference between each pair of terms.

47. What is the difference between the urethra and ureter?

48. What is the difference between the principal cells and the intercalated cells in the collecting duct?

49. What is the difference between tubular secretion and tubular reabsorption?

COMPLETE THE SENTENCES

Write one word in each blank to complete these sentences.

50. The location where the renal blood vessels, nerves, lymphatics, and ureter enter and exit the kidney is called the

_____.

51. The epithelial cells of the proximal convoluted tubule are the only renal tubular cells that have _____.

52. The _____ is the functional unit of the kidney; the _____ ones are highly important for concentrating urine.

53. Glomerular capillary blood flow is regulated in part by the contractile _____ cells and by vasoactive substances secreted by the endothelium.

54. The filtration fraction is the ratio of the glomerular filtration rate to _____ _____

_____.

Copyright © 2024 by Elsevier, Inc. All Rights Reserved.

Chapter **37** **Structure and Function of the Renal and Urologic Systems**

55. Renal arterioles are innervated by _____ nerves; increased firing of these nerves causes the arterioles to

_____.

56. Net glomerular filtration pressure is the sum of the forces that _____ filtration minus the forces that

_____ filtration.

57. The renal hormone _____ degrades catecholamines.

58. In response to hypoxia, the kidneys secrete _____, which circulates to bone marrow and stimulates

_____.

59. The term _____ refers to how much of a substance can be removed from the blood by the kidneys per a unit of time.

60. Plasma creatinine concentration _____ when the GFR decreases, but it takes 7 to 10 days for the level

to stabilize, so this measure is best for monitoring _____ renal disease.

61. The BUN level _____ when the GFR decreases, but also varies with dehydration, protein intake, and

protein _____, which may make it unreliable for monitoring renal function.

FINISH THE DESCRIPTIONS

Finish these descriptions of physiologic processes by writing or drawing in the spaces provided.

62. **Micturition reflex:** As the bladder fills with urine, it begins to stretch. Mechanoreceptors in the bladder wall send neural sensory messages of stretch to the spinal cord. What happens next?

63. **Renal autoregulation:** With arterial blood pressures between 80 and 180 mmHg, an increase of arterial blood pressure influences renal afferent arterioles in what way? Why is that important?

64. **Renin-angiotensin-aldosterone system:** Decreased blood flow through the renal artery stimulates the release of renin into the blood. What happens next? Describe the process until it has influenced renal function.

Copyright © 2024 by Elsevier, Inc. All Rights Reserved.

Write your response to each situation in the space provided.

65. Mr. Tyson, who is a plumber, says, "I understand that the ureters are tubes that carry urine from the kidney to the bladder. Gravity would move the urine down when a person is upright. But why does urine go through the ureters when a person is lying down?"

66. A nursing student asks, "If 20% of the arterial blood that enters the kidneys is filtered into the renal tubules at the glomerulus, what happens to the other 80% that stays in the glomerulus after it leaves the efferent arterioles? Does it just leave the kidney by way of veins?"

67. A medical assistant in a refugee camp working with protein-malnourished people says, "I am surprised that even when our new refugees obviously are dehydrated, they still do not have the small quantities of dark yellow urine I would expect. They make larger amounts of lighter yellow urine. Why?"

68. "I am learning how the kidneys work," says Mrs. Boulpaep. "It says here that the glomeruli in the kidneys filter about 180 liters per day. I know we do not have that much fluid in our bodies! Is this number an error, or if it is true, why aren't we dead from urinating out our body fluids?"

69. "I wake up every night needing to urinate," says a retired nurse, age 78. "I know that age-related nocturia is normal, but I forget what basic changes in the kidney make that happen. Please explain."

Copyright © 2024 by Elsevier, Inc. All Rights Reserved.

38 Alterations of Renal and Urinary Tract Function

MATCH THE DEFINITIONS

Match the word on the right with its definition on the left.

_____ 1. Dilation of a ureter by accumulated urine

A. Hydronephrosis

_____ 2. Enlargement of the renal pelvis and calyces by accumulated urine

B. Staghorn calculus

_____ 3. Narrowing of the lumen of a urethra

C. Hydroureter

_____ 4. Large urinary stone that has assumed the shape of the renal pelvis and calyces

D. Urethral stricture

CIRCLE THE CORRECT WORDS

Circle the correct word from the choices provided to complete these sentences.

5. In addition to relieving pain, rapid removal of an upper urinary tract obstruction is important because the accumulating urine causes back pressure that (damages, hyperstimulates) nephrons.

6. When one kidney develops irreversible damage, the other kidney (makes additional nephrons, undergoes hypertrophy of existing glomeruli and tubules).

7. An alkaline urinary pH significantly increases the risk for (calcium phosphate, uric acid) stone formation, whereas acidic urine increases the risk for a (calcium phosphate, uric acid) stone.

8. The technical term for bladder dysfunction due to neurologic disorders is (detrusor hyperreflexia, neurogenic bladder).

9. Cigarette smoking and exposure to occupational chemicals are risk factors for (renal, bladder) cancer, which is characterized by (painless, pain and) hematuria.

10. The most common route by which bacteria reach the bladder is (through the blood, retrograde up the urethra); the most common route by which bacteria reach the kidney is (through the blood, retrograde up a ureter).

11. The only manifestation of cystitis in an older adult may be development of (confusion, headache).

12. Acute pyelonephritis primarily affects the (glomeruli, renal pelvis and tubules) and is associated with sudden onset of fever, chills, and flank or groin (rash, pain); chronic pyelonephritis primarily involves inflammation and fibrosis of the renal (tubules, interstitium).

13. The terms *membranoproliferative glomerulonephritis* and *mesangial proliferative glomerulonephritis* refer to the (clinical course, histologic appearance) of the condition.

14. Proteinuria and angiotensin II contribute to (reversible, irreversible) renal damage in (acute kidney injury, chronic kidney disease).

15. Serum cystatin C is a biomarker used to detect changes in (tubular secretion and reabsorption, the glomerular filtration rate).

Copyright © 2024 by Elsevier, Inc. All Rights Reserved.

CATEGORIZE THE CAUSES

Write the type of acute kidney injury beside each cause. Choices: prerenal, intrarenal, postrenal.

_____ 16. Nephrotoxic antibiotics

_____ 17. Rapidly progressive glomerulonephritis

_____ 18. Massive hemorrhage

_____ 19. Renal ischemia during surgery

_____ 20. Very large pulmonary embolism

_____ 21. Bilateral renal calculi

_____ 22. Untreated enlarged prostate

ORDER THE STEPS

Sequence the events that occur to cause renal osteodystrophies.

23. Write the letters here in the correct order of the steps: _____
    A. GI calcium absorption decreases.
    B. Calcium is removed from bones.
    C. Plasma calcium concentration falls.
    D. Failing kidneys do not activate vitamin D.
    E. Parathyroid hormone secretion increases.

IDENTIFY THE EXAMPLES

Match the type of incontinence on the right with its example on the left.

_____ 24. A man was mildly confused, and his family brought him to adult day care during the week. He was incontinent there every day until a nurse suggested that they put a picture of a toilet on the bathroom door, and he became continent.

_____ 25. A woman has a bladder infection and is distressed to have episodes of a sudden, strong need to urinate that cause her to become incontinent.

_____ 26. A woman loses a small amount of urine involuntarily every time she sneezes.

_____ 27. A man with a cauda equina involvement in multiple sclerosis became incontinent when his caregiver was late and was not available to assist with the morning catheterization.

A. Urge incontinence

B. Stress incontinence

C. Overflow incontinence

D. Functional incontinence

DESCRIBE THE DIFFERENCES

Describe the difference between each pair of terms.

28. What is the difference between cystitis and pyelonephritis?

Copyright © 2024 by Elsevier, Inc. All Rights Reserved.

29. What is the difference between the abnormal urine contents in acute glomerulonephritis and in nephrotic syndrome?

30. What is the difference between azotemia and uremia?

COMPLETE THE SENTENCES

Write one word in each blank to complete these sentences.

31. Urinary stones, also called _____, most commonly are composed of _____ salts, but may have a different composition, depending on the individual's risk factors and the characteristics of the urine.

32. Obstructions to urine flow in the lower urinary tract include enlargement of the _____ in men and prolapse of the _____ _____ in women.

33. The most common renal cancers are renal cell _____ that arise from the renal tubular _____.

34. Uropathic strains of *E. coli* attach to the _____ with their type 1 fimbriae and resist being flushed from the bladder during _____.

35. Women who have symptoms of cystitis for more than 6 weeks with negative urine cultures may have _____ cystitis.

36. The primary cause of the damage in acute glomerulonephritis is the _____ system.

37. Two disease processes associated with chronic glomerulonephritis are lupus and _____.

38. Anuria is a urine output of less than _____ mL per 24 hours.

39. Oliguria is a urine output of less than _____ mL per 24 hours.

Copyright © 2024 by Elsevier, Inc. All Rights Reserved.

MATCH THE CLINICAL MANIFESTATIONS

Match the disorder on the right with its classic signs and symptoms on the left.

_____ 40. No symptoms in early stages; hematuria, dull flank pain, weight loss, anemia in late stages

_____ 41. Sudden onset of hematuria, red blood cell casts, mild proteinuria, plus edema, hypertension, and oliguria if severe; may be asymptomatic

_____ 42. Severe colicky flank pain radiating to the groin, nausea and vomiting, some hematuria

_____ 43. Urgency, with or without urge incontinence, associated with frequency and nocturia; no bacteria in urine

_____ 44. Frequency, urgency, dysuria, suprapubic and low back pain, cloudy urine

_____ 45. Massive proteinuria, hypoproteinemia, hyperlipidemia, edema

_____ 46. Sudden onset of oliguria with elevated plasma BUN and plasma creatinine levels

A. Calculus lodged in ureter

B. Acute cystitis

C. Overactive bladder

D. Renal cancer

E. Acute kidney injury

F. Acute glomerulonephritis

G. Nephrotic syndrome

COMPLETE THE TABLE

Complete this table to figure out aspects of the uremic syndrome.

Normal Renal Function	Result of Impaired Function in the Uremic Syndrome
Excrete nitrogenous wastes	
Excrete potassium ions	
Excrete metabolic acids	
Excrete phosphate	
Activate vitamin D	
Secrete erythropoietin	
Excrete sodium and water	

TEACH PEOPLE ABOUT PATHOPHYSIOLOGY

Write your response to each situation in the space provided.

47. "I heard the medical student tell the doctor there are casts in my urine," says Mrs. Masterson, who has pyelonephritis. "What are casts?"

48. "I have a bladder infection," says Mrs. Barr, who is pregnant for the first time. "Why did my obstetrician tell me to call her office immediately if I get chills and fever?"

219

Copyright © 2024 by Elsevier, Inc. All Rights Reserved.

49. "Why am I so tired all the time?" asks Mr. Rao, who has newly diagnosed end-stage chronic kidney disease. "Is that part of my kidney disease?"

50. "Why did the dialysis nurse tell me not to eat a lot of strawberries?" asks Mr. Snyder, who has end-stage chronic kidney disease. "I love strawberry shortcake!"

51. "The nephrologist said my kidneys are damaged," says Mr. Lee, who has diabetes. "But I make so much urine that I get up three times in the night to urinate. She must be wrong."

52. "The doctor said I have hydronephrosis," says Mr. Boulet. "I thought I had a big kidney stone in my ureter. What is going on?"

53. Mrs. Patel has severe acute glomerulonephritis. "I understand that my glomerulus filters are injured and they let some red blood cells into my urine. But why am I making so much less urine than usual? Why doesn't a lot of water leak out through the injured places as well?"

54. "My patient has acute tubular necrosis," says a nurse. "I took care of him for over 2 weeks, and he had oliguria. After my days off, I come back and find that he has mild polyuria. I am really worried at this change, but no one else is. What is going on?"

55. "Why did the doctor say that it is possible for my husband to recover from his kidney problem?" asks Mrs. Empire, whose husband has acute tubular necrosis after hemorrhage from a motor vehicle accident. "My cousin who had diabetes got a kidney problem, and her doctor said her kidneys would not recover. He was right. She died after several years of dialysis treatments. Is my husband's doctor not being honest with me?"

56. Mr. Roswell has acute glomerulonephritis. He says, "A nurse told me I have blood in my urine. Why is my urine a smoky brown color? Why isn't it pink like my wife's urine was when she had blood in her urine from a bladder problem?"

 Copyright © 2024 by Elsevier, Inc. All Rights Reserved.

57. "Why do people who have nephrotic syndrome have so much protein in their urine?" asks a nurse who is new to the renal unit. "Do they have big holes in their glomeruli?"

58. A woman approaches a physician assistant at a community blood pressure screening. "I need to know what stress incontinence is," she says. "Tell me first, and then I shall explain why I ask."

59. Mrs. Hixon, who has type 2 diabetes, has newly diagnosed end-stage chronic kidney disease. A nurse who enters Mrs. Hixon's hospital room sees a big box of raisins on the bedside table. Mrs. Hixon smiles and says, "My physician said I am anemic, so I asked my husband to bring me some raisins. That is what I ate years ago when I got anemic from menstruating so heavily. That cured it!" How should the nurse respond?

60. A newly employed nurse at a neurologic injury rehabilitation facility says, "Please help me make sense of the bladder dysfunctions after neurologic injury. Some of our patients have underactive bladders, and others have overactive bladders. What makes the difference?"

CLINICAL SCENARIOS

Mr. Flores worked for a roofing company and spent long days in the sun nailing shingles. One very hot week, he lost the water bottle he usually clipped to his belt and became quite dehydrated because his supervisor yelled at him every time he climbed down the ladder to get a drink. On Friday afternoon, Mr. Flores began to experience severe pain in his left flank that came and went in rhythmic waves. The pain was so severe that he could not even climb the ladder and he became very nauseated. All he could do was lie on the ground, moaning. The other workers convinced his supervisor to take Mr. Flores to the emergency department, where he received appropriate care.

61. *Complete the sentence by choosing from the lists of options.*

Mr. Flores most likely had _____(1)_____ that was precipitated by _____(2)_____.

Options for 1	Options for 2
pyelonephritis	heat exhaustion
renal calculi	bacteria ascending from his bladder
oliguria	dehydration causing concentrated urine

62. Why did Mr. Flores experience the severe flank pain in rhythmic waves rather than as a steady pain?

Copyright © 2024 by Elsevier, Inc. All Rights Reserved.

63. What teaching is important to preventing such situations in the future?

Amira went to a neighborhood clinic because she was experiencing dysuria and urinary frequency and urgency. As she had suspected, she had a bladder infection. The nurse practitioner prescribed an antibiotic.

64. What is dysuria?

65. What is urinary frequency?

66. What is urgency?

67. Knowing that antibiotics are not effective treatment for viral infections, why are antibiotics prescribed so routinely for bladder infections?

68. What technical term do health care professionals use to indicate "bladder infection"?

Copyright © 2024 by Elsevier, Inc. All Rights Reserved.

39 Alterations of Renal and Urinary Tract Function in Children

MATCH THE CONGENITAL ABNORMALITIES

Match the congenital abnormality on the right with its description on the left.

_____ 1. Congenital counterclockwise twist of the penile shaft

_____ 2. Ventral bend of the penis

_____ 3. Congenital herniation of the urinary bladder through the abdominal wall

_____ 4. Congenital condition in which the urethral meatus is located on the ventral surface of the penis

_____ 5. Membrane that blocks the urethral lumen

_____ 6. Small kidney with decreased number of nephrons

_____ 7. Absence of one or both kidneys

A. Chordee

B. Urethral valve

C. Exstrophy of the bladder

D. Hypoplastic kidney

E. Penile torsion

F. Renal agenesis

G. Hypospadias

CIRCLE THE CORRECT WORDS

Circle the correct word from the choices provided to complete these sentences.

8. If the neonate is not premature, (all of the, half of the) nephrons are present at birth; the kidneys typically reach adult size by (age 40; adolescence).

9. Urine formation begins by the (third, eighth) month of gestation; the glomerular filtration rate (decreases, increases) at birth and attains adult levels by (6 months, 2 years) of age.

10. Renal vascular resistance is (high, low) in neonates and infants and the GFR (increases, decreases) until around age 2, when it reaches adult levels.

11. Bladder infection, also known as (cystitis, bladderitis), causes detrusor muscle hyperactivity that (increases, decreases) bladder capacity.

12. Symptoms of urinary tract infections in children are (specific, nonspecific); one indicator is that UTI in a previously toilet-trained child may cause (enuresis, hyperactivity).

13. Differentiating between bladder and kidney infection in children is (easy, difficult).

14. Most children acquire bladder control before (2, 5) years of age; incontinence after that age when no structural or neurologic abnormalities are found is called (enuretic, functional) incontinence.

15. Primary nephrotic syndrome also is known as (functional, idiopathic) nephrotic syndrome and occurs in the (presence, absence) of preexisting renal disease.

Copyright © 2024 by Elsevier, Inc. All Rights Reserved.

16. Presence of a urethral valve obstructs the (bladder outlet, kidney outflow).

17. IgA nephropathy is (a congenital, an autoimmune) disease in which immune complexes are deposited in the (glomerulus, distal tubules), triggering injury.

EXPLAIN THE PICTURES

Examine the pictures and answer the questions about them.

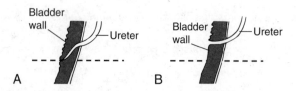

18. These pictures show the insertion of a ureter into the bladder wall. What is the difference in the angle at which the ureter travels through the bladder wall in picture B compared with picture A?

19. Which picture shows the normal anatomy? _____

20. The abnormal insertion angle of the ureter is associated with what condition?

    _____

21. What happens when the bladder muscle contracts in this condition?

22. How does this condition predispose to cystitis and pyelonephritis?

DESCRIBE THE DIFFERENCES

Describe the difference between each pair of terms.

23. What is the difference between hypospadias and epispadias in males?

Copyright © 2024 by Elsevier, Inc. All Rights Reserved.

24. What is the difference between a hypoplastic kidney and a dysplastic kidney?

25. What is the difference between primary incontinence and secondary incontinence?

26. What is the difference between chordee and penile torsion?

COMPLETE THE SENTENCES

Write one word in each blank to complete these sentences.

27. When kidneys fuse in the midline as they ascend during development, the U-shaped kidney is called a _____ kidney.

28. Failure of the abdominal muscles and anterior bladder to fuse in the midline with subsequent exposure of the posterior bladder mucosa is called _____ of the bladder.

29. Blockage of the tapered point where the renal pelvis transitions into the ureter is called _____ _____ obstruction and causes _____ in neonates.

30. When a kidney contains both renal and nonrenal tissues, the condition is called renal _____.

31. Autosomal dominant polycystic kidney disease arises from inherited mutations of the _____ gene and becomes apparent in late childhood or adulthood when multiple _____ form in the kidneys, interfering with renal function.

32. Another name for Wilms tumor is _____, a tumor of the _____ that usually presents as an enlarging, firm, nontender, smooth mass on one side of the _____.

33. Nephrotic syndrome is characterized by proteinuria, _____, hyperlipidemia, and edema, which often is _____ in the morning and more evident in the abdomen and lower extremities later in the day.

34. Minimal change nephropathy is one of the common histopathology patterns of _____ _____ in children.

Copyright © 2024 by Elsevier, Inc. All Rights Reserved.

Write your response to each situation in the space provided.

35. "Why is Keely's urine foamy?" asks Keely's mother. "Is that part of her nephrotic syndrome?"

36. "My mother had polycystic kidney disease too," says Jason Frei, age 15, who has just learned that he has the condition. "I have always wondered what 'polycystic' means."

37. Mrs. Garrow's infant died a few hours after birth due to Potter syndrome. "The doctor said my baby had no kidneys and that is why his lungs went bad," she says. "Please explain that."

38. Tami McArdle, age 13, who has polycystic kidney disease, went to her first dialysis session. There she met Mrs. Singleton, age 53, who also has polycystic kidney disease and who began dialysis at age 50. Tami asks, "Because we both have polycystic kidney disease, why did I end up in dialysis so much faster than she did?"

39. Molly Culkins, age 3, developed hemolytic uremic syndrome after eating a contaminated hamburger from a fast-food restaurant. She is recovering after a stay in an intensive care unit. "Tell me again how the *E. coli* damaged her kidneys," says her father. "I know it was not a direct infection."

CLINICAL SCENARIO

Read the clinical scenario and answer the questions to explore your understanding of glomerulonephritis.

Shane Nye, age 9, had a severe sore throat that was diagnosed as "strep throat" at a clinic visit. His mother was given a prescription for an antibiotic, which she did not fill because she received notice that her electricity would be cut off if she did not pay her overdue bill immediately. After paying her electric bill, she had no money left. Ten days later, Shane's urine became smoky brown, and he did not feel well. His ankles were slightly swollen, so his mother took him to a free clinic. Shane's diagnosis is acute poststreptococcal glomerulonephritis.

40. "Did the strep infect Shane's kidneys?" asks Mrs. Nye. "I did not have the money for that antibiotic." What should the clinic nurse respond?

Copyright © 2024 by Elsevier, Inc. All Rights Reserved.

41. Why is Shane's urine smoky brown?

42. Why did Shane's ankles swell?

43. What is an immune complex? What role do immune complexes play in the pathophysiology of acute poststreptococcal glomerulonephritis?

Copyright © 2024 by Elsevier, Inc. All Rights Reserved.

40 Structure and Function of the Digestive System

MATCH THE DEFINITIONS

Match each word on the right with its definition on the left.

_____	1. Waves of sequential relaxations and contractions of the gastrointestinal muscles	A. Segmentation
_____	2. The functional units of the small intestine	B. Chyme
_____	3. An iron-binding protein	C. Peristalsis
_____	4. Localized, rhythmic contractions of intestinal circular smooth muscles that are not peristalsis	D. Villi
_____	5. Partially digested food in the stomach and intestine	E. Transferrin

MATCH THE CELLS

Match the cell on the right with its function on the left.

_____	6. Metabolize nutrients, detoxify chemicals, secrete bile, synthesize albumin and clotting factors, and other functions	A. Kupffer cells
_____	7. Remove bacteria and foreign particles from blood in the hepatic sinusoids	B. Pancreatic acinar cells
_____	8. Secrete digestive proenzymes	C. Pancreatic ductal epithelium
_____	9. Secrete bicarbonate-rich fluid	D. Hepatocytes
_____	10. Secrete gastrin	E. Enterochromaffin-like cells
_____	11. Secrete hydrochloric acid and intrinsic factor	F. Chief cells
_____	12. Secrete gastric histamine	G. G cells
_____	13. Secrete gastric somatostatin	H. Parietal cells
_____	14. Secrete pepsinogen	I. D cells

CIRCLE THE CORRECT WORDS

Circle the correct word from the choices provided to complete these sentences.

15. Gastrin and motilin (stimulate, delay) gastric emptying; secretin and cholecystokinin (stimulate, delay) gastric emptying.

16. The (gallbladder, liver) produces bile, which is slightly (acidic, alkaline).

Copyright © 2024 by Elsevier, Inc. All Rights Reserved.

17. The composition of saliva depends on the rate of (eating, **its secretion**).

18. Saliva contains (lymphocytes, **immunoglobulin A**), which can help prevent infection.

19. Stretching the esophagus or intestine by a bolus of food causes (**peristalsis**, relaxation).

20. Fatty foods (stimulate, **delay**) gastric emptying; hypertonic gastric contents (stimulate, **delay**) gastric emptying.

21. The intestinal brush border is the collection of (villi, **microvilli**); enzymes in the brush border hydrolyze (**oligopeptides**, amino acids).

22. Most of the water that enters the gastrointestinal tract each day is absorbed in the (**small**, large) intestine; sugars are absorbed primarily in the (**initial**, terminal) portions of the (**small**, large) intestine.

23. The intestinal tract is (**sterile**, partially colonized) at birth and becomes well colonized within 3 to 4 (**days**, weeks).

24. A choleretic agent is a substance that stimulates the (pancreas, **liver**) to secrete (**bile**, glucagon).

25. Pancreatic proteases are secreted in (active, **inactive**) form; pancreatic amylases are secreted in (**active**, inactive) form; pancreatic lipases are secreted in (**active**, inactive) form.

26. As age increases, gastrointestinal motility tends to (increase, **decrease**), liver blood flow and enzyme activity (increase, **decrease**) with age, and liver function tests (show dysfunction, **remain normal**) in an older adult who does not have overt liver disease.

CATEGORIZE THE STIMULI

Write the action of each stimulus on secretion of gastric acid. Choices: increase, decrease.

_____ 27. Histamine

_____ 28. Cholecystokinin

_____ 29. Gastrin

_____ 30. Increased vagal stimulation

_____ 31. Ghrelin

_____ 32. Caffeine

ORDER THE STEPS

Ending with the formation of bile, sequence the events that occur with the heme when an aged erythrocyte is destroyed in the spleen.

33. Write the letters here in the correct order of the steps: _____
    A. Unconjugated bilirubin binds to albumin and circulates to the liver.
    B. Aged erythrocyte is destroyed by macrophages in the spleen.
    C. Unconjugated bilirubin enters the liver sinusoids and then the hepatocytes.
    D. Macrophages separate heme from the remainder of the hemoglobin, converting it to biliverdin.
    E. Hepatocytes conjugate bilirubin and secrete it into bile.
    F. Macrophages convert biliverdin to unconjugated bilirubin.

Copyright © 2024 by Elsevier, Inc. All Rights Reserved.

Examine the picture and answer the questions about it.

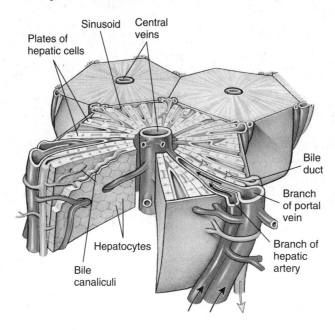

34. This drawing shows the internal architecture of what organ? _____

35. What term is used to describe the structure that surrounds the central veins? (Hint: This drawing shows three of these structures.)

    _____

36. What structures lie between sheets of hepatocytes?

    _____

37. What is the source of the blood that enters the sinusoids?

    _____

38. The sinusoids drain into what blood vessels?

    _____

39. Why is it important that the sinusoids are lined with highly permeable endothelium?

    _____

40. The hepatocytes secrete bile into what structures?

    _____

Copyright © 2024 by Elsevier, Inc. All Rights Reserved.

DESCRIBE THE DIFFERENCES

Describe the difference between each pair of terms.

41. What is the difference between the esophageal wall muscles in the upper third and the lower third of the esophagus?

42. What is the difference between the visceral and parietal peritoneum?

43. What is the difference between the gastric antrum and fundus?

44. What is the difference between a micelle and a chylomicron?

MATCH THE ENZYMES

Match the enzyme on the right with its description on the left.

_____	45. Pancreatic enzyme that digests proteins	A. Lipase
_____	46. Gastric enzyme that digests proteins	B. Amylase
_____	47. Salivary enzyme that digests carbohydrates	C. Maltase
_____	48. Pancreatic enzyme that digests carbohydrates	D. Ptyalin
_____	49. Intestinal enzyme that digests disaccharides	E. Trypsin
_____	50. Pancreatic enzyme that digests fats	F. Pepsin

COMPLETE THE SENTENCES

Write one word in each blank to complete these sentences.

51. Branches of the _____ artery provide most of the blood to the stomach; the _____ _____ artery provides most of the blood to the small intestine.

52. The three segments of the small intestine, in order, are _____, _____, and _____.

53. The center of every villus has a lymphatic capillary that is known as a _____ that is important for absorption of _____ molecules.

54. In the intestines, _____ occurs in the crypts, and _____ occurs at the tops of the villi.

Copyright © 2024 by Elsevier, Inc. All Rights Reserved.

55. The _____ sphincter marks the junction between the stomach and duodenum; the sphincter of _____ marks the junction between the bile duct and the duodenum.

56. Hepcidin is synthesized by the _____ and prevents enterocytes from taking up _____.

57. The _____ valve marks the junction between the terminal ileum and the large intestine; this valve normally is _____ to prevent the retrograde flow of intestinal contents.

58. The four parts of the colon, in order, are the ascending colon, _____ colon, _____ colon, and _____ colon.

59. The internal anal sphincter contains _____ muscle; the external anal sphincter contains _____ muscle.

60. The _____ ligament is the remnant of the umbilical vein; the _____ ligament separates the right and left lobes of the liver and attaches the liver to the anterior _____ wall.

61. Hepatocytes synthesize the primary bile acids from _____; the body recycles bile acids through the process of _____ circulation.

62. The enzyme _____ activates trypsinogen in the duodenum.

63. The layers of the stomach and intestinal walls, in order beginning at the lumen, are the mucosa, _____, _____, and serosa.

64. The _____ nervous system lies within the gastrointestinal tract and consists of neurons of the submucosal plexus, the _____ plexus, and the subserosal plexus.

TEACH PEOPLE ABOUT PATHOPHYSIOLOGY

Write your response to each situation in the space provided.

65. Mr. Hazzard learned that ibuprofen, his favorite analgesic, decreases the mucus in the stomach. He asks, "Why should I care about mucus in the stomach?"

66. Frank, age 17, is learning about digestion. He asks, "Why doesn't the pepsin from the stomach digest the protein in the walls of the small intestine?"

67. Mrs. Easton, a retired chemist, has a prescription for iron supplements because she has iron-deficiency anemia. She asks, "Why did the physician assistant tell me to take vitamin C when I take my iron pill?"

Chapter **40** **Structure and Function of the Digestive System**   Copyright © 2024 by Elsevier, Inc. All Rights Reserved.

68. Mrs. Hamilton's son has appendicitis. "I know the appendix is in the belly," she says, "but where is it attached?"

69. Mrs. Lee says, "My nurse practitioner told me to go sit on the toilet right after eating to take advantage of the gastro-colic reflex. What is that?"

70. Mr. Thomas, a butcher, says, "Every time I see a gallbladder, I wonder if bile has any good purpose? Can you tell me?"

Copyright © 2024 by Elsevier, Inc. All Rights Reserved.

Use the clues to complete the puzzle, demonstrating your knowledge of important technical terms.

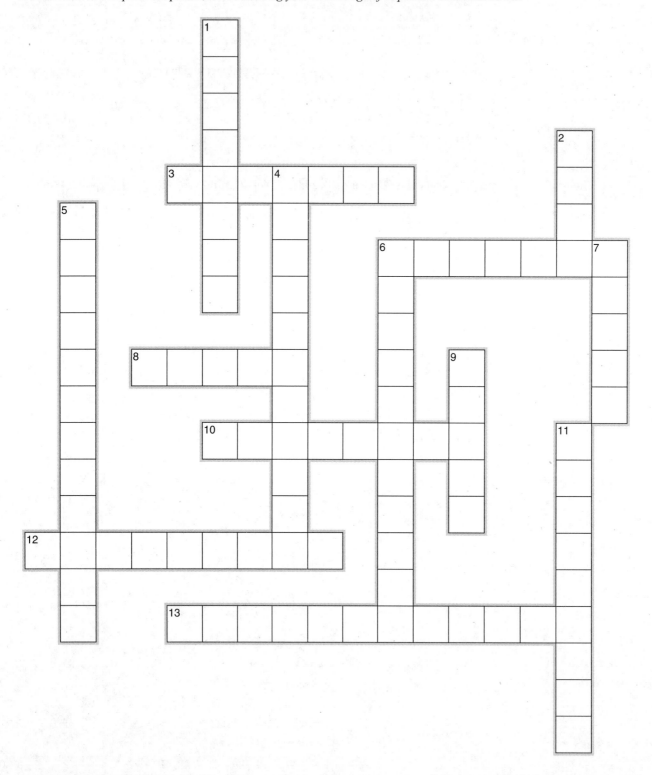

Copyright © 2024 by Elsevier, Inc. All Rights Reserved.

Across

3. Substance secreted by gastric G cells
6. Valve between the stomach and duodenum
8. Gastric cells that secrete pepsinogen
10. Gastric cells that secrete hydrochloric acid
12. Substance secreted by gastric enterochromaffin-like cells
13. Substance secreted by gastric D cells

Down

1. Phase of gastric acid secretion involving anticipation and swallowing
2. Sphincter through which bile enters the intestine
4. An iron-binding protein
5. Localized rhythmic contractions of intestinal circular smooth muscles that are not peristalsis
6. Waves of sequential relaxations and contractions of the gastrointestinal muscles
7. Partially digested food in the stomach and intestine
9. The functional units of the intestine
11. Factor necessary for the intestinal absorption of vitamin B_{12}

Copyright © 2024 by Elsevier, Inc. All Rights Reserved.

Chapter **40 Structure and Function of the Digestive System**

Alterations of Digestive Function

MATCH THE DEFINITIONS

Match the word on the right with its definition on the left.

_____ 1. Difficulty swallowing

_____ 2. Accumulation of fluid in the peritoneal cavity

_____ 3. Loss of appetite

_____ 4. Vomiting of blood

_____ 5. Dark, tarry stools

_____ 6. Frank bleeding from the rectum

_____ 7. Formation of gallstones

_____ 8. Physical wasting with weight loss, muscle atrophy, fatigue, and weakness

_____ 9. The muscular event of vomiting without the expulsion of vomitus

_____ 10. Distended, tortuous, collateral veins

A. Melena

B. Anorexia

C. Cholelithiasis

D. Dysphagia

E. Retching

F. Ascites

G. Cachexia

H. Hematochezia

I. Varices

J. Hematemesis

CIRCLE THE CORRECT WORDS

Circle the correct word from the choices provided to complete these sentences.

11. People who have GERD have (increased, decreased) resting tone of the (upper, lower) esophageal sphincter; the symptoms include heartburn and chronic (constipation, cough).

12. The most common type of hiatal hernia is (paraesophageal, sliding); this type (is, is not) associated with gastroesophageal reflux.

13. Acute obstruction high in the small intestine causes (vomiting, constipation) first; acute obstruction low in the small intestine causes (vomiting, constipation) first.

14. With acute mesenteric arterial insufficiency, the damaged intestinal mucosa cannot produce enough mucus to protect itself from (acid, digestive enzymes); bacteria invade the (healthy, necrotic) intestinal wall, eventually causing (peritonitis, malabsorption).

15. Eosinophilic esophagitis is (an acute, a chronic) condition that involves (immune, metaplastic) cells that are different from those found with GERD.

16. Esophageal cancers associated with GERD are (squamous cell carcinomas, adenocarcinomas); esophageal cancers associated with smoking tobacco and chronic alcohol consumption are (squamous cell carcinomas, adenocarcinomas).

Copyright © 2024 by Elsevier, Inc. All Rights Reserved.

17. Cirrhosis and hepatitis can cause (posthepatic, intrahepatic) portal hypertension; severe right heart failure can cause (posthepatic, intrahepatic) portal hypertension.

18. The most accepted theory of ascites formation involves the combination of portal (vasodilation, hypertension) and splanchnic (vasodilation, hypertension); ascites can be complicated by (bacterial, viral) peritonitis.

19. The (blue, yellow) tint of jaundice usually appears first in the (skin, sclera of the eye).

CATEGORIZE THE CLINICAL MANIFESTATIONS

Write the major cause beside each clinical manifestation of cirrhosis. Choices: portal hypertension, hepatocyte dysfunction.

_____ 20. Esophageal varices

_____ 21. Jaundice

_____ 22. Hepatic encephalopathy

_____ 23. Hemorrhoids

_____ 24. Splenomegaly

_____ 25. Caput medusae

_____ 26. Hypoalbuminemia

ORDER THE STEPS

Sequence the events that occur with an acute obstruction of the small intestine.

27. Write the letters here in the correct order of the steps: _____
    A. Decreased venous flow contributes to decreased arterial flow in the intestinal wall.
    B. Fluid and gas accumulate proximal to the obstruction, causing distention.
    C. Increased capillary permeability facilitates bacterial and fluid movement into peritoneal cavity.
    D. Intestinal lumen becomes obstructed acutely.
    E. Edema and ischemia of intestinal wall occur.
    F. Prolonged increase of tension in the intestinal wall collapses veins in the wall.
    G. Hypovolemia and peritonitis are likely.

CHARACTERIZE THE TYPES OF HEPATITIS

Characterize the types of hepatitis by completing this table.

Characteristic	Hepatitis A Infection	Hepatitis B Infection	Hepatitis C Infection	Hepatitis D Infection	Hepatitis E Infection
Routes of transmission					
Acute or chronic?					
Carrier state (Yes or No)					

Copyright © 2024 by Elsevier, Inc. All Rights Reserved.

DESCRIBE THE DIFFERENCES

Describe the difference between each pair of terms.

28. What is the difference between GERD and NERD?

29. What is the difference between type A and type B chronic gastritis?

30. What is the difference between maldigestion and malabsorption?

31. What is the difference between alcoholic cirrhosis and biliary cirrhosis (primary biliary cholangitis)?

MATCH THE DISORDERS

Match the disorder on the right with its description on the left.

_____ 32. Absence of an enzyme causes bloating, crampy pain, diarrhea, and flatulence after ingesting milk

_____ 33. A disorder of brain-gut interaction characterized by recurrent abdominal pain with altered bowel habits

_____ 34. Rapid gastric emptying of hypertonic chyme causes tachycardia, hypotension, pallor, diaphoresis, cramping, nausea, and diarrhea

_____ 35. Asymptomatic presence of sac-like outpouchings that are continuous with the GI tract lumen

_____ 36. Gastrin-secreting tumor causes gastric and duodenal ulcers, gastroesophageal reflux with abdominal pain, and diarrhea

_____ 37. Inflammation of sac-like outpouchings that are continuous with the GI tract lumen

_____ 38. Increased bilirubin, predominantly conjugated, in the blood due to obstruction of the common bile duct

_____ 39. Increased bilirubin, both conjugated and unconjugated, in the blood due to failure of liver cells to conjugate bilirubin and of bilirubin to pass from liver to intestine

_____ 40. Necrosis of liver cells without preexisting liver disease or cirrhosis, often due to acetaminophen overdose

A. Zollinger-Ellison syndrome

B. Lactase deficiency

C. Obstructive jaundice

D. Dumping syndrome

E. Diverticulitis

F. Diverticulosis

G. Irritable bowel syndrome

H. Acute liver failure

I. Hepatocellular jaundice

238

Copyright © 2024 by Elsevier, Inc. All Rights Reserved.

Complete the sentences

Write one word in each blank to complete these sentences.

41. Functional dysphagia caused by loss of esophageal innervation is called _____.

42. Protrusion of the upper part of the stomach through the diaphragm and into the thorax is called _____ _____.

43. People who have acute obstruction high in the small intestine are at risk for metabolic _____, but those with prolonged obstruction or acute obstruction low in the small intestine are at risk for metabolic _____.

44. Acute gastritis often heals within a few _____, especially when injurious agents such as NSAIDs and alcohol are stopped.

45. Gastric ulcers and duodenal ulcers both are called _____ ulcers; risk factors include *H.* _____ and chronic use of NSAIDs.

46. Although pancreatic insufficiency causes poor digestion of all nutrients, maldigestion of _____ because of lack of _____ is the chief problem.

47. Diverticula involve herniation of the mucosa and submucosa through the _____ layers; the most common location where diverticula develop is the _____.

48. Pain from appendicitis typically moves from the epigastric or _____ region to the _____ _____ quadrant.

49. Hepatitis _____ virus depends on hepatitis B virus in order to replicate.

50. Jaundice in viral hepatitis occurs during the _____ phase; when jaundice resolves, the _____ phase begins.

51. Cholecystitis occurs when a gallstone lodges in the _____ duct; the most common type of gallstone is made of _____.

52. An important diagnostic marker for acute pancreatitis is elevated serum _____ or amylase; chronic pancreatitis most commonly is associated with chronic _____ abuse, but does have other risk factors.

53. Fatty liver is associated with chronic use of _____ or with _____ and metabolic syndrome; although fatty liver is asymptomatic, persons who have it may develop steatohepatitis and may progress to _____, liver failure, or liver cancer.

Copyright © 2024 by Elsevier, Inc. All Rights Reserved.

COMPLETE THE CHART

Compare and contrast Crohn's disease and ulcerative colitis by completing this table.

Characteristics	Crohn's Disease	Ulcerative Colitis
Family history		
Location of lesions		
Nature of lesions		
Fistulas and abscesses		
Narrowed lumen, possible obstruction		
Recurrent episodes of diarrhea		
Blood in stools		
Clinical course		

MATCH THE RISK FACTORS

Match the cancer on the right with its risk factor(s) on the left.

_____ 54. Familial adenomatous polyposis   A. Esophageal cancer

_____ 55. *H. pylori*, high salt intake, nitrates, nitrites   B. Gastric cancer

_____ 56. Cirrhosis, chronic hepatitis B or C   C. Primary liver cancer

_____ 57. Alcohol and tobacco use, reflux   D. Colon cancer

TEACH PEOPLE ABOUT PATHOPHYSIOLOGY

Write your response to each situation in the space provided.

58. A nurse asks, "What is the difference between alcoholic hepatitis and alcoholic cirrhosis?"

59. "What is Barrett esophagus?" asks Mrs. Cloude. "Is that like heartburn with GERD?"

60. "Why do the enzymes digest the pancreas in pancreatitis?" asks Mx. Tran. "I thought the pancreas normally makes those enzymes all the time."

Copyright © 2024 by Elsevier, Inc. All Rights Reserved.

61. "My wife is in ICU, and now she is bleeding from stress ulcers!" exclaims Mr. Wang. "She is unconscious; how can she have stress? I am the one who has stress!"

62. Mr. Higgins had a gastrectomy last year after being diagnosed with gastric cancer. Now he has developed sustained epigastric pain that worsens after eating and is not relieved by antacids. His gastroenterologist diagnosed alkaline reflux gastritis. "My doctor said that I do not have enough stomach left to make a lot of acid," says Mr. Higgins. "What damaged my stomach remnant?"

63. Mr. Jetson has cirrhosis with severe hepatic encephalopathy. His partner says, "I know that his liver is not working well, but how does that cause him to be so drowsy and confused?"

64. A nurse says, "All of our cirrhosis patients have low albumin. How does cirrhosis cause hypoalbuminemia?"

CLINICAL SCENARIOS

Read the clinical scenarios and answer the questions to explore your understanding of some gastrointestinal disorders.

Mary Hawk, age 28, has had episodes of diarrhea and cramping abdominal pain for several months. Recently, she developed bloody stools, fatigue, and weight loss.

Family History

- Ms. Hawk's mother had ulcerative colitis and colon cancer.

Physical Examination

- Vital signs, cardiac, and neurologic examinations normal

- Bowel sounds normal, abdomen flat with mild diffuse tenderness but no rebound tenderness

Laboratory and Diagnostic Tests

- Stool on glove after rectal examination is positive for occult blood

- Complete blood count showed decreased hemoglobin and hematocrit

- Stool sample negative for *C. difficile* toxin, positive for fecal white blood cells

- Colonoscopy reveals inflammation and multiple small bleeding ulcers throughout the rectum and sigmoid colon; biopsy confirmed the lesions to be ulcerative colitis

Copyright © 2024 by Elsevier, Inc. All Rights Reserved.

Ms. Hawk's diagnoses are ulcerative colitis and mild anemia.

65. *Complete the sentence by choosing from the lists of options.*

Inflammatory bowel disease involves _____(1)_____ and abnormal _____(2)_____ reactions to intestinal _____(3)_____

Options for 1	Options for 2	Options for 3
chronic substance abuse	eosinophil	nutrients
genetic predisposition	B-cell	microbiota
NSAID use	T-cell	

66. Why did the nurse practitioner test for rebound tenderness when he examined Ms. Hawk's abdomen?

67. Why is it important to monitor Ms. Hawk's red cell count?

68. Why did the nurse practitioner order a colonoscopy before making the diagnosis?

69. Why was it important to ask Ms. Hawk about her family history of bowel disorders?

70. Why is it important for Ms. Hawk to have periodic colonoscopies to monitor for development of colon cancer?

71. Why should a nurse teach Ms. Hawk to increase her intake of fluid and salt during active episodes of ulcerative colitis?

 Copyright © 2024 by Elsevier, Inc. All Rights Reserved.

Mr. Blue was in the midst of a divorce and living alone in his home. For several years, he had consumed four beers every evening. One Saturday morning, Mr. Blue started drinking and finished almost two cases of beer by Sunday evening, when he fell asleep in front of the television. He awoke Monday morning with nausea and vomiting. Although he had vomited occasionally after drinking in the past, this time was different. He felt such severe pain in his upper abdomen that he was bent over and could not stand upright. Medicating himself with the last swallows of beer that were left in his bottle did not help.

Fortunately for Mr. Blue, his neighbor came over to return a hedge trimmer and discovered Mr. Blue lying on the floor and moaning. The neighbor called an ambulance that took Mr. Blue to the hospital.

Complete the following sentences by choosing from the lists of options.

72. Mr. Blue's situation is consistent with a diagnosis of _____(1)_____ which in his case, probably arose from _____(2)_____ causing cellular changes that activated _____(3)_____ in the organ that synthesizes it, leading to autodigestion and inflammation.

Options for 1	Options for 2	Options for 3
acute pancreatitis	beer	HMG Co-A reductase
acute appendicitis	ethanol metabolites	glucagon
cirrhosis	bacteria	trypsin

73. In the emergency department, laboratory results showed that serum _____(1)_____ and _____(2)_____ were elevated, which is characteristic of this condition.

Options for 1	Options for 2
magnesium	amylase
lipase	cholesterol
troponin	alkaline phosphatase

74. Mr. Blue now has high risk of developing _____(1)_____, which can cause _____(2)_____.

Options for 1	Options for 2
Hyperkalemia	Tetany
Hypocalcemia	Respiratory acidosis
Hyperventilation	Constipation

75. In addition to signs and symptoms and complications of his painful condition, Mr. Blue should be monitored during the first few days of his hospitalization for what other condition?

Copyright © 2024 by Elsevier, Inc. All Rights Reserved.

42 Alterations of Digestive Function in Children

MATCH THE DEFINITIONS

Match the word on the right with its definition on the left.

_____ 1. Chronic scarring of the liver in response to inflammation and tissue damage   A. Atresia

_____ 2. Abnormal narrowing of an opening or lumen   B. Volvulus

_____ 3. Absence of a normal body opening or passageway   C. Stenosis

_____ 4. Twisting of loops of intestine on themselves, which obstructs the lumen   D. Cirrhosis

CIRCLE THE CORRECT WORDS

Circle the correct word from the choices provided to complete these sentences.

5. Neonates who have a congenital anomaly should be examined for the presence of (infection, other anomalies).

6. Children who have cleft palate may have difficulty (feeding, crying) and should be evaluated for loss of (hearing, smell).

7. In children, chronic hepatitis most often occurs from hepatitis viruses (B and C, A and C); childhood chronic hepatitis often has (no, severe) symptoms.

8. In intestinal malrotation, (a congenital, an acquired) condition, the cecum and initial portion of the colon reside in the upper (right, left) quadrant of the abdomen, and (intussusception, volvulus) can lead to clinical manifestations of acute bowel obstruction.

9. Stenosis of a segment of bowel causes (collapse, dilation) of the lumen proximal to the obstruction and (collapse, dilation) distal to it.

10. A child who has a low weight/height ratio (over time, at 12 months) is likely to have (malnutrition, faltering growth), previously known as failure to thrive.

11. A neonate who has meconium ileus should be evaluated for (cystic fibrosis, necrotizing enterocolitis).

12. Rotavirus is a leading cause of (acute infectious diarrhea, necrotizing enterocolitis) in infants and young children.

CATEGORIZE THE CONDITIONS

Write the type of condition beside each name. Choices: congenital, acquired.

_____ 13. Imperforate anus

_____ 14. Esophageal atresia

_____ 15. Hepatitis A

_____ 16. Cleft lip

Copyright © 2024 by Elsevier, Inc. All Rights Reserved.

_____ 17. Tracheoesophageal fistula

_____ 18. Intussusception

_____ 19. Eosinophilic esophagitis

_____ 20. Hirschsprung's disease

_____ 21. Cirrhosis

_____ 22. Necrotizing enterocolitis

ORDER THE STEPS

Sequence the events that occur when intussusception occurs.

23. Write the letters here in the correct order of the steps: _____
    A. Constriction of the attached mesentery obstructs venous flow.
    B. Bowel wall becomes ischemic and necrotic.
    C. Proximal intestine telescopes into distal intestine in the direction of peristaltic flow.
    D. Capillaries become engorged, causing edema that compresses arterioles.
    E. Bowel may bleed or perforate.

EXPLAIN THE PICTURE

Examine the picture and answer the questions about it.

24. This picture shows congenital anomalies. What is the technical name of the anomaly labeled A? _____

25. Why is maternal polyhydramnios associated with this condition?

26. What is the technical name of the anomaly labeled B? _____

27. Given the anatomy of anomaly B, what mechanisms put this infant at high risk for pneumonia?

DESCRIBE THE DIFFERENCES

Describe the difference between each pair of terms.

28. What is the difference between marasmus and kwashiorkor?

Copyright © 2024 by Elsevier, Inc. All Rights Reserved.

29. What is the difference between physiologic jaundice and pathologic jaundice in infants?

MATCH THE RISK FACTORS

Match the risk factor on the right with the condition on the left.

_____ 30. Cleft lip

_____ 31. Distal intestinal obstruction syndrome

_____ 32. Esophageal atresia

_____ 33. Hepatitis A infection

A. Cystic fibrosis

B. Daycare personnel who do not practice good hand hygiene

C. Maternal vitamin B deficiency

D. Maternal exposure to methimazole for hyperthyroidism

COMPLETE THE SENTENCES

Write one word in each blank to complete these sentences.

34. Cleft lip arises from processes that begin during the fourth _____ of gestation.

35. Wilson's disease is an autosomal-_____ defect of _____ accumulation in the _____, that also damages the brain, eyes, and kidneys.

36. In biliary atresia, some of the extrahepatic _____ ducts are absent or obstructed, which leads to development of portal _____ and cirrhosis.

37. Gluten-sensitive enteropathy, also called _____ disease or _____ _____, is an autoimmune disease in which autoreactive _____ lymphocytes mediate damage to the intestinal _____.

38. In kwashiorkor, generalized edema occurs because of decreased plasma _____; the liver accumulates _____ because of lack of amino acids to make lipoproteins.

39. Children who have marasmus do not have the subcutaneous _____ seen with kwashiorkor, and they have muscle wasting but not _____.

40. Brain damage caused by high bilirubin levels is known as _____.

41. The immature mucosal barrier of a premature infant's gastrointestinal tract is an important factor in the development of _____ _____, which can lead to abdominal distention, _____ perforation, sepsis, and _____.

   Copyright © 2024 by Elsevier, Inc. All Rights Reserved.

42. Many infants who have gastroesophageal reflux outgrow the condition by age _____ months.

43. Cystic fibrosis is characterized by deficiency of _____ enzymes, thick respiratory _____, and increased sodium and chloride in _____.

MATCH THE SIGNS AND SYMPTOMS

Match the condition on the right with its typical signs and symptoms on the left.

_____ 44. Chronic constipation, poor weight gain, and progressive abdominal distention; may develop small volume diarrhea

_____ 45. Infant who previously has fed well and gained weight develops repeated projectile vomiting and wants to eat again soon after each vomiting episode

_____ 46. Enlarged spleen, bloody emesis or melena, and ascites

_____ 47. Abdominal pain, bloating, flatulence, and diarrhea after drinking milk

_____ 48. Jaundice, enlarged liver, clay-colored feces, failure to gain weight

A. Portal hypertension

B. Biliary atresia

C. Hirschsprung's disease

D. Pyloric stenosis

E. Lactose intolerance

TEACH PEOPLE ABOUT PATHOPHYSIOLOGY

Write your response to each situation in the space provided.

49. The Herrera's neonate has meconium ileus and is receiving a therapeutic enema. Mr. Herrera asks, "Why does he have meconium rather than a real bowel movement? And why is his meconium so thick?"

50. Travis, age 13 months, had painless rectal bleeding and was diagnosed with Meckel diverticulum. "Why would a little pouch on the intestine bleed?" asks his mother. "And why was that doctor talking about an ulcer?"

51. Diego has been diagnosed with Hirschsprung's disease. "I understand that 'megacolon' means big bowel," says his mother. "But what does that other word, 'aganglionic,' mean?"

52. Diego's mother has another question about Hirschsprung's disease. "But if the bowel contents do not move because the bowel is not contracting, why did Diego have a bit of diarrhea?"

Copyright © 2024 by Elsevier, Inc. All Rights Reserved.

53. Nina has gluten-sensitive enteropathy. "I understand that we need to avoid gluten in her diet," says her mother, "but I do not understand why Nina did not grow like she should have. A nurse said there was 'flattening of villi' in her intestine, but what does that really mean?"

54. Nina's mother has another question about gluten-sensitive enteropathy. "Did the lack of nutrients in her body also cause that diarrhea that Nina had?"

Copyright © 2024 by Elsevier, Inc. All Rights Reserved.

43 Structure and Function of the Musculoskeletal System

MATCH THE DEFINITIONS

Match each word on the right with its definition on the left.

_____ 1. The narrow tubular portion of a long bone

_____ 2. The broad end of a tubular bone

_____ 3. Substance that gives synovial fluid its viscous quality

_____ 4. Muscle protein that stores oxygen

_____ 5. Connective tissue that attaches muscle to bone

_____ 6. Connective tissue that attaches bone to another bone

A. Hyaluronate

B. Myoglobin

C. Ligament

D. Tendon

E. Epiphysis

F. Diaphysis

MATCH THE CELL FUNCTIONS

Match each cell on the right with its function on the left.

_____ 7. Secrete hyaluronate into joint fluid

_____ 8. Can differentiate into multiple cell types, including chondrocytes and osteoblasts

_____ 9. Help maintain bone by signaling osteoblasts and osteoclasts

_____ 10. Repair or regenerate skeletal muscle

_____ 11. Secrete collagen and other components of cartilage

_____ 12. Lay down a new bone

_____ 13. Resorb bone

A. Osteoclasts

B. Chondrocytes

C. Osteoblasts

D. Mesenchymal stem cells

E. Type B synovial cells

F. Osteocytes

G. Satellite cells

CIRCLE THE CORRECT WORDS

Circle the correct word from the choices provided to complete these sentences.

14. Spongy bone is also called (compact, cancellous) bone.

15. The small channels that connect the osteocytes in bone are called (lacunae, canaliculi); the spaces in which the osteocytes reside in bone are called (lacunae, canaliculi).

249

Copyright © 2024 by Elsevier, Inc. All Rights Reserved.

16. In utero, most bones are formed by the process of (intramembranous bone formation, endochondral ossification), which (does, does not) require a cartilage framework.

17. Articular cartilage has (numerous, no) nerves and therefore (will, does not) generate pain when injured.

18. In utero, (myotubes, myoblasts) fuse with each other to become (myotubes, myoblasts), which eventually develop into muscle fibers.

19. In muscle, the greater the innervation ratio of a particular organ, the greater its (speed of contraction, endurance); higher innervation ratios (prevent fatigue, provide precision of movement), and lower innervation ratios (prevent fatigue, provide precision of movement).

20. Ryanodine receptors are located in skeletal muscle (sarcoplasmic reticulum membranes, sarcomere H bands) and are (potassium, calcium) ion channels.

21. A muscle contracts more forcefully by (causing each motor unit to contract more forcefully, recruiting more motor units).

22. With a dynamic contraction, the muscle maintains a constant (length, tension) as it contracts; with an isometric contraction, the muscle maintains a constant (length, tension) as (length, tension) increases.

CATEGORIZE THE SUBSTANCES

For each substance, write its effect on bone resorption beside its name. Choices: inhibits, facilitates.

_____ 23. Osteoprotegerin (OPG)

_____ 24. Prostaglandin E_2 (PGE_2)

_____ 25. RANKL

_____ 26. Interleukin-6 (IL-6)

_____ 27. Estrogen

_____ 28. Tumor necrosis factor-a (TNF-α)

ORDER THE STEPS

Sequence the events that occur in bone remodeling.

29. Write the letters here in the correct order of the steps: _____
    A. Osteoclasts receive stimulus to begin resorption.
    B. Osteoblasts lay down layers of bone.
    C. Osteoclasts secrete hydrochloric acid and cathepsin K to create resorption cavity.

Sequence the events that occur in bone healing after a fracture.

30. Write the letters here in the correct order of the steps: _____
    A. Osteoblasts form woven bone (callus).
    B. Fibroblasts, capillary buds, and osteoblasts move into the wound; granulation tissue (procallus) and cartilage are formed.
    C. Callus is replaced with a stronger bone.
    D. Bone is reshaped through remodeling.
    E. Hematoma forms.

Copyright © 2024 by Elsevier, Inc. All Rights Reserved.

Sequence the events that occur in muscle contraction and then relaxation.

31. Write the letters here in the correct order of the steps: _____
    A. Ryanodine receptors open, and calcium ions flow into the cytoplasm.
    B. Myosin hydrolyzes ATP, and actin–myosin cross-bridges form, causing actin filaments to slide toward myosin filaments, thus shortening the sarcomere.
    C. Muscle fiber action potential spreads along the sarcolemma.
    D. An active transport process moves calcium back into the sarcoplasmic reticulum.
    E. Action potential in motor nerve reaches the neuromuscular junction.
    F. Troponin moves back to its previous position, which closes the active sites on actin.
    G. Calcium ions bind to troponin, causing a structural change that opens active sites on actin filaments.
    H. Cross-bridging stops, sarcomeres lengthen.

EXPLAIN THE PICTURES

Examine the pictures and answer the questions about them.

32. The item marked A is _____ cartilage; the major type of collagen it contains

    is _____.

33. The item marked B is _____ bone; what substance does its spaces contain?

    _____

34. The item marked C is the _____ cavity; what substance does it contain?

    _____

35. The item marked D is _____ bone; another name for this type of bone is

    _____ bone because it surrounds the other type of bone.

36. The item marked E is the _____; it is made of what type of tissue?

    _____

37. The narrow shaft of a long bone, part of which is marked by letter F in the picture,

    is called the _____.

38. Which two letters mark locations where osteocytes are found? _____

39. Which letter marks a location where trabeculae are found? _____

40. Which letter marks a location where haversian canals are found? _____

Copyright © 2024 by Elsevier, Inc. All Rights Reserved.

41. Which band in the picture of the striated muscle fiber contains actin?

_____

42. Which band contains myosin? _____

43. Which band will shorten the most when this muscle fiber contracts?

_____

|—— A band ——| |—— Titin ——|

|‾H band‾| |——I band——| Z disk   M line

RELAXED STRIATED MUSCLE FIBER

DESCRIBE THE DIFFERENCES

Describe the difference between each pair of terms.

44. What is the difference between compact bone and cancellous bone?

45. What is the difference between a diarthrosis, a synarthrosis, and an amphiarthrosis?

46. What is the difference between osteoid and bone?

47. What is the difference between a synovial joint and a symphysis?

COMPLETE THE SENTENCES

Write one word in each blank to complete these sentences.

48. Members of the transforming growth factor-β (TGF-β) family are known as _____ _____ proteins because they play important roles in initiation, differentiation, and commitment of precursor cells into

_____.

   Copyright © 2024 by Elsevier, Inc. All Rights Reserved.

49. Articular cartilage is an organized system of _____ fibers and proteoglycans; the _____ act as a pump that controls the amount of fluid in the cartilage during and after weight bearing.

50. The bone directly underneath articular cartilage is called _____ bone; the calcified layer of cartilage that attaches to it is called the _____.

51. The connective tissue framework that surrounds a skeletal muscle is called the _____.

52. The most important proteins in the sarcomeres are actin and _____.

53. An anterior horn neuron, its axon, and the muscle fibers innervated by it are called a _____ _____.

54. The description of muscle contraction is called the _____ theory.

55. Oxygen _____ is the amount of oxygen needed to convert the buildup of _____ acid to glucose and replenish ATP and phosphocreatine stores.

56. Dual-photon absorptiometry (DXA) is a way to measure bone _____ and risk for _____.

57. Loss of skeletal muscle mass with increasing age is known as _____; aging muscle loses more type _____ muscle fibers than type _____ fibers.

COMPARE AND CONTRAST THE MUSCLE FIBERS

Compare and contrast type I and type II muscle fibers by completing this chart.

Characteristic	Type I Fibers	Type II Fibers
Speed of Contraction		
Intensity of Contraction		
Type of Metabolism		
Number of Mitochondria		
Amount of Myoglobin		
Color		
Capillary Supply		

TEACH PEOPLE ABOUT PATHOPHYSIOLOGY

Write your response to each situation in the space provided.

58. A nursing student says, "I know about osteoclasts and osteoblasts, but what are osteocytes?"

Copyright © 2024 by Elsevier, Inc. All Rights Reserved.

Chapter **43 Structure and Function of the Musculoskeletal System**

59. Jamal, a 22-year-old soccer player, asks, "If my knee cartilage has no blood supply, how does it get its nourishment?"

60. Ms. Jackson, age 37, asks, "What is the difference between striated muscle and skeletal muscle?"

61. A beginning physical therapy student says, "I was so busy memorizing the names of the little tubules that I lost the big picture. Why do muscle fibers need a sarcotubular system?"

62. Mr. Taylor says, "At the gym I hear people talk about building lean body mass. What exactly does that mean?"

63. "A lot of athletes I know are taking creatine supplements for their muscles," says Mr. Young. "What do muscles do with creatine?"

    Copyright © 2024 by Elsevier, Inc. All Rights Reserved.

Alterations of Musculoskeletal Function

MATCH THE DEFINITIONS

Match the word on the right with its definition on the left.

_____ 1. A break in the continuity of a bone

_____ 2. Failure of fractured bone ends to grow together

_____ 3. Inflammation of a tendon where it attaches to a bone

_____ 4. Inflammation in small fluid-filled sacs located between tendons, muscles, and bony prominences

_____ 5. Band of connective tissue that attaches skeletal muscle to bone

_____ 6. Band of connective tissue that connects two bones

A. Bursitis

B. Fracture

C. Tendon

D. Ligament

E. Nonunion

F. Epicondylitis

CIRCLE THE CORRECT WORDS

Circle the correct word from the choices provided to complete these sentences.

7. Two relatively unstable joints that dislocate fairly easily are the knee and (hip, shoulder); the key symptoms of this latter dislocation are pain and inability to (bear full weight, elevate the arm).

8. A tear in a ligament is known as a (strain, sprain); a tear in a tendon is known as a (strain, sprain).

9. Bony prominences at the end of a bone where tendons or ligaments attach are called (epicondyles, bursa).

10. Tennis elbow and golfer's elbow are examples of (bursitis, epicondylopathy).

11. In young people, (tendons, muscles) are ruptured more often than (tendons, muscles), but in older adults, (tendons, muscles) are ruptured more often than (tendons, muscles).

12. Compartment syndromes occur when (venous, arterial) pressure increases, causing eventual ischemia and edema that cause (redness, pain) out of proportion to the injury.

13. Rhabdomyolysis is characterized by (skeletal muscle, chest) pain, weakness, (bloody, dark) urine, and increased serum (creatine kinase, alkaline phosphatase); a main treatment goal is to prevent damage to the (liver, kidneys).

14. The most common microorganisms that cause osteomyelitis are (fungi, bacteria); an area of dead bone that is separated from the viable bone in osteomyelitis is called (involucrum, sequestrum).

15. In ankylosing spondylitis, the primary pathologic problem is uncontrolled bone (destruction, formation) rather than bone (destruction, formation).

16. People who have McArdle disease are unable to (synthesize, break down) glycogen; people who have acid maltase deficiency accumulate glycogen in their (mitochondria, lysosomes).

17. The most common cause of toxic myopathy is (alcohol, autoimmunity).

Copyright © 2024 by Elsevier, Inc. All Rights Reserved.

CATEGORIZE THE CHARACTERISTICS

Write the type of arthropathy beside each characteristic. Choices: osteoarthritis, rheumatoid arthritis.

_____ 18. Subchondral bone sclerosis

_____ 19. Antibodies against citrullinated proteins

_____ 20. Severe joint deformities

_____ 21. Osteophyte formation

_____ 22. Nodule formation in soft tissue

_____ 23. Pannus

_____ 24. Autoimmune disease

_____ 25. Loss of articular cartilage

_____ 26. Joint pain relieved by rest

_____ 27. Joint stiffness for first hour after awakening

ORDER THE STEPS

Sequence the events that occur when a broken bone heals.

28. Write the letters here in the correct order of the steps: _____
    A. Bone is remodeled over time.
    B. Hematoma forms beneath the periosteum around the broken area.
    C. Unnecessary callus is resorbed and trabeculae form.
    D. Osteoblasts in procallus synthesize collagen and matrix, which become mineralized into callus.
    E. Necrotic tissue stimulates an inflammatory response.
    F. Vascular tissue invades the fracture area, creating granulation tissue.
    G. Bone-forming cells become activated and produce procallus beneath the periosteum.
    H. Leukocytes release cytokines and other factors that promote healing.

EXPLAIN THE PICTURES

Examine the pictures and answer the questions about them.

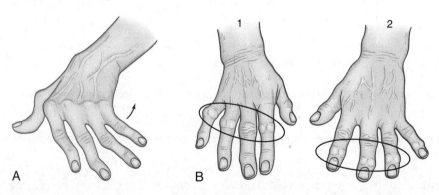

29. What two-word technical term describes the finger deformities in picture A? _____

30. What disease process causes hands to look like picture A? _____

Copyright © 2024 by Elsevier, Inc. All Rights Reserved.

31. In addition to the joint deformities, picture A shows muscle wasting. What caused it?

32. What causes the joint swelling in this condition?

33. Why does this condition have systemic manifestations as well as joint ones?

34. What disease process causes hands to look like picture B? _____

35. The nodes that are circled in hand number 1 are called _____ nodes.

36. The nodes that are circled in hand number 2 are called _____ nodes.

37. What causes these nodes?

38. What is the role of matrix metalloproteinases in this disease process?

MATCH THE FRACTURES

Match each type of fracture with its description on the left.

_____ 39. Fracture with intact skin overlying the bone	A. Linear
_____ 40. Break on only one cortex of bone with splintering of inner bone surface	B. Spiral
_____ 41. Fracture line parallel to long axis of bone	C. Transverse
_____ 42. Fracture with communicating wound between bone and skin	D. Closed
_____ 43. Fracture where bone is weakened by disease	E. Open
_____ 44. Fracture line at an angle (but not perpendicular) to long axis of bone	F. Greenstick
_____ 45. Fragment of bone connected to a ligament or tendon breaks off from the main bone	G. Impacted
_____ 46. Fracture with one, both, or all fragments out of normal alignment	H. Comminuted
_____ 47. Fracture with multiple bone fragments	I. Oblique
_____ 48. Fracture line encircles bone while ascending	J. Displaced
_____ 49. Fracture fragments are pushed into each other	K. Avulsion
_____ 50. Fracture line perpendicular to long axis of bone	L. Pathologic

Copyright © 2024 by Elsevier, Inc. All Rights Reserved.

DESCRIBE THE DIFFERENCES

Describe the difference between each pair of terms.

51. What is the difference between delayed union and malunion?

52. What is the difference between dislocation and subluxation?

53. What is the difference between tendinitis and tendinosis?

54. What is the difference between rhabdomyolysis and myoglobinuria?

MATCH THE PATHOPHYSIOLOGIES

Match the disease on the right with its pathophysiologies on the left.

_____ 55. Increased metabolic activity in bone causing abnormal and excessive bone remodeling that enlarges and softens bones

_____ 56. Syndrome involving high levels of uric acid in body fluids, precipitation of urate crystals, and recurrent monoarticular arthritis

_____ 57. Inflammation and symmetrical weakness of muscles, often in pelvic and shoulder girdles

_____ 58. A metabolic disease of adults characterized by inadequate and delayed mineralization of osteoid in mature bone

_____ 59. Chronic inflammatory joint disease characterized by stiffening and fusion of the spine and sacroiliac joints

_____ 60. Chronic musculoskeletal syndrome characterized by widespread chronic pain, fatigue, and non-restorative sleep

A. Osteomalacia

B. Ankylosing spondylitis

C. Fibromyalgia

D. Paget disease

E. Polymyositis

F. Gout

COMPLETE THE SENTENCES

Write one word in each blank to complete these sentences.

61. Realigning the fragments of a broken bone is called _____; subsequent surgical placement of screws, plates, or other devices to immobilize the site is called internal _____.

Copyright © 2024 by Elsevier, Inc. All Rights Reserved.

62. The term _____ _____ denotes abnormal bone formation in soft tissue that occurs after localized muscle injury.

63. Inadequate or delayed mineralization of osteoid in children, often due to vitamin _____ deficiency, is known as _____.

64. In Paget disease, thickening of the _____ can compress the _____ or cranial nerves.

65. Primary bone cancer is rare, but _____ cancer often affects bone; the most common primary bone cancer in young adults is _____.

66. Classification of bone tumors is based on the cell type and the type of _____ _____ synthesized by the tumor cells.

67. In gout, accumulation of urate crystals in subcutaneous tissue causes formation of white nodules known as _____.

68. Failure of a muscle to generate force is called _____; failure of a muscle to sustain force is called _____.

69. Abnormal muscle shortening is called a _____.

70. Tension headaches are due in part to a feedback cycle with the reticular activating system and muscle _____.

71. Chronic fatigue syndrome, preferably known as _____ encephalomyelitis, is characterized by unexplained persistent _____ fatigue and unrestful sleep.

72. Prolonged inactivity from bed rest or a cast causes _____ atrophy.

73. Myotonic channelopathies are characterized by delayed muscle _____, whereas an episode of periodic paralysis is characterized by inability to initiate muscle _____.

MATCH THE TUMOR CHARACTERISTICS

Match the tumor type on the right with its characteristic(s) on the left.

_____ 74. Cartilage-forming malignant tumor that does not ossify and typically seeds in surrounding tissue

_____ 75. Benign solitary tumor originating from osteoclasts that is associated with pathologic fractures due to extensive bone resorption

_____ 76. Aggressive malignant bone-forming tumor that typically produces periosteal reaction

_____ 77. Malignant tumor of skeletal muscle that metastasizes rapidly

_____ 78. Collagen-forming solitary malignant tumor that may be a secondary complication of radiation therapy

A. Fibrosarcoma

B. Osteosarcoma

C. Giant cell tumor

D. Chondrosarcoma

E. Rhabdomyosarcoma

Copyright © 2024 by Elsevier, Inc. All Rights Reserved.

Write your response to each situation in the space provided.

79. "The doctor said I have a compound fracture in my leg," says Mr. Reilly. "Does that mean it is infected? I know the doctor is worried about infection."

80. Mr. Tay has osteomyelitis in his lower fibula. He asks, "How did my leg bone get infected? The only break in my skin is this oozing diabetes sore on my ankle."

81. Mr. Vargas says, "It has been 3 weeks, and I want this leg cast off now! I have to go back to work! I cannot wait another 3 weeks! My kids are hungry!"

82. "What makes these ugly lumps on my knuckles?" asks Mrs. Boult. "The doctor called them Heberden nodes, but he was busy writing prescriptions for my hip arthritis drugs, and I did not ask him."

83. Mr. Crabbe is undergoing treatment for osteosarcoma. He says, "I understand why they do scans to look at my bones, but why do they take blood to monitor bone cancer? Why not just look at the bones?"

CLINICAL SCENARIO

Read the clinical scenario and answer the questions to explore your understanding of osteoporosis.

Mrs. Lottner, age 61, visited a nurse practitioner because she was developing "bent-over posture, just like my mother." History revealed physical inactivity.

Physical Examination

- Vital signs normal except blood pressure 150/88 mmHg

- Heart and lung sounds normal

- Kyphotic posture

The nurse practitioner ordered a bone mineral density test and repeat blood pressure at a different time. Repeat blood pressure measurements confirmed the diagnosis of hypertension. DXA scan confirmed the diagnosis of postmenopausal osteoporosis.

84. What is the difference between osteopenia and osteoporosis?

85. What relationship between bone formation and bone resorption is responsible for osteoporosis?

86. Why does Mrs. Lottner have a kyphotic posture?

87. At what age did Mrs. Lottner most likely have her peak bone mass? _____

88. What happens to bone mineral density between peak mass and menopause? _____

89. Describe the pattern of change in bone mineral density after menopause.

90. How does lack of estrogen after menopause contribute to osteoporosis?

91. Why did the nurse practitioner encourage Mrs. Lottner to walk every day?

Copyright © 2024 by Elsevier, Inc. All Rights Reserved.

Use the clues to complete the puzzle, demonstrating your knowledge of important technical terms.

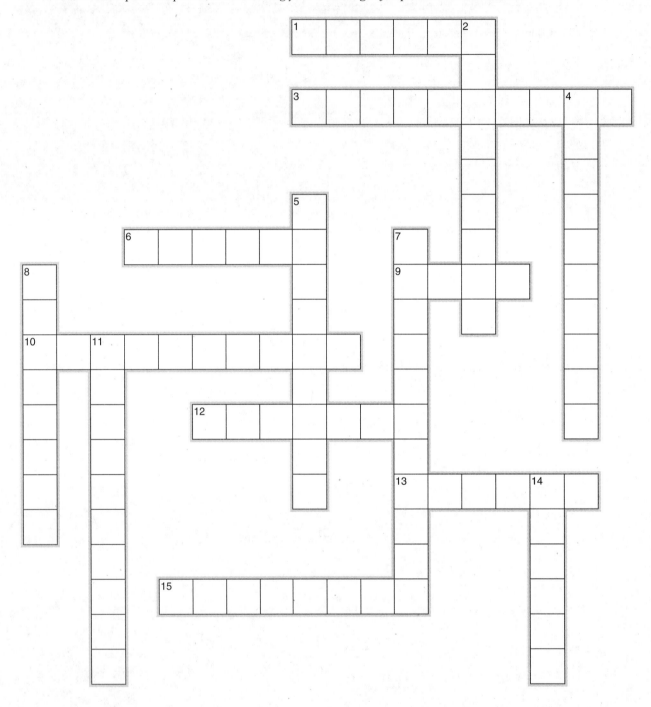

Copyright © 2024 by Elsevier, Inc. All Rights Reserved.

Across

1. Fracture with intact skin overlying the bone

3. Break on only one cortex of bone with splintering of inner bone surface

6. Fracture line parallel to long axis of bone

9. Fracture with communicating wound between bone and skin

10. Fracture where bone is weakened by disease

12. Fracture line at an angle (but not perpendicular) to long axis of bone

13. Microfracture

15. Fragment of bone connected to a ligament or tendon breaks off from the main bone

Down

2. Fracture with one, both, or all fragments out of normal alignment

4. Fracture with multiple bone fragments

5. Fracture caused by low-level trauma

7. Vertebra collapsed into a wedge shape

8. Fracture fragments are pushed into each other

11. Fracture line perpendicular to long axis of bone

14. Fracture line encircles bone while ascending

Copyright © 2024 by Elsevier, Inc. All Rights Reserved.

Chapter **44** Alterations of Musculoskeletal Function

45 Alterations of Musculoskeletal Function in Children

MATCH THE DEFINITIONS

Match the word on the right with its definition on the left.

_____ 1. Webbing of the fingers	A. Genu valgum
_____ 2. Layer of cartilage between the metaphysis and epiphysis	B. Genu varum
_____ 3. Adduction deformity of the forefoot	C. Equinovarus
_____ 4. Knock knees	D. Syndactyly
_____ 5. Bowlegs	E. Physeal plate
_____ 6. Clubfoot	F. Metatarsus adductus
_____ 7. Flatfoot	G. Scoliosis
_____ 8. Lateral curvature of the spinal column	H. Dorsiflexion
_____ 9. Bending of the foot upward and backward	I. Plantar flexion
_____ 10. Bending of the foot downward and forward	J. Pes planus

CIRCLE THE CORRECT WORDS

Circle the correct word from the choices provided to complete these sentences.

11. Bone mass peaks in the mid- to late (20s, 40s); bone remodeling (stops at, continues after) that time.

12. At birth, the facial muscles are (poorly, well) developed; pelvic muscles take (weeks, years) to develop fully.

13. Osteosarcoma commonly is located at the (midshaft, ends) of bones, whereas Ewing sarcoma commonly is located at the (midshaft, ends) of bones.

14. "Corner" metaphyseal fractures, caused by a (twisting, pulling) force, are (rarely, almost always) associated with abuse.

15. (Osteomyelitis, Septic arthritis) in children can cause permanent (bone, joint) injury because the articular cartilage of (bones, joints) is unable to repair itself after injury from infection.

16. The pathophysiology of Legg-Calvé-Perthes disease occurs at the (tibial tubercle, head of the femur).

17. The pathophysiology of Osgood–Schlatter disease occurs at the (tibial tubercle, head of the femur).

Copyright © 2024 by Elsevier, Inc. All Rights Reserved.

Examine the picture and answer the questions about it.

18. The skull, rib cage, and vertebral column in the picture are the _____ skeleton.

19. The rest of the bones in the picture are the _____ skeleton.

20. Which grows faster during childhood, the bones in question 18 or the bones in question 19? _____

21. Look the letters on the tibia.

    Location(s) of the primary ossification center(s): _____

    Technical name of this area: _____

    Location(s) of the secondary ossification center(s): _____

    Technical name of this area: _____

22. Which letter marks the location where scoliosis occurs? _____

23. In which age group does idiopathic scoliosis develop most commonly? _____

24. Which letter marks the location where Legg-Calvé-Perthes disease occurs? _____

25. What is the basic pathophysiology of Legg-Calvé-Perthes disease?

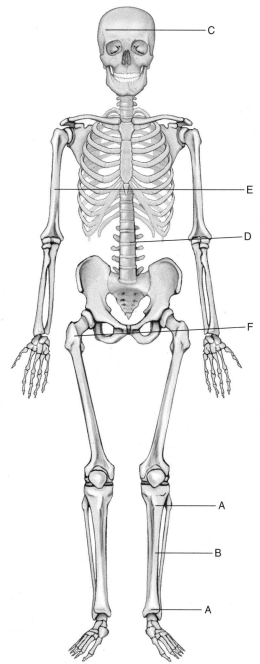

Copyright © 2024 by Elsevier, Inc. All Rights Reserved.

DESCRIBE THE DIFFERENCES

Describe the difference between each pair of terms.

26. What is the difference between intramembranous formation of bone and endochondral formation of bone?

27. What is the difference between osteosarcoma and osteochondroma?

28. What is the difference between osteomyelitis and septic arthritis?

29. What is the difference between septic arthritis and juvenile idiopathic arthritis?

COMPLETE THE SENTENCES

Write one word in each blank to complete these sentences.

30. Developmental dysplasia of the hip typically is associated with a shallow _____; if the condition is not corrected, the child likely will develop a _____ gait.

31. Infants who have _____ skin folds at the groin should be evaluated for developmental dysplasia of the hip.

32. Idiopathic scoliosis is _____ scoliosis with no known cause.

33. Rickets is caused by deficiency or lack of function of vitamin _____; it causes skeletal deformities because bones do not become _____ effectively.

34. Diseases caused by an insufficient blood supply to growing bones are called _____.

35. The two most common malignant bone tumors of childhood are osteosarcoma and _____ sarcoma; the most common presenting symptom of both cancers is _____.

36. The most common type of soft tissue sarcoma in children is _____, which arises in _____ muscle; the tumor usually is noticed by the presence of a palpable, painless _____.

Copyright © 2024 by Elsevier, Inc. All Rights Reserved.

TEACH PEOPLE ABOUT PATHOPHYSIOLOGY

Write your response to each situation in the space provided.

37. Mrs. Rivera is concerned about her son, age 20 months. "My baby is bowlegged! If I take him to a doctor, can they splint his little legs and make them straight?"

38. A nurse manager of a hospital pediatric unit learns that an 18-month-old boy with osteogenesis imperfecta is being admitted to her unit. What basic facts about osteogenesis imperfecta should the nurse manager teach her staff so that they will give safe care?

39. Alex, age 13, has just been diagnosed with Osgood–Schlatter disease. He asks, "Why did part of my tibia die? Will it grow back?"

40. A physician assistant asks, "The father said his 6-month-old baby fell off the sofa. Why did you report suspected abuse when that baby had a fractured tibia and some bruises? And why did the physician order full body radiographs?"

41. Kiley Norman, age 7 months, had impetigo and developed osteomyelitis. Now she has septic arthritis. Her nurse asks, "Why do infants get septic arthritis with osteomyelitis more commonly than older children do?"

CLINICAL SCENARIO

Read the clinical scenario and answer the questions to explore your understanding of a genetic disorder.

Tommy Lewis, age 3, was brought to a pediatrician's office by his mother, who said, "Tommy is clumsy, falls frequently, and has difficulty climbing stairs."

Physical Examination

- Vital signs normal

- Waddling gait, appears to walk on his toes

- Positive Gower's sign

- Calf muscles proportionately larger than other lower extremity muscles

Copyright © 2024 by Elsevier, Inc. All Rights Reserved.

Laboratory Results

- Serum creatine phosphokinase (CPK) level is 14 times normal

- Serum LDH, AST (SGOT), and aldolase all above normal

- Genetic testing confirmed the diagnosis

Complete the sentences by choosing from the lists of options.

42. Tommy's assessment is consistent with a diagnosis of _____(1)_____, which involves mutation of the _____(2)_____ gene.

Options for 1	Options for 2
spinal muscular atrophy	dystrophin
myotonic muscular dystrophy	DMPK or ZNF9
Duchenne muscular dystrophy	4q35 locus

43. Muscle weakness in Tommy's _____(1)_____ muscles causes his waddling gait; muscle weakness in his _____(2)_____ muscles causes him to appear to walk on his toes.

Options for 1	Options for 2
spinal	spinal
pelvic girdle	pelvic girdle
anterior tibial and peroneal	anterior tibial and peroneal

44. Why does classic Duchenne muscular dystrophy occur only in boys?

45. What is the normal function of the protein that is lacking in Tommy's condition?

46. What is the Gower's sign? Why does Tommy have this sign?

Copyright © 2024 by Elsevier, Inc. All Rights Reserved.

47. What makes his serum CPK and other enzymes elevated?

48. What caused Tommy's calf muscles to enlarge? Are they strong like hypertrophied muscles?

49. Given his diagnosis, what is the expected clinical course?

Copyright © 2024 by Elsevier, Inc. All Rights Reserved.

46 Structure, Function, and Disorders of the Integument

MATCH THE DEFINITIONS

Match the word on the right with its definition on the left.

_____ 1. Hives

_____ 2. The nail bed

_____ 3. Wart

_____ 4. Bacterial infection of a hair follicle; a boil

_____ 5. The subcutaneous layer of the skin

_____ 6. Hair loss

_____ 7. Itching

_____ 8. Diffuse bacterial infection of the dermis and subcutaneous tissue

_____ 9. Acute bacterial infection of the upper dermis

_____ 10. Excessive hair growth, especially male pattern of hair growth in women

A. Alopecia

B. Pruritus

C. Urticaria

D. Hirsutism

E. Erysipelas

F. Folliculitis

G. Hyponychium

H. Hypodermis

I. Verruca

J. Cellulitis

CIRCLE THE CORRECT WORDS

Circle the correct word from the choices provided to complete these sentences.

11. Sweat glands, sebaceous glands, and hair follicles are located in the (epidermis, dermis).

12. Blood vessels, lymphatic vessels, and nerves are located in the (epidermis, dermis).

13. Blood supply to the skin is regulated by (sympathetic, parasympathetic) nerves to (epidermal, dermal) arterioles.

14. As a person ages, the skin becomes (thinner, thicker), drier, (less, more) elastic, and wrinkled, with (fewer, more) sweat glands.

15. Irritant contact dermatitis (is, is not) mediated by T lymphocytes.

16. Pityriasis rosea may be associated with a (virus, fungus), begins as a single lesion known as a (rete peg, herald patch), and is a benign self-limited condition except during (pregnancy, old age).

17. Discoid lupus erythematosus manifests with (skin, systemic) signs and symptoms in genetically susceptible adults.

270

 Copyright © 2024 by Elsevier, Inc. All Rights Reserved.

18. Erythema multiforme produces lesions that appear target-like with alternating rings of (edema, necrosis) and (vesicles, inflammation).

19. Lyme disease is caused by a (virus, bacterium) transmitted by (flea, tick) bites.

20. Androgenic and female-pattern alopecia are similar in that they both involve hair loss in the (frontotemporal, central) area of the scalp, but androgenic alopecia also includes the (frontotemporal, central) area.

21. Frostbite is characterized by formation of (ice crystals, nodules) in the tissues and progresses from (distal to proximal, proximal to distal).

CATEGORIZE THE DISORDERS

Write the type of disorder beside each name. Choices: autoimmune, bacterial infection, viral infection, fungal infection.

_____ 22. Erysipelas

_____ 23. Tinea pedis

_____ 24. Lichen planus

_____ 25. Impetigo

_____ 26. Candidiasis

_____ 27. Alopecia areata

_____ 28. Onychomycosis

_____ 29. Pemphigus

_____ 30. Lupus erythematosus

_____ 31. Vitiligo

ORDER THE LAYERS AND NOTE THEIR FUNCTIONS

Put the layers of the epidermis in order within the table and indicate the function of each layer.

Latin Name of Epidermal Layer	Function of Epidermal Layer
Put the top layer here	

Copyright © 2024 by Elsevier, Inc. All Rights Reserved.

Examine the pictures and answer the questions about them.

Answer the two questions underneath each picture and then identify the lesions.

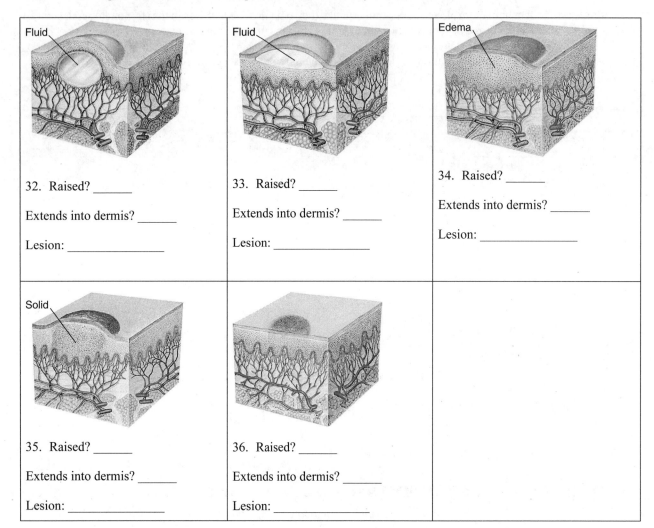

32. Raised? _____

Extends into dermis? _____

Lesion: _____

33. Raised? _____

Extends into dermis? _____

Lesion: _____

34. Raised? _____

Extends into dermis? _____

Lesion: _____

35. Raised? _____

Extends into dermis? _____

Lesion: _____

36. Raised? _____

Extends into dermis? _____

Lesion: _____

37. How would the picture of the vesicle need to change to make it depict a bulla?

38. How would the picture of the macule need to change to make it depict a patch?

39. The picture from which question number shows a lesion associated with allergic reactions? _____

40. The picture from which question number shows a lesion associated with shingles? _____

Copyright © 2024 by Elsevier, Inc. All Rights Reserved.

DESCRIBE THE DIFFERENCES

Describe the difference between each pair of terms.

41. What is the difference between a furuncle and a carbuncle?

42. What is the difference between apocrine sweat glands and eccrine sweat glands?

43. What is the difference between a hypertrophic scar and a keloid?

44. What is the difference between acne vulgaris and acne rosacea?

MATCH THE FUNCTIONS

Match the cell type on the right with its function(s) on the left.

_____ 45. Assist with sensation of touch

A. Melanocytes

_____ 46. Process and present antigens to lymphocytes

B. Fibroblasts

_____ 47. Secrete pigment that gives color to skin and protects it against ultraviolet radiation

C. Merkel cells

_____ 48. Release histamine; play roles in inflammation and in hypersensitivity reactions in the skin

D. Langerhans cells

_____ 49. Provide the barrier function of the skin

E. Mast cells

_____ 50. Secrete the connective tissue matrix and collagen

F. Keratinocytes

COMPLETE THE SENTENCES

Write one word in each blank to complete these sentences.

51. The term _____ can be used interchangeably with the term *eczema* to describe an inflammatory response in the skin involving pruritus, lesions with indistinct borders, and epidermal changes.

52. Allergic _____ dermatitis from poison ivy is caused by a type _____ hypersensitivity reaction, also called _____ hypersensitivity.

53. Dermatitis that occurs on the legs as a result of chronic venous stasis is called _____ dermatitis; dermatitis that involves scaly, yellowish, inflammatory plaques is called _____ dermatitis.

Copyright © 2024 by Elsevier, Inc. All Rights Reserved.

Chapter **46** Structure, Function, and Disorders of the Integument

54. In psoriasis, excessive proliferation of _____ causes abnormal thickened patches of the skin; rapid _____ shedding time causes the lesions to be scaly; remissions and _____ are characteristic of psoriasis.

55. In addition to concern about the appearance of their skin, people who have lichen planus are distressed by severe _____.

56. The irreversible bulbous appearance of the nose that occurs in acne rosacea is known as _____.

57. An autoimmune blistering disease known as _____ has several forms, all of which involve _____ against proteins involved in adhesion of the epidermis to the dermis.

58. Candidiasis can occur on the skin, on mucous membranes, and in the _____ _____.

59. Cold sores and genital herpes are caused by the herpes _____ virus, which has two types; although _____ usually causes the cold sores and _____ usually causes genital herpes, either type can cause lesions in either site.

60. The _____ _____ virus causes warts; some strains of this virus predispose to cervical _____.

61. Many types of skin cancer are associated with damage from _____ exposure, but _____ _____ is associated with herpesvirus type 8.

MATCH THE TUMORS

Match the tumor type on the right with the tumor name on the left.

_____ 62. Basal cell carcinoma

_____ 63. Seborrheic keratosis

_____ 64. Squamous cell carcinoma

_____ 65. Malignant melanoma

_____ 66. Nevus

_____ 67. Actinic keratosis

_____ 68. Cutaneous lymphoma

_____ 69. Keratoacanthoma

A. Benign tumor arising from cutaneous basal cells

B. Malignant tumor arising from cutaneous basal cells

C. Benign lesion formed from melanocytes

D. Malignant tumor arising from melanocytes

E. Premalignant lesion with aberrant proliferation of epidermal keratinocytes

F. Benign tumor arising from a hair follicle

G. Malignant tumor arising from the epidermis

H. Malignant tumor arising from T cells or B cells

Copyright © 2024 by Elsevier, Inc. All Rights Reserved.

TEACH PEOPLE ABOUT PATHOPHYSIOLOGY

Write your response to each situation in the space provided.

70. "The doctor said my husband has vitiligo," says Mrs. Watson. "Is that contagious?"

71. Mrs. Burkhardt says, "Now that I have a lot of gray hair, I would like to know some details of why hair gets gray as we age. Please explain."

72. "My doctor said I have psoriasis. Is that a fungal infection?" asks Mrs. Marks. "I am afraid to hug my son because I might give it to him. Is it contagious?"

73. "We are going to take care of my mother at our house when she is released from the hospital," says Mr. Turner. "A nurse told me to be sure to make sure she does not lie in one position all day to prevent pressure injury. How can lying in a bed cause pressure injury?"

74. "I heard that nurse tell the doctor I have wheals on my chest and arms, probably from the penicillin," says Mr. Tier. "They look like hives to me. What is the difference?"

75. "My aunt has scleroderma, and she does not even smile at me anymore," says Agnes Walker, age 11. "Do you think she is mad at me or just sad about having a disease?"

CLINICAL SCENARIO

Read the clinical scenario and answer the questions to explore your understanding of shingles.

Mrs. Maxwell was having financial difficulties during stressful divorce proceedings and was not sleeping well. She was trying to find a second job to support her children and was behind on her rent payments. She developed painful blisters on one side of her chest and went to a nurse practitioner.

Copyright © 2024 by Elsevier, Inc. All Rights Reserved.

Chapter **46 Structure, Function, and Disorders of the Integument**

Physical Examination

- Vital signs normal

- Reddish wheals on the left chest in dermatome distribution (see photo)

Mrs. Maxwell's diagnosis is shingles.

Complete the sentences by choosing from the lists of options.

76. The technical term for shingles is _____(1)_____;
    it is caused by _____(2)_____.

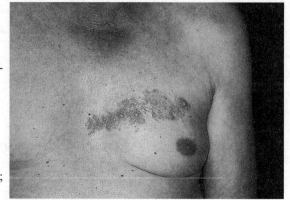

(Courtesy Department of Dermatology, School of Medicine, University of Utah.)

Options for 1	Options for 2
varicella	human herpesvirus 8
herpes zoster	HSV-1
verruca	varicella-zoster virus

77. The virus infects _____(1)_____ nerves; after the lesions disappear, _____(2)_____ might develop.

Options for 1	Options for 2
sensory	weakness or paralysis
motor	postherpetic neuralgia

78. Was this Mrs. Maxwell's first exposure to the virus? Explain your answer.

79. Why do the lesions have this distribution? Why do they not cross the midline?

80. Why might Mrs. Maxwell have developed the shingles now?

Copyright © 2024 by Elsevier, Inc. All Rights Reserved.

Alterations of the Integument in Children

MATCH THE DEFINITIONS

Match the word on the right with its definition on the left.

_____ 1. A congenital malformation of the dermal capillaries

_____ 2. Fungi that thrive on keratin

_____ 3. Benign tumor formed from rapid growth of vascular endothelial cells that causes formation of extra blood vessels

_____ 4. Fungal infections

A. Dermatophytes

B. Mycoses

C. Port wine stain

D. Hemangioma

CIRCLE THE CORRECT WORDS

Circle the correct word from the choices provided to complete these sentences.

5. The pathophysiology of atopic dermatitis involves interplay between an abnormal (epidermal, lymphatic) barrier and a dysregulated response of the (endocrine, immune) system.

6. Impetigo is a (mildly, highly) contagious infection of the skin with streptococci or (gonococci, staphylococci); the lesions begin as (macules, vesicles) that rupture to form a honey-colored (crust, ulcer).

7. In staphylococcal scalded-skin syndrome, the toxin (circulates to, is produced in) the skin.

8. Roseola infantum, also known as (herpes zoster, exanthema subitum), causes a (pruritic, nonpruritic) rash that appears (before, after) a high fever, primarily in (infants, adolescents).

9. Infantile hemangiomas tend to (shrink, grow) during the first few years of life and then (shrink, grow).

10. Cutaneous vascular malformations grow proportionately with the child and (then, do not) regress.

CATEGORIZE THE INFECTIONS

Write the type of infection beside each name. Choices: bacterial, viral, fungal.

_____ 11. Tinea capitis

_____ 12. Impetigo

_____ 13. Thrush

_____ 14. Molluscum contagiosum

_____ 15. Herpes zoster

_____ 16. Tinea corporis

_____ 17. Chickenpox

_____ 18. Measles

Copyright © 2024 by Elsevier, Inc. All Rights Reserved.

Examine the picture and answer the questions about it.

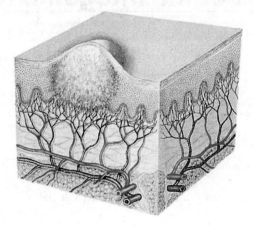

19. This picture shows an acne lesion in cross-section. What substance fills the lesion?

_____

20. What age group most commonly has this type of lesion?

_____

21. A single acne lesion is a comedo. What is the plural of this term?

_____

22. This lesion is closed at the surface of the skin. Is it a blackhead or a whitehead?

_____

23. Name a type of hormone and a bacterium that contribute to the development of acne.

_____

DESCRIBE THE DIFFERENCES

Describe the difference between each pair of terms.

24. What is the difference between atopic dermatitis and diaper dermatitis?

25. What is the difference between rubeola and rubella?

Copyright © 2024 by Elsevier, Inc. All Rights Reserved.

26. What is the difference between variola and varicella?

27. What is the difference between the cause of hand, foot, and mouth disease and the cause of scabies?

COMPLETE THE SENTENCES

Write one word in each blank to complete these sentences.

28. Children who have atopic dermatitis often have elevated levels of the antibody _____ and often also have _____, which also involves this antibody.

29. The technical name for ringworm is _____ _____; this condition is spread by direct or indirect contact with infected persons, kittens, or _____.

30. *Candida albicans* penetrates the epidermal barrier more easily than other microorganisms because it secretes keratolytic _____ and other enzymes.

31. Children who have chickenpox have a risk for developing _____ _____, also known as _____, later in life.

32. Low-flow vascular malformations involve capillaries, _____, and lymphatics; high-flow malformations involve _____.

33. Two blood-sucking parasites are _____, which are nocturnal, and _____, which attach their eggs (also known as _____) to hair shafts.

34. **Miliaria** is caused by occlusion of the _____ ducts in infants.

35. Erythema toxicum _____ is a benign, erythematous accumulation of macules, papules, and pustules that appear at birth or 3 to 4 days after birth and then spontaneously resolve within a few _____.

36. The technical term for lice infestation is _____.

Copyright © 2024 by Elsevier, Inc. All Rights Reserved.

MATCH THE CLINICAL MANIFESTATIONS

Match the disorder on the right with its classic signs and symptoms on the left.

_____ 37. Erythematous, round or oval scaling patches that spread peripherally with clearing in the center, primarily on nonhairy parts of the face, trunk, and limbs in asymmetrical distribution

_____ 38. Acute pruritic vesicles that rupture with a honey-colored serum and form yellow to white-brown crusts or pustular lesions

_____ 39. Recurrent pruritic red, scaly, crusted lesions on cheeks, knees, ankles, and elbows, or may be more widespread

_____ 40. Pruritic linear lesions that itch more at night; may also have vesicles and papules

_____ 41. Redness and tenderness of skin that becomes widespread, followed by painful blisters, bullae, and sloughing of skin

_____ 42. White plaques or spots in the mouth that lead to shallow ulcers that may bleed when the plaques are removed; may spread to the groin or other areas

A. Impetigo

B. Staphylococcal scalded-skin syndrome

C. Thrush

D. Tinea corporis

E. Scabies

F. Atopic dermatitis

TEACH PEOPLE ABOUT PATHOPHYSIOLOGY

Write your response to each situation in the space provided.

43. "My grandson has impetigo," says Mrs. Grey. "What is that? Is it like chickenpox?"

44. "I am not used to working with children," says Nurse Singh. "I need a quick reminder of the characteristics of the rash in chickenpox and in measles."

45. A pediatric nurse says, "I saw a child with strange dome-like structures on their skin. The pediatrician said it was molluscum contagiosum, but they did not prescribe any treatment. Why not treat it?"

46. Mrs. Chin says, "If rubella is such a mild illness, why do we vaccinate against it?"

Copyright © 2024 by Elsevier, Inc. All Rights Reserved.

47. Mrs. Dreyer's son Donny, age 6, had a high fever, enlarged cervical lymph nodes, runny nose, and a "barking" cough. She took him to a pediatric nurse practitioner, who told her that Donny probably had measles and would break out in a rash in a day or two. The rash came the very next day. "Donny has measles, just as the nurse practitioner said. All she did was take Donny's temperature, feel his neck, and look carefully in his mouth," says Mrs. Dreyer. "How did she know he had measles?"

CLINICAL SCENARIO

Read the clinical scenario and answer the questions to explore your understanding of scabies.

Angie Sherwood, age 11, kept scratching her hands, her armpits, and her elbow creases until her mother took her to an urgent care facility. When asked, Angie reported that the itching is worse at night.

Physical Examination

- Linear erythematous lesions, with a few papules in webs of fingers, elbow creases, and anterior axillary folds

- No other abnormal findings

Laboratory Examination

- Microscopic examination of skin scrapings revealed eggs and an adult mite

Angie's diagnosis is scabies.

48. What causes the linear lesions of scabies?

49. What causes the itching of scabies infestation?

50. What is the major complication of scabies?

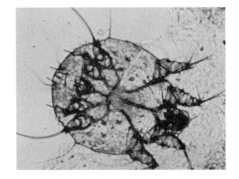

51. Why did the physician assistant at the urgent care facility instruct Angie's mother to wash Angie's clothes, bed linen, and towels with hot water and dry them on the hottest cycle, even though they were clean already?

52. Angie's mother says, "Our dog has fleas. Maybe Angie has flea bites instead of scabies. Do the bites look different?" How should the physician assistant respond?

Copyright © 2024 by Elsevier, Inc. All Rights Reserved.

48 Shock, Multiple Organ Dysfunction Syndrome, and Burns in Adults

MATCH THE DEFINITIONS

Match the word on the right with its definition on the left.

_____ 1. Failure of at least two organs caused by uncontrolled inflammatory response to a severe illness or injury

A. SIRS

_____ 2. Life-threatening organ dysfunction caused by a dysregulated host response to infection

B. MODS

C. Bacteremia

_____ 3. A systemic response to inflammation, defined clinically by specific changes from baseline temperature, heart rate, respiratory rate, and WBC parameters

D. Sepsis

_____ 4. Presence of viable bacteria in the blood

CIRCLE THE CORRECT WORDS

Circle the correct word from the choices provided to complete these sentences.

5. Fever in septic shock makes tissue hypoxia worse by (increasing, decreasing) cellular oxygen demand.

6. Anaerobic metabolism (increases, decreases) intracellular pH, which causes enzyme dysfunction; eventually blood pH (increases, decreases), causing metabolic (acidosis, alkalosis).

7. In addition to inadequate oxygen delivery in shock, there is inadequate delivery of (cortisol, glucose), which causes hormonal release and cellular metabolism changes in order to generate (fuel for survival, metabolic wastes).

8. Body glycogen stores are depleted in about (3, 10) hours in shock; after that the liver cells rely on (glycolysis, gluconeogenesis) to provide a glucose supply.

9. Breakdown of (fat, protein) to provide material for gluconeogenesis contributes to organ failure and decreases capillary (hydrostatic, colloid osmotic) pressure, thus contributing to edema.

10. A burn that blisters immediately is a (first, second) -degree burn; a burn that will heal without any scarring is a (first, second) -degree burn.

11. Fluid resuscitation after a burn (does, does not) return the decreased cardiac output to pre-burn levels; the most reliable criterion for adequate resuscitation of burn shock is (blood pressure, urine output).

12. Burns produce an inflammatory (hypometabolic, hypermetabolic) state and cause (excessive bleeding, hypercoagulability).

Copyright © 2024 by Elsevier, Inc. All Rights Reserved.

CATEGORIZE THE CAUSES

Write the type of shock beside each causative factor. Choices: cardiogenic, hypovolemic, neurogenic, anaphylactic, septic.

_____ 13. Massive hemorrhage

_____ 14. Acute heart failure

_____ 15. Severe pro-inflammatory response to gram-positive bacterial infection

_____ 16. Acute myocardial infarction

_____ 17. Extreme persistent sympathetic understimulation

_____ 18. Inadvertent peanut ingestion in a person with severe peanut allergy

_____ 19. Burns with inadequate fluid replacement

_____ 20. Dilated cardiomyopathy

_____ 21. Untreated diabetes insipidus

_____ 22. Insulin overdose

_____ 23. Bee stings in a person with severe allergy to bee venom

_____ 24. Severe pro-inflammatory response to fungal infection

SELECT THE ORDER

In order to demonstrate your understanding of the processes of shock, circle the answer within each pair that happens first.

25. Which happens first in any type of shock?
    A. Less ATP is available for cell function
    B. Cell shifts to anaerobic metabolism

26. Which happens first in neurogenic shock?
    A. Cardiac output falls
    B. Widespread vasodilation

27. Which happens first in neurogenic shock?
    A. Widespread vasodilation
    B. Decreased sympathetic stimulation

28. Which happens first in cardiogenic shock?
    A. Cardiac output falls
    B. Blood pressure decreases

29. Which happens first in cardiogenic shock?
    A. Cardiac output falls
    B. Renin-angiotensin-aldosterone system is activated

30. Which happens first in hypovolemic shock?
    A. Cardiac output falls
    B. Heart rate increases

31. Which happens first in hypovolemic shock?
    A. Heart rate increases
    B. Catecholamine release increases

Copyright © 2024 by Elsevier, Inc. All Rights Reserved. Chapter **48 Shock, Multiple Organ Dysfunction Syndrome, and Burns in Adults**

32. Which happens first in anaphylactic shock?
    A. Cardiac output falls
    B. Widespread vasodilation and increased capillary permeability

33. Which happens first in anaphylactic shock?
    A. Widespread vasodilation and increased capillary permeability
    B. Allergen attaches to IgE and causes mast cell degranulation

34. Which happens first in septic shock?
    A. Endothelial dysfunction
    B. Blood pressure decreases

35. Which happens first in septic shock?
    A. Increase of proinflammatory cytokines
    B. Release of toxic microbial products

DESCRIBE THE DIFFERENCES

Describe the difference between each pair of terms.

36. What is the difference between bacteremia and sepsis?

37. What is the difference between sepsis and septic shock?

38. What is the difference between a first-degree burn and a second-degree burn?

MATCH THE SPECIFIC CLINICAL MANIFESTATIONS

Match the type of shock on the right with the specific clinical manifestations on the left.

NOTE: These clinical manifestations are in addition to hypotension, tachycardia, and other general manifestations of shock from any cause.

_____ 39. Chest pain, dyspnea, feeling of impending doom, jugular venous distention, crackles, pulmonary edema, low ejection fraction

_____ 40. Very low systemic vascular resistance, possible initial bradycardia, high ejection fraction, fresh spinal cord or brainstem injury, hypoglycemia, anesthetics, or overdose of other CNS depressants

_____ 41. Poor skin turgor, thirst, dry mucous membranes

_____ 42. Pruritus, rash, urticaria, laryngeal edema, angioedema of face or other areas, wheezing, dyspnea

_____ 43. Low systemic vascular resistance, normal or elevated cardiac output, body temperature instability, elevated blood cytokine levels, possible manifestations of infection and of organ dysfunction

A. Anaphylactic shock

B. Septic shock

C. Cardiogenic shock

D. Hypovolemic shock

E. Neurogenic shock

Copyright © 2024 by Elsevier, Inc. All Rights Reserved.

COMPLETE THE SENTENCES

Write one word in each blank to complete these sentences.

44. Neurogenic shock also is called _____ shock.

45. Anaphylactic, neurogenic, and septic shock are similar in that they all involve widespread _____ that creates relative _____; these three types are categorized as _____ shock.

46. Persistent hypotension and tissue hypoperfusion caused by cardiac dysfunction in the presence of adequate intravascular volume and left ventricular filling pressure is the definition of _____ _____.

47. Progressive dysfunction of two or more organ systems resulting from an uncontrolled inflammatory response to a severe illness or injury is the definition of _____ _____ _____ _____, often called by its acronym _____.

48. A full-thickness burn destroys epidermis, dermis, and _____ _____.

49. The term _____ _____ is used to identify the point at which capillary permeability has normalized and burn shock has ended.

50. The accumulation of activated _____ in organs is thought to play a key role in the pathogenesis of MODS; with failure of five or more organs, mortality is nearly _____ percent.

51. During the first 24 hours, the clinical manifestations of developing MODS are _____; the first organ to show signs of failure typically is the _____.

TEACH PEOPLE ABOUT PATHOPHYSIOLOGY

Write your response to each situation in the space provided.

52. "My wife is in the intensive care unit, and they said something about her being in shock," says Mr. Abel. "What is shock?"

53. A nurse says, "I know that systemic vascular resistance increases in cardiogenic shock patients but not in neurogenic shock patients. Why are these responses different?"

54. Mr. Lund received some superficial and deep partial-thickness burns on his hands from a chemical explosion. "This is confusing," he says. "Sometimes they talk about 'partial-thickness burns' and sometimes they say 'second-degree burns.' So which is it?"

Copyright © 2024 by Elsevier, Inc. All Rights Reserved.

55. An intensive care unit nurse says, "I know that neutrophils play an important role in MODS, but how does neutrophil accumulation in various organs actually contribute to organ dysfunction?"

CLINICAL SCENARIO

Read the clinical scenario and answer the questions to explore your understanding of burn pathophysiology.

Mr. Eisner, age 43, sustained severe burns while welding an automobile gasoline tank that he had removed from a truck. He had full-thickness burns on his face and bald head and on both of his arms and hands, as well as a mixture of superficial and deep partial-thickness burns on his anterior trunk. His genital area, lower extremities, and posterior body were not burned.

Mr. Eisner was transported to a regional burn center for care.

56. Using the rule of nines (see diagram), calculate Mr. Eisner's approximate percentage of total body surface area that was burned.

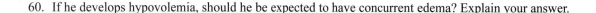

57. Should blisters be expected to appear on Mr. Eisner's bald head? Why or why not?

58. Which of Mr. Eisner's burns should cause him the most pain? Why?

59. Why is Mr. Eisner at high risk for hypovolemia?

60. If he develops hypovolemia, should he be expected to have concurrent edema? Explain your answer.

61. Which burn areas have the greatest risk for scarring?

62. If he survives, will Mr. Eisner need any skin grafts? Provide the reason for your answer.

Copyright © 2024 by Elsevier, Inc. All Rights Reserved.

49 Shock, Multiple Organ Dysfunction Syndrome, and Burns in Children

MATCH THE DEFINITIONS

Match the word on the right with its definition on the left.

_____ 1. Concurrent failure of at least two organs resulting from a systemic inflammatory response after a single cause, such as a severe illness or injury

A. NPMODS

B. MODS

_____ 2. A systemic response to inflammation, defined clinically by specific changes from baseline temperature, heart rate, respiratory rate, and WBC parameters

C. SIRS

_____ 3. Dysfunction of one or fewer organs on day 1 of sepsis recognition with subsequent development of two or more concurrent organ failures at any time during treatment

CIRCLE THE CORRECT WORDS

Circle the correct word from the choices provided to complete these sentences.

4. Children can be in shock and still have an adequate (systolic, mean) blood pressure.

5. Initial assessment of a child who may be in shock should include three items: (consciousness, pupil reaction to light), (urine output, breathing), and (blood pressure, color).

6. With a child in a warm environment, (mottling, darkening) of the skin may indicate poor tissue perfusion.

7. The most common type of shock in children is (cardiogenic, hypovolemic).

8. Newborns often develop (hypothermia, fever) as a sign of infection and may develop (bradycardia, tachycardia) instead of the usual heart rate change in older children.

9. An increase in serum lactate is a (poor, sensitive) indicator of inadequate systemic perfusion in children.

10. One of the causes of MODS is damage to endothelial cells in the (large arteries, microvasculature) by (oxygen free radicals, lactic acid).

11. In a neonate, bradycardia is a heart rate below (50, 100) bpm, and tachycardia is a heart rate above (100, 180) bpm; in school-aged children, these numbers are (higher, lower).

12. Although adults who have septic shock typically have peripheral (vasodilation, vasoconstriction) and (low, high) cardiac output, many children with septic shock have severe peripheral (vasodilation, vasoconstriction) and (low, high) cardiac output.

13. The rule of nines to calculate the percentage of total body surface area that is burned (is, is not) accurate in children.

14. (Flame, Scald) burns are more common in young children, but (flame, scald) burns are more common in older children.

Copyright © 2024 by Elsevier, Inc. All Rights Reserved.

CATEGORIZE THE CAUSES

Write the type of pediatric shock beside each cause. Choices: hypovolemic, cardiogenic, distributive, obstructive.

_____ 15. Hemorrhage after trauma

_____ 16. Anaphylaxis from severe peanut allergy

_____ 17. Severe aortic stenosis

_____ 18. Spinal cord injury

_____ 19. Pulmonary embolus

_____ 20. Repeated emesis with inadequate fluid replacement

_____ 21. Sepsis from bacterial infection

_____ 22. Myocarditis

DESCRIBE THE DIFFERENCES

Describe the difference between each pair of terms.

23. What is the difference between compensated and hypotensive shock in children?

24. What is the difference between primary and secondary MODS?

25. What is the difference between the ebb and flow phases of metabolism after a burn injury?

26. What is the difference between SIRS and sepsis?

COMPLETE THE SENTENCES

Write one word in each blank to complete these sentences.

27. The term _____ *shock* encompasses septic, neurogenic, and anaphylactic shock.

28. The term _____ *shock* can be used for conditions such as cardiac tamponade, pneumothorax, or
    pulmonary _____ that provide a mechanical block to blood flow through the heart.

Copyright © 2024 by Elsevier, Inc. All Rights Reserved.

29. The most common cause of bradycardia in young children is _____, which often indicates impending cardiovascular _____ and is the most common _____ cardiac rhythm observed in children.

30. Because a child's heart is small, the main determinant of cardiac output in children is _____ _____.

31. Invasive catheters, burns, and immunocompromise are risk factors for development of _____.

32. During sepsis, changes in the endothelium promote an antifibrinolytic and _____ state that gives rise to microthrombi in the microcirculation.

33. If a child with sepsis develops signs of _____ dysfunction, septic shock is present.

34. Pediatric patients with _____ injury also may have inhalation injury, which increases mortality.

35. The typical burn pattern from nonaccidental trauma involving hot liquid immersion is _____ or hand with a clear boundary.

36. A major complication of healing burns is _____ because eschar provides a fertile environment for _____ to grow.

TEACH PEOPLE ABOUT PATHOPHYSIOLOGY

Write your response to each situation in the space provided.

37. "I am used to working with adults," says a nurse. "If children can have shock and still have adequate systolic pressure, what defines them as being in shock?"

38. "My son's skin is warm," says Mrs. Landau, whose son has neurogenic shock after a spinal cord injury sustained in a diving accident. "They said he is in shock, but people on television who are in shock have cool skin. I watch all those medical shows, and I remember that. Is he really in shock?"

39. Devon, age 6, has SIRS. His parents ask, "What does SIRS mean?"

40. Carly, age 18 months, sustained extensive partial-thickness burns when she knocked over a large kettle of boiling apple cider. She is in a pediatric burn unit in a large medical center. Her mother asks, "Why are you giving her so much IV fluid? When I had an accident and was in the hospital, they gave me IV fluid for 2 days, but Carly has had IVs for 5 days now. Why?"

Copyright © 2024 by Elsevier, Inc. All Rights Reserved.

41. A child rescued from a burning car after an automobile accident was brought to the emergency department. The burned area has some blood drainage. What should the experienced emergency department personnel teach a new employee about interpreting this assessment finding?

42. Austin, age 3, was discharged from the hospital after staying a month in the burn unit. His father says, "Now that Austin's burns have healed, why did the burn doctor tell us that we need to have more appointments to watch his scars?"

CLINICAL SCENARIO

Read the clinical scenario and answer the questions to explore your understanding of shock in infants.

Kiley, age 5 months, spent a 3-day weekend with a babysitter when her parents went camping. Her parents returned to find Kiley very weak. The babysitter said, "I used up almost all of the disposable diapers; she has had diarrhea since you left. During the last 12 hours, I used at least eight diapers, and she filled them with watery poop." Kiley's parents called the pediatrician, who told them to take Kiley to the emergency department.

Physical Examination

- Lethargic

- Depressed anterior fontanel, sunken eyes

- HR 176 bpm; BP 90/58 mmHg; respirations 56 breaths/minute

- Capillary refill delayed; peripheral pulses weak

- Skin mottled and cool to touch

Complete the sentences by choosing from the lists of options.

43. Kiley's history and signs and symptoms are consistent with _____(1)_____ and she needs immediate _____(2)_____.

Options for 1	Options for 2
cardiogenic shock	cardiopulmonary resuscitation (CPR)
distributive shock	volume resuscitation
hypovolemic shock	antibiotics

 Copyright © 2024 by Elsevier, Inc. All Rights Reserved.

44. The mottling of Kiley's skin indicates _____(1)_____ and should _____(2)_____ when she is treated successfully.

Options for 1	Options for 2
infection	remain the same
poor tissue perfusion	become worse
parasympathetic nervous system activation	disappear

45. Why did Kiley develop hypovolemic shock?

46. What physiologic compensatory mechanisms are maintaining Kiley's blood pressure within the normal range for her age?

47. What is the importance of Kiley's tachycardia?

48. What physiologic mechanism is causing Kiley's skin to be cool?

49. Fluid replacement with isotonic sodium-containing fluid is ordered. Will the route be oral or intravenous? Why?

50. What assessments will indicate that Kiley's shock is being treated effectively?

51. How could development of this condition have been prevented in this case?

Copyright © 2024 by Elsevier, Inc. All Rights Reserved.

Answer Key

CHAPTER 1

Identify Cellular Structures and Their Functions
1. B; mitochondrion
2. F; ribosome
3. C; Golgi apparatus
4. G; nucleus
5. E; endoplasmic reticulum
6. H; nucleolus
7. D; vesicle
8. A; lysosome

Describe the Differences
9. A eukaryote has numerous organelles and a membrane surrounding its nucleus, but a prokaryote does not have organelles, and its genetic material is not organized into a nucleus.
10. The nucleolus is a small, dense structure within the nucleus.
11. Microtubules are small, somewhat rigid, single, unbranched protein tubes, but microfilaments are smaller, more flexible fibrils of actin that usually occur in bundles. Both are part of the cytoskeleton.
12. A hydrophilic substance attracts water, but a hydrophobic substance repels water.
13. Lysosomes and peroxisomes contain different enzymes. Lysosomes contain digestive enzymes that break down molecules to their component parts, whereas peroxisomes contain oxidative enzymes that are important in producing hydrogen peroxide and other reactive oxygen species.

Complete the Sentences
14. histones
15. peroxisomes
16. raft
17. fibroblasts
18. hydrostatic
19. isotonic
20. basement
21. Connective
22. muscle

Order the Steps
23. C, A, E, B, D
24. C, B, D, A

Circle the Correct Words
25. G_1

26. differentiation
27. solute
28. oxygen
29. water molecules
30. Paracrine; diffusion
31. the citric acid cycle
32. Active transport
33. proteins
34. an anion

Write Your Definitions
35. A substance that binds to a receptor
36. Tiny flask-shaped pits in the outer surface of the plasma membrane that may be important locations for receptors or for entry of molecules into the cell
37. Carbohydrate coating on the exterior of the cellular plasma membrane
38. A molecule that has both a hydrophobic part and a hydrophilic part
39. Infolding of the plasma membrane to form a vesicle that enters the cell

Choose the Direction
40. A
41. B
42. A
43. B
44. A

Teach People about Cellular Biology
45. Gap junctions synchronize contractions of heart muscle cells through ionic coupling.
46. Cell surface receptors use second messengers because the ligand (the first messenger) cannot enter the cell. Intracellular receptors do not need second messengers because the ligand enters the cell.
47. During interphase (the G_1, S, and G_2 phases), the cell increases its mass by producing DNA, RNA, protein, lipids, and other substances, and duplicates its chromosomes. These processes are necessary to prepare the cell for mitosis and cytokinesis.

CHAPTER 2

Match the Definitions
1. E
2. D
3. G
4. H

Copyright © 2024 by Elsevier, Inc. All Rights Reserved.

5. F
6. B
7. C
8. A

Categorize the Clinical Examples
9. Hyperplasia
10. Hypertrophy
11. Atrophy
12. Metaplasia
13. Hypertrophy
14. Atrophy
15. Hyperplasia

Circle the Correct Words
16. necrosis; apoptosis
17. atypical
18. calcium
19. less; more
20. storage
21. superoxide radicals; membranes
22. do not involve
23. brain; hydrolases
24. hypoxia; bacterial invasion

Describe the Differences
25. Hypertrophy increases tissue mass by keeping the same number of cells and making each individual cell larger, but hyperplasia increases tissue mass by increasing the number of cells.
26. Suffocation occurs when oxygen fails to reach the blood, but strangulation occurs when neck pressure collapses blood vessels, stopping blood flow to the brain.
27. An abrasion is a scrape in which superficial skin layers have been removed, but a laceration is a jagged or irregular tearing of tissues.
28. Dystrophic calcification occurs in dying and dead tissues, but metastatic calcification occurs in normal tissues when plasma calcium concentration is too high.
29. With a penetrating gunshot wound, the bullet remains in the body, but with a perforating gunshot wound, the bullet has exited the body.

Order the Steps
30. B, C, A, E, G, H, F, D

Complete the Sentences
31. caspases
32. oxygen
33. caseous; liquefactive
34. apoptotic bodies; phagocytosis
35. acetaldehyde
36. oxidative stress
37. somatic
38. melanocytes; keratinocytes
39. greenhouse; heat

Respond to Clinical Situations
40. When cells undergo necrosis, enzymes normally found inside cells are released and enter the blood. The enzyme creatine kinase normally occurs inside skeletal muscle. Mr. Turino's injuries caused a lot of skeletal muscle necrosis.
41. After death, when blood is no longer circulating, gravity causes blood to settle in the lowest (most dependent) tissues. Pooling of blood caused the purple discoloration of her skin. That purple discoloration is called *livor mortis* or *postmortem lividity*.
42. After death, the muscles are relaxed at first, and then they get stiff after several hours.
43. A very large excess of reactive oxygen species (ROS) tends to cause necrosis, but a smaller excess of ROS can cause apoptosis.

Draw Your Answers
44.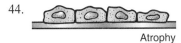
Atrophy

45.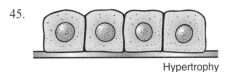
Hypertrophy

(**Questions 43 and 44,** From Lewis SM, Heitkemper MM, Dirksen SR: *Medical-surgical nursing: assessment and management of clinical problems,* ed 6, St Louis, 2004, Mosby.)

Identify the Characteristics
46. B and E

Teach People about Pathophysiology
Compare your answers with these sample answers.

47. Kenesha, when your arm comes out of the cast, it probably will look smaller than your other arm because the cast kept you from using it. When we do not use our muscles, they get smaller and weaker. The good news is that when we do use our muscles, they get bigger and stronger. So if you use your arm again, it can get back to normal size after a few weeks.
48. If you lift weights, your muscles eventually will get bigger and stronger because they are working harder than usual. The same thing happens with the heart muscle if it works harder. Your heart has to work harder than usual to pump against high blood pressure, so your heart muscle got bigger.
49. When the tissue at the ends of your toes died, it was exposed to the air and dried out, making it black and hard. If your dad's toes were swollen and mushy before they were amputated, they might have been infected. Your blackened toes did not get infected.

Copyright © 2024 by Elsevier, Inc. All Rights Reserved.

Work with the Clinical Scenario

50. His left upper arm looked shrunken when compared with his right arm.
51. The shoulders and biceps increased in size as he continued his workouts.
52. The left foot developed a callus where his shoe rubbed it.
53. Not applicable
54. Not applicable

Puzzle Out These Technical Terms

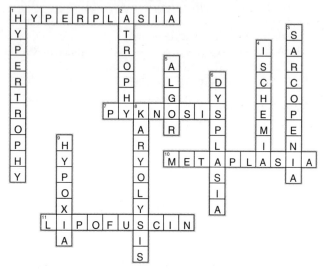

CHAPTER 3

Match the Definitions

1. D
2. F
3. A
4. B
5. C
6. E

Circle the Correct Words

7. the same as; freely
8. Albumin
9. osmoreceptors; hypothalamus
10. hypervolemia
11. slow; fast
12. filtration; osmosis
13. carbon dioxide
14. heart

Categorize the Causes of Edema

15. Lymphatic obstruction
16. Increased capillary hydrostatic pressure
17. Increased capillary permeability
18. Increased capillary hydrostatic pressure
19. Decreased plasma oncotic pressure
20. Increased capillary permeability
21. Increased capillary hydrostatic pressure

Select the Greater

22. A lean woman
23. An infant
24. A man
25. A 56-year-old man
26. Intracellular fluid
27. Extracellular fluid
28. The pH of an alkaline solution
29. The respiratory rate during metabolic acidosis

Explain the Pictures

30. Hypotonic; hypertonic
31. When the extracellular fluid became hypotonic, the osmolality of the intracellular fluid was greater; osmosis then pulled water into the cell to equalize the osmolalities in the two fluids.
32. Lethargy, confusion, seizures, and coma
33. In both cases, the neurons do not function well. The clinical manifestations are non-specific indicators of cerebral dysfunction.

Characterize the Hormones

34. E, 2
35. C, 3
36. D, 1
37. A, 5
38. B, 4

Describe the Differences

39. Interstitial fluid is a component of extracellular fluid. Extracellular fluid consists of the fluid inside the blood vessels (intravascular fluid) and the fluid between the cells (interstitial fluid), as well as minor components such as lymph and various secretions (transcellular fluids).
40. A volatile acid (carbonic acid) is excreted by the lungs, but a non-volatile acid (metabolic acid) is excreted by the kidneys.
41. Acidemia is the state in which the pH of arterial blood is less than 7.35, but acidosis is the condition of having too much acid or too little base, regardless of pH.
42. Correction of an acid–base imbalance returns the bicarbonate and carbonic acid concentrations to normal, but compensation for an acid–base imbalance returns the bicarbonate-to-carbonic acid ratio to normal (20:1) while the actual bicarbonate and carbonic acid concentrations are abnormal.

Complete the Sentences

43. extracellular; intracellular
44. 42
45. edema
46. isotonic
47. respiratory; metabolic
48. 20:1
49. acid; conjugate base
50. acidosis
51. hyperphosphatemia; decrease

Answer Key

Copyright © 2024 by Elsevier, Inc. All Rights Reserved.

Work with These Patients

52. Isotonic fluid excess and hypokalemia; Dependent edema, weight gain, distended neck veins when upright, skeletal muscle weakness, constipation, abdominal distention
53. Respiratory alkalosis; Paresthesias of fingers, lightheadedness, confusion
54. Respiratory acidosis; Slow, shallow respirations; blood pH less than 7.35; blood $PaCO_2$ increased
55. Isotonic fluid deficit, hypokalemia, metabolic alkalosis; Tachycardia; rapid weight loss; decreased urine output; skeletal muscle weakness; slow, shallow respirations; lethargy
56. Hypercalcemia; Fatigue, weakness, anorexia, constipation, lethargy

Choose the Direction

57. A
58. A
59. A
60. B

Teach People about Pathophysiology

Compare your answers with these sample answers.

61. Inflammation does cause swelling, but that is not the reason your ankles are swollen. They are not inflamed. They are swollen because your body is overloaded with fluid, and that makes extra outward pressure in your smallest blood vessels. Adding the effects of gravity to that outward pressure makes the swelling appear in your ankles.
62. The location varies with body position. Dependent edema means swelling in the lower-most portion of the body. If your husband has been walking or sitting in a chair with his feet hanging down, then look at his ankles for swelling. If he has been lying on his back in bed all day, then look at the area in the back just above his buttocks.
63. Your body makes metabolic acids from the foods that you eat. That is a normal part of what we call cellular metabolism, the processes by which our cells break down nutrients and use them for energy. You got metabolic acidosis because your body keeps making those metabolic acids, even though your kidneys are no longer able to excrete them. That is why you receive dialysis now.
64. Her fast and deep breathing is her body protecting her from the effects of the ketoacids. When her kidneys could not get rid of the ketoacids fast enough, her breathing sped up to remove another kind of acid called *carbonic acid*. The important thing to remember is that her fast breathing means that her body is responding normally to protect her, and it is not a lung problem.
65. You can figure out the fluid and electrolyte imbalances in oliguric end-stage renal disease patients if you remember that the kidneys normally excrete water and sodium, potassium, magnesium, phosphate, and metabolic acids. With oliguria, these will not be excreted and will accumulate in the body. Therefore, you can expect isotonic fluid excess, hyperkalemia, metabolic acidosis, possibly hypermagnesemia, and hyperphosphatemia.

Clinical Scenario

66. Isotonic fluid deficit. Supporting data: history of diarrhea for 3 weeks, possible orthostatic hypotension (fell when stood up, although muscle weakness might have contributed), tachycardia, weak pulse, low BP when supine, flat neck veins when supine, normal serum sodium.
67. Hypokalemia. Although there are other causes for these manifestations, she has muscle weakness and constipation, which are characteristic of hypokalemia. Hypokalemia also causes orthostatic hypotension.
68. Hypocalcemia and/or hypomagnesemia. Both of these imbalances are caused by decreased intestinal absorption, which could have occurred with her chronic diarrhea; both of them cause muscle cramping, which she has.
69. Metabolic acidosis. Supporting data: history of diarrhea for 3 weeks (loss of bicarbonate in diarrhea), her slowness in responding to questions, and her deep, rapid respirations (might be compensation for metabolic acidosis).
70. Isotonic sodium-containing fluid will expand her extracellular fluid volume, which will correct her isotonic fluid deficit. The fluid will replace her deficient electrolytes as well.

CHAPTER 4

Match the Definitions

1. I
2. E
3. H
4. F
5. A
6. B
7. D
8. C
9. G

Complete the Sentences

10. karyotype
11. 23
12. frameshift
13. recessive
14. Alzheimer
15. Klinefelter
16. translocation

Copyright © 2024 by Elsevier, Inc. All Rights Reserved.

Interpret a Pedigree Chart

17. None; the two affected individuals are girls.
18. Mating between two close relatives (consanguineous mating)
19. The symbol for identical twins is:

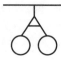

Describe the Differences

20. Heterozygous means that the two genes at the same locus on both chromosomes are not identical, but homozygous means that the two genes are identical.
21. Monosomy means that one of the chromosomes in somatic cells has only one copy instead of the normal two copies, but trisomy means that one of the chromosomes in somatic cells has three copies.
22. A genotype is an individual's genetic makeup, but a phenotype is the outward appearance of an individual.
23. In mitosis, a diploid cell makes a copy of itself, but in meiosis, a haploid cell is created from a diploid cell.

Order the Steps

24. D, B, E, C, A

Categorize the Clinical Examples

25. Single-gene disorder
26. Chromosomal disorder
27. Chromosomal disorder
28. Chromosomal disorder
29. Single-gene disorder
30. Chromosomal disorder
31. Single-gene disorder

Circle the Correct Words

32. diploid cell
33. single genes
34. males; females
35. DNA
36. amino acids
37. triploidy
38. Loss
39. X; female

Interpret a Punnett Square

40. A

Write Your Definitions

41. A cell that has only 23 chromosomes; a gamete (sperm or egg)
42. A pair of identical chromosomes
43. Condition in which cells have more than two copies of each chromosome
44. An error during meiosis or mitosis in which homologous chromosomes or sister chromatids fail to separate normally

45. An individual who has a disease-causing allele but is phenotypically normal, often because the allele is recessive and the individual is a heterozygote

Teach People about Pathophysiology

Compare your answers with these sample answers.

46. We have two copies of most genes. You and Mrs. Medlow each have one PKU gene and one normal gene. PKU is an autosomal recessive disease, which means that a person must have two PKU genes in order to have the disease. You have one PKU gene, so you do not have the disease. Kira has two PKU genes, so she has the disease.
47. Autosomal means any chromosome that is not an X or Y chromosome. As you may remember, the X and Y chromosomes are the sex chromosomes. All of the other chromosomes are called *autosomal.*
48. Yes, cystic fibrosis is autosomal recessive, as PKU is. It is caused by a defective gene, and a person must have two copies of the defective gene to have cystic fibrosis.
49. Having two copies of the PKU gene keeps Kira from processing the amino acid phenylalanine, so you manage it by keeping phenylalanine out of her diet. The cystic fibrosis gene makes an abnormal transporter protein in cell membranes, and all of the body's secretions become too thick. That problem cannot be managed with a special diet.

CHAPTER 5

Match the Definitions

1. E
2. C
3. A
4. B
5. D

Calculate the Rates

6. 16,500/150,000 = 11%
7. 4050/150,000 = 2.7%
8. 3.3/1.5 = 2.2

Circle the Correct Words

9. liability
10. In contrast
11. more than
12. multifactorial
13. more

Complete the Sentences

14. bell-shaped
15. empirical
16. proband
17. identical
18. 1 (one)

Copyright © 2024 by Elsevier, Inc. All Rights Reserved.

Interpret the Table

19. Measles is unlikely to be influenced markedly by genes.
20. Spina bifida has a sizable genetic component.
21. Bipolar disorder has a sizable genetic component.

Match the Gene Variants

22. B
23. C
24. E
25. A
26. D

Teach People about Pathophysiology

Compare your answers with these sample answers.

27. High blood pressure is not caused by a specific mutated gene, as PKU is. High blood pressure is what we call a multifactorial genetic disorder, which means that it is caused by mutations in several genes and is affected by environmental factors such as diet and exercise. You are doing a great job with managing your diet and exercise!
28. No, dizygotic does not mean anything bad or abnormal. It simply means that your boys are fraternal twins rather than identical twins. They are twins, but they will not look exactly alike.
29. The good news is that although heart attacks have a genetic component, they also have an environmental component. That means that you are not doomed. Your health behaviors, such as choosing to stop smoking and to exercise regularly, can make a difference and reduce your heart attack risk.

CHAPTER 6

Match the Definitions

1. D
2. A
3. B
4. C

Circle the Correct Words

5. not caused by
6. silencing
7. are
8. imprinting
9. mRNA; miRNA
10. Some
11. progression

Explain the Pictures

12. A
13. A
14. B
15. Transcription is less likely to occur because the chromatin stays tightly wound and transcription factors are not able to reach the promoter regions of genes to initiate transcription.

16. Transcription does not occur because transcription factors are not able to bind the hypermethylated promoter regions of genes.

Complete the Sentences

17. promoter
18. oncomirs
19. housekeeping
20. transgenerational
21. epigenetic

Teach People about Pathophysiology

Compare your answers with these sample answers.

22. Hypermethylation silences a gene, so if tumor suppressor genes are silenced, that would encourage development of cancer.
23. You probably learned that messenger RNA carries the genetic code from DNA to the areas of the cell (ribosomes) that make proteins. There are other types of RNA that do not perform this function. They are called *noncoding* because they do not carry the genetic code for making proteins. Instead, they participate in other functions, such as regulating which genes become active at any one time.
24. As the cells differentiate, epigenetic silencing of certain genes occurs. The DNA is the same, but some genes are silenced by mechanisms such as DNA methylation. The genes that remain active are the genes that are needed for that particular cell type.

Clinical Scenario

25. Prader-Willi; father
26. Some of the genes on chromosome 15 inherited from the mother are imprinted (transcriptionally silenced). Because those same genes are deleted from the chromosome inherited from the father, no products are produced from those genes during development, causing Prader-Willi syndrome.
27. Imprinting of those genes on the mother's chromosome 15 is normal. The deletion of those genes from the father's chromosome is abnormal.
28. Some of the genes in the critical region of chromosome 15 normally are read only from the chromosome inherited from the father; other genes in that region normally are read only from the chromosome inherited from the mother. If a deletion of the critical region occurs on the chromosome inherited from the father, the child develops Prader-Willi syndrome. If the deletion occurs in the chromosome inherited from the mother, the child develops Angelman syndrome.

CHAPTER 7

Match the Definitions

1. D
2. A
3. B
4. C

Copyright © 2024 by Elsevier, Inc. All Rights Reserved.

Match the Functions
5. C
6. E
7. A
8. B
9. D

Circle the Correct Words
10. anatomic barriers
11. collectins
12. microbiome
13. Defensins; kinins
14. pattern recognition receptors
15. complement; cell lysis

Complete the Overview Table
16. B
17. C
18. A

Categorize the Immune Cells
19. Nonphagocytic innate
20. Adaptive
21. Phagocytic innate
22. Phagocytic innate

Order the Steps
23. B, E, C, D, A, F
24. G, C, A, H, D, B, E, F

Describe the Differences
25. A PAMP is a molecular pattern that is associated with pathogenic microorganisms, but a DAMP is a molecular pattern that is associated with injured or stressed host cells.
26. Innate immunity is non-specific, meaning that one cell or other element will defend against many different types of antigens, but adaptive immunity is specific, meaning that one cell will defend against only one particular antigen.
27. Opsonins are molecules that mark antigens for destruction by innate immune cells, but cytokines are signaling molecules that influence the behavior of immune and other types of cells.

Explain the Pictures
28. Diapedesis
29. They move by chemotaxis to the area where the chemotactic cytokines are in the highest concentration.
30. Polymorphonuclear neutrophil
31. B
32. Macrophages
33. To secrete collagen, which forms the scar tissue
34. After

Complete the Sentences
35. innate
36. granuloma
37. cascades
38. keloid
39. dehiscence
40. complement
41. capillaries
42. degranulation; synthesizing

Complete the Table

Characteristics of Immune Defenses

Aspect	Barrier Function of Innate Immunity	Inflammatory Response of Innate Immunity	Adaptive Immunity
43. How soon does this defense begin working after first contact with a pathogen?	Already working before pathogen contact	Very rapidly	After some delay
44. Does this defense remember the pathogen and act more rapidly upon subsequent exposure?	No	No	Yes
45. Does one cell or other component of this defense work against many different antigens or only one antigen?	Many different antigens	Many different antigens	Only one antigen

Characterize the Exudates
46. C
47. E
48. D
49. B
50. A

Use Knowledge in Clinical Situations
51. D
52. D
53. A
54. C
55. A

Copyright © 2024 by Elsevier, Inc. All Rights Reserved.

Teach People about Pathophysiology

Compare your answers with these sample answers.

56. Innate immunity is a type of immunity that you have even before you are vaccinated. It is not a specific kind of immunity like a vaccination provides, but it is a general type of immunity. You have skin to keep out invading microorganisms, innate immune cells that defend against many different microorganisms, and some chemical defenses that help protect you.

57. The red color means your body is taking care of you. When you fell and scraped your knee, the top skin was injured, so your body sent more good red blood to your knee to help fix the injury. The blood brings some helpful cleanup cells that will help your knee get better.

58. When you sprain your ankle, the injured tissue puts out chemical messengers that act on the nearby blood vessels. They expand and let more blood flow into the injured tissue, and the blood vessels become leaky. The leaky blood vessels allow fluid from the blood to leak into the tissues, which makes them swell.

59. Yes, white blood cells are in the blood, but when a mosquito bite gets infected, the injured area sends out chemical distress signals. Some of the white blood cells leave the blood and follow the chemical signals, which get stronger the closer they get to the mosquito bite. That is how white blood cells know to come and help get rid of the infection.

60. I think you misunderstood what she said. Nurses use the term *secondary intention* to describe how a pressure ulcer heals. Healing by secondary intention means that the ulcer gradually fills up with new tissue until it heals completely. Healing your ulcer is our first priority for your care, and I know it is your top priority also.

61. The term *normal microbiome* means the good bacteria and other microorganisms that normally live on your skin and in areas of your body such as the gastrointestinal tract. These normal microbiome microorganisms help keep disease-causing microorganisms, such as that fungus, from causing an infection. When the penicillin killed off some of the normal microbiome, the fungus had an opportunity to grow in their place.

62. An acute phase reactant is a normal protein that the liver makes when there is inflammation in the body. An increased amount of C-reactive protein in the blood tells us that you have inflammation somewhere in your body.

63. Mr. Moreno; wound infection

Assessment Finding	Normal Tissue Healing	Possible Wound Infection
64. Cuts very red and swollen on their edges, which are not fully approximated		X
65. Cuts slightly red and swollen on their edges; no discharge and fully approximated	X	
66. Open crater; light red and not weeping	X	
67. Cut oozing a thick whitish liquid		X

CHAPTER 8

Match the Definitions

1. D
2. E
3. A
4. C
5. B

Complete the Overview

6. B lymphocytes (Humoral), T lymphocytes (Cell-mediated)

Circle the Correct Words

7. HLA
8. MHC I; both MHC I and MHC II
9. Dendritic cells
10. IgM
11. Th2
12. T lymphocyte differentiation

Categorize the Clinical Examples

13. Passive
14. Active
15. Active
16. Passive

Order the Steps

17. B, D, E, A, C

Describe the Differences

18. In central tolerance, lymphocytes with receptors against self-antigens are eliminated, but in peripheral tolerance, these cells are suppressed by regulatory T cells and other mechanisms.

19. Antibodies defend against bacteria and viruses, but cytotoxic T cells defend against virus-infected cells and host cells that have become abnormal.

20. MHC class I molecules are located on all nucleated cells and platelets, but MHC class II molecules are located only on antigen-presenting cells, B lymphocytes, and some epithelial cells.

Copyright © 2024 by Elsevier, Inc. All Rights Reserved.

Explain the Pictures

21. A
22. The Fab fragment is the portion that binds the antigen.
23. B
24. Phagocytic innate immune cells bind the Fc fragment with their Fc receptors, which enables them to grasp and phagocytize the antigen that is bound on the other end of the immunoglobulin.
25. The words *antibody titer* indicate that adaptive immunity is involved.
26. Curves in section B
27. Memory cells respond quickly to a previously experienced antigen.

Complete the Sentences

28. epitope
29. adjuvant
30. lipid
31. II; I
32. memory
33. cellular; humoral; inflammation; suppress
34. IgM
35. perforins; granzymes
36. cytokines (IFN-gamma also is correct)

Characterize the Immunoglobulins (Igs)

37. C
38. D
39. A
40. E
41. B

Teach People about Pathophysiology

Compare your answers with these sample answers.

42. A plasma cell is a cell that makes antibodies. Antibodies are a protective part of the immune system and normally defend us against bacteria and viruses. The long word *immunoglobulin* means antibody. Antibodies have several parts called *heavy chains* and *light chains*, so immunoglobulin light chains are pieces of antibodies.
43. Antibodies in your blood attach to invading organisms like viruses and bacteria that could make you sick. They help your immune cells to kill the invaders and keep you healthy.
44. Yes, antibodies are proteins, but infants have immature gastrointestinal tracts, and they absorb some proteins whole without them being digested.
45. NK cells are natural killer cells. They do not make antibodies. They attack cells that are infected with virus so that the virus cannot reproduce and spread.

CHAPTER 9

Match the Definitions

1. D
2. C
3. B
4. A

Circle the Correct Words

5. sensitized
6. T; B
7. phagocytosis
8. autoimmunity
9. donors; no A and B antigens
10. MHC
11. immunocompromised
12. H1
13. only specific

Categorize the Clinical Examples

14. Type I (IgE-mediated)
15. Type IV (cell-mediated)
16. Type IV (cell-mediated)
17. Type II (tissue-specific)
18. Type I (IgE-mediated)

Order the Steps

19. I, C, A, E, B, G, F, D, H

Explain the Picture

20. C
21. They are destroyed in the blood, often by phagocytes.
22. The tissue-bound immune complexes activate the complement cascade, and chemotactic complement fragments (C5a) are produced.
23. Neutrophils bind the Fc ends of the immune complexes, attempting to phagocytize them, and damage the tissue in the process with destructive enzymes and reactive oxygen species.

Complete the Sentences

24. self-antigens
25. sensitization
26. opsonin
27. B
28. T
29. T; thymus
30. activate; block
31. deficiency
32. urticaria

Teach People about Pathophysiology

Compare your answers with these sample answers.

33. You are correct that phagocytic cells normally dispose of immune complexes when they form. However, in situations when immune complexes are of a certain intermediate size, they are not phagocytized as effectively. Those immune complexes are the ones that deposit in various tissues and cause type III, or immune complex-mediated, hypersensitivity reactions.
34. *Combined* refers to two parts of the immune system that do not work in SCID: the antibody part, also called *humoral immunity,* and the T lymphocyte part, also called *cell-mediated immunity.* In some other immunodeficiencies, one or the other of the parts does not work, but because both parts are not working in SCID, it is called a *combined immunodeficiency.*

Answer Key

Copyright © 2024 by Elsevier, Inc. All Rights Reserved.

35. Calling it a secondary immunodeficiency does not mean that it is unimportant. It means that the immunodeficiency was caused by something outside your immune system, rather than being a problem that started with your immune system. As you know, the cancer drugs suppressed your immunity. That is why we call it secondary immunodeficiency. We think it is very important also and are working to protect you from infection.

36. It takes 1 to 3 days for any reaction to develop, so we would not see any response in an hour. The type of response that causes a positive test is called a *delayed hypersensitivity response* because it arises so slowly. It is important for you to have a qualified person look at it later this week. Let us talk about how you can arrange that.

Clinical Scenario

37. The malar rash of SLE commonly is called a *butterfly rash* because it has the shape of a butterfly with extended wings.

38. Photosensitivity is common with SLE. Her rash is most prominent on sun-exposed areas of her skin.

39. Her elevated BUN and creatinine and urine protein indicate renal dysfunction, which is common with SLE.

40. Remissions and exacerbations of symptoms, arthralgia, pleurisy (pleural friction rub), anemia and mild thrombocytopenia, and positive ANA and anti-DNA antibodies all can occur with SLE.

41. Antinuclear antibodies (antibodies against normal nuclear antigens) are important autoantibodies that participate in the pathophysiology of SLE.

42. SLE is an autoimmune disease, with antibodies against self-antigens causing type III hypersensitivity reactions and other autoimmune processes in many different body tissues.

43. Type III hypersensitivity is an immune complex-mediated reaction in which an antigen–antibody complex lodges in tissue, activating complement, and attracting phagocytes that cause tissue damage.

CHAPTER 10

Match the Definitions
1. B
2. D
3. A
4. C

Circle the Correct Words
5. emerging
6. mechanical
7. one person to another
8. Exotoxins, endotoxins
9. colonization
10. capsule
11. avoid recognition by the host

Categorize the Microorganisms
12. Fungus
13. Bacterium
14. Fungus
15. Parasite
16. Fungus
17. Bacterium
18. Fungus
19. Bacterium
20. Parasite
21. Bacterium
22. Bacterium

Order the Steps
23. B, G, A, F, D, E, H, C

Explain the Pictures
24. B
25. Yeast
26. Window period
27. Virus multiplies in mucosa and lymphoid tissue and spreads widely; the adaptive immune system eventually recognizes it and begins to make antibodies against it, which ends the window period.
28. Clinical latency
29. None

Describe the Differences
30. Endemic refers to diseases that constantly have a relatively stable infection rate in a particular population, but epidemic refers to diseases that have a much greater infection rate than usual in a particular population.
31. Epidemic refers to diseases that have a much greater infection rate than usual in a particular population, but pandemic refers to diseases that have a much greater infection rate than usual in a very large area such as a continent or the entire world.
32. Pathogenicity is the ability of an organism to cause disease, but immunogenicity is the ability of an organism to induce an immune response.
33. Biological vectors transmit infectious microorganisms through bites and stings, but mechanical vectors transmit them passively.

Complete the Sentences
34. pili; fimbriae also is correct
35. prodromal
36. negative; endotoxin
37. incubation
38. biofilms
39. CD4
40. mycoses
41. erythrocytes; anemia
42. disseminated
43. ß-lactamase
44. zoonotic

Copyright © 2024 by Elsevier, Inc. All Rights Reserved.

Teach People about Pathophysiology

Compare your answers with these sample answers.

45. You are correct that viruses reproduce inside cells. However, a virus must reach the cell and attach to it before it can go inside and reproduce. If you have antibodies against a flu virus, the antibodies can bind to the virus outside the cells and keep it from attaching and entering cells. That way the virus will not be able to reproduce and will not make you sick.

46. The term your doctor used is *opportunistic infection*, which does sound a lot like opportunity infection. That means an infection with a microorganism that does not cause infection in persons whose immune system are functioning fully but that can cause infection in persons whose immune system are suppressed like yours. The microorganism seizes the opportunity when the immune defenses are low.

47. The white blood cell soldiers that protect you from measles need to be reminded to do their job from time to time. This shot is a reminder shot. The shot you had when you were a baby caused your white blood cell soldiers to be alert for measles and protect you then, but now you are a big boy, and they need a reminder.

48. HIV does destroy CD4$^+$ cells, but right now your body is able to produce them as fast as the virus destroys them. That is why your CD4$^+$ cell count is normal.

49. Nurses follow universal precautions that are expected for all bodily fluids. Bowel movements can transmit other organisms. If there is blood in the bowel movement, it can transmit HIV, hepatitis B and C, and other blood-borne infections as well.

50. What you have is HIV infection, not AIDS. There is a difference between HIV infection and AIDS. Your positive test tells us that you are infected with the virus but you do not have the low CD4$^+$ cell count or infections that characterize AIDS. You do not have AIDS; you have HIV infection. You can fight your HIV infection by taking the antiretroviral pills that the doctor prescribed. Would you like me to explain these pills to you now?

51. Kaposi sarcoma initially is visible as a skin cancer, but it can spread inside the body. Because your immune system is suppressed, your immune cells cannot destroy abnormal cells as well as they should, so Kaposi sarcoma can arise and spread internally.

Clinical Scenario

52. Because he is immunosuppressed, his immune system did not detect and eliminate the abnormal cells, as a fully functional immune system does.

53. HIV destroys infected CD4$^+$ T cells by reproducing inside them and destroys uninfected CD4$^+$ T cells as well, by inducing apoptosis.

54. CD4$^+$ T cells are helper T cells, the type of adaptive immune cells that secrete the cytokines that activate and regulate innate immune cells as well as other adaptive immune cells. With fewer helper T cells available, the entire immune system is impaired. Microorganisms that the immune system normally keeps in check will multiply, establishing an opportunistic infection such as *Pneumocystis* pneumonia.

55. More than 6 years; likely 8 to 10 years.

56. The initial acute clinical manifestations of HIV infection are mild and non-specific (muscle aching, fatigue, low-grade fever). Years of clinical latency follow, with no signs and symptoms. Because he did not have his blood tested, Mr. Hohner did not know that he had HIV infection until it progressed to AIDS.

Assessment Finding	Kaposi Sarcoma	Pneumocystis Pneumonia
57. Shortness of breath and cough		X
58. Reddish-brown, flat lesions on chest and arms	X	
59. Elevated respiratory rate		X
60. Crackles in the lower half of lung fields, with inspiratory and expiratory rhonchi		X

CHAPTER 11

Match the Definitions

1. D
2. B
3. A
4. C

Identify the Effects of Sympathetic Nervous System Activation

5. Increased
6. Increased
7. Increased
8. Decreased
9. Decreased
10. Increased
11. Increased

Circle the Correct Words

12. non-specific; Hans Selye
13. memory; anticipation
14. leads directly to
15. dementia
16. increases

Answer Key

Copyright © 2024 by Elsevier, Inc. All Rights Reserved.

17. anabolic; catabolic
18. increases; increases
19. cortisol
20. uncontrollable

Categorize the Clinical Situations
21. Reactive
22. Reactive
23. Anticipatory
24. Reactive
25. Reactive
26. Anticipatory

Explain the Picture
27. A = Corticotropin-releasing hormone (CRH); B = Adrenocorticotropic hormone (ACTH); C = cortisol
28. Circles 1 through 4 are + (plus; activating); circles 5 and 6 are – (minus; inhibitory).
29. Negative feedback
30. Circle 4

Identify the Effects of Coping Strategies
31. Beneficial
32. Beneficial
33. Maladaptive
34. Maladaptive
35. Beneficial

Complete the Sentences
36. systemic
37. stress
38. catecholamines
39. corticotropin; HPA
40. adrenergic
41. fibroblasts
42. increased; increased
43. allostatic
44. oxytocin
45. stimulate; suppress
46. cortisol
47. anti-inflammatory

Teach People about Pathophysiology
Compare your answers with these sample answers.

48. The response to stimuli such as the sight of an oximeter depends on the individual's perception. An individual who perceives it as a threat will have a stress response, but an individual who perceives it as non-threatening will not have that response.
49. Immune cells have a lot of receptors in their cell membranes that make them responsive to circulating hormones like epinephrine and to other chemical messengers that increase during the stress response.
50. When we are frightened, our brains turn on the signals that make our hearts beat faster and more strongly. That is a normal response to a scary event. What can I do to help make your chemo less scary? Do you want to watch a video?
51. When you are stressed, your immune cells increase their antibody-making activity and decrease some other activities. That shift in function can make your allergies worse.

Work with the Clinical Scenario
52. Blood glucose, plasma free fatty acids, heart rate, blood pressure
53. B

CHAPTER 12

Name the Neoplasms
1. E
2. A
3. I
4. G
5. H
6. C
7. B
8. F
9. J
10. D

Circle the Correct Words
11. regrow
12. multiple
13. proto-oncogene; oncogene
14. liver
15. heterogeneous
16. oxidative phosphorylation; glycolysis
17. genes
18. Chronic

Match the Definitions
19. E
20. F
21. A
22. C
23. D
24. B

Categorize the Changes
25. Procancer effect
26. Procancer effect
27. Anticancer effect
28. Procancer effect
29. Procancer effect
30. Procancer effect
31. Anticancer effect
32. Procancer effect
33. Procancer effect

Order the Steps
34. D, B, F, C, A, G, E

Copyright © 2024 by Elsevier, Inc. All Rights Reserved.

Complete the Chart

Characteristic	Benign Tumors	Malignant Tumors
Appearance of the Cells	Well differentiated	Poorly differentiated
Usual Rate of Growth	Slow	Rapid
Presence of Capsule	Yes	No
Vascularization	Slight	Neovascularization through angiogenesis
Mode of Growth	Expansile	Invasive
Ability to Metastasize	No	Yes

Explain the Picture

35. T = Tumor (size and extent of tumor); N = Nodes (lymph node involvement); M = Metastases (extent of distant metastases)
36. Stage
37. T3 N2 M1

Describe the Differences

38. A proto-oncogene is a normal gene that codes for proteins that stimulate cell proliferation appropriately, but an oncogene is a proto-oncogene that is mutated in such a way that its proteins are inappropriately active, accelerating cell proliferation.
39. A proto-oncogene codes for proteins that stimulate cell proliferation, but a tumor-suppressor gene codes for proteins that suppress cell proliferation.
40. A driver mutation is important for cancer progression, but a passenger mutation is a random mutation that probably does not contribute to cancer progression.

Complete the Sentences

41. telomerase
42. angiogenic
43. in situ
44. genomic; increases
45. autocrine
46. independence
47. macrophages
48. HPV

Teach People about Pathophysiology

Compare your answers with these sample answers.

49. Cancer cells often secrete chemicals, such as parathyroid hormone-related peptide, that circulate to bone and cause bone resorption, which releases calcium into the blood.
50. Cancer starts in one location, and then cancer cells can break off and travel to a new location, where they form another tumor, in a process called *metastasis*. The first place where cancer starts is called the *primary tumor.* So the cancer in your uncle's body started in his liver. The cancer in your mother's body started in another location, and cells from that primary tumor broke off and moved to your mother's liver. That is why her liver cancer is called *metastatic.*

51. Some cancers release substances into the blood that cause effects elsewhere in the body. Those effects are called *paraneoplastic syndromes.* Your husband's cancer cells release a substance called *antidiuretic hormone (ADH)* into the blood that is causing a paraneoplastic syndrome. The word *ectopic* means that the hormone ADH is released from an abnormal place, your husband's lung cancer. Normally, the pituitary gland releases ADH, but feedback controls keep it from making too much ADH. The cancer cells do not have feedback controls, so they keep releasing too much ADH.
52. The Warburg effect describes how cancer cells derive their energy for rapid cellular growth by metabolizing large amounts of glucose rapidly by glycolysis, even in the presence of oxygen (aerobic glycolysis). That is different from normal cells, which rely on glycolysis for most of their energy only when there is not enough oxygen (anaerobic glycolysis).
53. No, the reverse Warburg effect does not involve cancer cells making glucose. They need energy to fuel their rapid growth. The reverse Warburg effect involves cancer cells influencing tumor-associated fibroblasts to use glycolysis, even in the presence of oxygen (aerobic glycolysis). The tumor-associated fibroblasts then secrete metabolites that the cancer cells can use for fuel.

Clinical Scenarios

54. Bronchogenic carcinoma arises in the lining of the airways and can cause an obstruction as it grows inward into the lumen.
55. Her cancer arose in her lung. The term *bronchogenic* means that the tumor arose in the bronchi.
56. Obstruction to airflow due to the tumor in the airway and compression of lung tissue from an expanding tumor both can contribute to dyspnea in persons who have bronchogenic carcinoma.
57. Repeated exposure to cigarette smoke causes squamous metaplasia in the bronchi, which means that the normal pseudostratified columnar epithelial cells are replaced with squamous cells that can survive more easily in the harsh environment. One or more of these squamous cells eventually accumulated enough mutations to become malignant.

Copyright © 2024 by Elsevier, Inc. All Rights Reserved.

58. Bronchogenic carcinoma frequently metastasizes to the liver.

59. Bronchogenic carcinoma usually does not cause symptoms in its early stages; by the time the cancer is discovered, the tumor may be advanced, and there has been time for metastasis to occur.

60. They look at the size of the tumor, how many lymph nodes it has involved, and if it has spread to distant locations in the body.

61. Metastasis. That means the cancer cells have traveled in the blood or the lymph and have formed a new tumor distant from the primary one. The liver is a common place for cancer metastasis.

62. No, cancer can arise in the liver, just as it can arise in the colon. Cancer arises when the genetic material in the cells develops mutations that cause the cells to multiply in an uncontrolled fashion and develop the characteristics of cancer cells.

63. Chemotherapy drugs kill cells that are dividing rapidly. That kills cancer cells, but it also kills some normal cells like the cells in the lining of your mouth. So the drugs that helped get rid of the cancer also made those painful sores. Now that you are no longer receiving chemotherapy, your body has repaired the lining of your mouth.

64. No, chemotherapy drugs usually do not kill red blood cells, but they can kill the rapidly dividing cells in your bone marrow that make the red blood cells. Normally, we make new red blood cells all the time to replace the old ones; during your chemo treatment, you were not making enough new red blood cells. Now that you have recovered, your bone marrow is able to make enough red blood cells.

65. Pain usually does not occur until a cancer is advanced. Your cancer was detected early, before the tumor had grown big enough to put pressure on nerves or cause a lot of tissue destruction and inflammation.

CHAPTER 13

Match the Definitions
1. C
2. A
3. B

Circle the Correct Words
4. silence; methylation
5. immune
6. cell phones
7. decrease
8. xenobiotics
9. myokines; decrease
10. methylation
11. increases

Categorize the Dietary Factors
12. anticancer
13. anticancer
14. procancer
15. anticancer
16. procancer

Complete the Sentences
17. carcinogens
18. environmental
19. nutrigenomics
20. plasticity
21. weight
22. adipokines
23. Ultraviolet; basal; melanoma
24. Ionizing
25. Asbestos; radon
26. activating; deactivating

Match the Microorganisms
27. B
28. D
29. A
30. C

Teach People about Pathophysiology
Compare your answers with these sample answers.

31. Examples of similar foods to avoid are sausages and meats that are smoked or cured, such as bacon. After you eat them, nitrites get changed into chemicals that can damage the genetic material inside your cells and encourage development of cancer.

32. Actually, drinking a lot of beer can increase your cancer risk. Whether you drink beer or vodka does not matter because both contain alcohol (ethanol, to use the technical word). The alcohol itself is what increases the risk for cancer.

33. The good news is that HPV does not infect the bones. If you have had anal or oral sex, then you might want to have those areas checked, but HPV will not cause cancer in your bones.

34. The term *bystander effects* does not mean that a person was exposed to radiation. What it means is that cells near the irradiated cells also can be affected, even if they do not receive radiation directly.

35. Transgenerational effects of a carcinogen occur in germline cells, which affects future generations of people. Multigenerational effects involve simultaneous direct exposure of people from multiple generations to the same carcinogen.

Work with This Scenario
36. Mr. Ortiz works in the dye department of a textile factory. He lives 3 blocks from a petrochemical plant. Several times a week, he goes to a bar with his friends after their work shift, and drinks beer until closing time. He usually eats hot dogs or sausages at the bar for dinner. He does not smoke cigarettes, but the bar is smoky from others who do smoke. Mr. Ortiz cannot afford a cell phone or a car. If he needs to ask a friend to drive him somewhere that is not within walking distance, he repays them by helping remove old siding and flooring from abandoned houses they are trying to make livable.

Copyright © 2024 by Elsevier, Inc. All Rights Reserved.

CHAPTER 14

Describe the Cancers
1. D
2. A
3. C
4. B

Categorize the Cancers
5. Adults
6. Children/adolescents
7. Children/adolescents
8. Adults
9. Children/adolescents
10. Children/adolescents

Circle the Correct Words
11. more
12. leukemia
13. rapidly
14. less than 5 years; 15-19 years
15. proto-oncogenes; oncogenes
16. blast

Match the Risks
17. D
18. A
19. B
20. C

Complete the Sentences
21. leukemia
22. testicular
23. leukemia
24. Kaposi; lymphoma
25. multifactorial
26. tumor suppressor

Teach People about Pathophysiology
Compare your answers with these sample answers.

27. Mr. Johnson, it takes a long time for cancer to develop after exposure to the chemicals that are linked to adult cancers. We have not seen strong linkages between environmental chemicals and neuroblastoma in children. Cancers that have the term *blast* in their name arise from immature cells that are unable to mature fully. We are not sure why that happens, but it is very unlikely that chemicals in your home caused your daughter's cancer.
28. Before a baby is born, when it first is growing and developing in the uterus, there are different areas that give rise to different parts of the body. Cancers in children often arise from the area called the *mesodermal germ layer*. The term *germ* does not mean bacteria or other germs. It means the original place from which the body parts develop.
29. Mr. Talison, your son's diagnosis is not a death sentence. More than 80% of the children who are diagnosed with cancer are cured. We shall talk together with your cancer care team and look at the treatment options and the supports that are available for your family.
30. A useful way to think about such studies is the concept of multiple causation or multifactorial etiology. This concept carries the idea that cancer develops because environmental factors interact with predisposing characteristics of the individual. So it is not the pesticides alone that cause leukemia, but the interaction of the pesticides and particular characteristics of the children.
31. Most adult carcinomas are caused by environmental exposure to carcinogens. Children have not lived long enough to be exposed to carcinogens with subsequent malignant transformation of cells, so childhood carcinomas are much less common.

CHAPTER 15

Match the Definitions
1. D
2. F
3. J
4. H
5. C
6. A
7. I
8. B
9. G
10. E

Categorize the Physiologic Effects
11. Sympathetic
12. Sympathetic
13. Parasympathetic
14. Sympathetic
15. Parasympathetic
16. Parasympathetic
17. Sympathetic
18. Sympathetic
19. Sympathetic
20. Sympathetic
21. Parasympathetic

Explain the Pictures
22. D
23. B
24. C
25. Axon hillock

Copyright © 2024 by Elsevier, Inc. All Rights Reserved.

26.

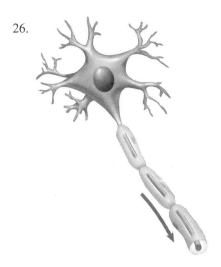

27. Multipolar
28. Node of Ranvier
29. Allows rapid conduction velocity, through saltatory conduction
30. D
31. F
32. Axons
33. Area A is the gray matter, which contains cell bodies of interneurons, and area B is the white matter, which contains tracts of axons, many of which are myelinated.

Circle the Correct Words

34. do not need
35. plasticity
36. divergence
37. potential; real
38. extrapyramidal
39. gray; skeletal
40. sympathetic; parasympathetic
41. sympathetic; postganglionic

Order the Structures

42. A, J, C, G, E, H, F, D, B, I

Match the Functions

43. D
44. F
45. C
46. E
47. A
48. G
49. B

Describe the Differences

50. Efferent nerves carry impulses away from the central nervous system (CNS), but afferent nerves carry impulses toward the CNS.
51. The somatic nervous system consists of sensory pathways and motor pathways that govern voluntary motor control of skeletal muscle, but the autonomic nervous system consists of sensory and motor pathways that regulate primarily involuntary function of body organ systems.
52. A gyrus is a convolution of the cerebral cortex; a sulcus is a shallow groove between adjacent gyri; and a fissure is a deeper groove between adjacent gyri.
53. The cranial nerves arise from the brain and pass through foramina (openings) in the skull, but the spinal nerves arise from the spinal cord and pass through intervertebral foramina of the vertebrae.
54. An excitatory postsynaptic potential (EPSP) is a small depolarization that occurs in a postsynaptic neuron and promotes creation of an action potential, but an inhibitory postsynaptic potential (IPSP) is a small hyperpolarization that occurs in a postsynaptic neuron and inhibits creation of an action potential.

Complete the Sentences

55. 31; cranial
56. neuroglia
57. neuron
58. oligodendroglia; Schwann cells
59. ganglia; nuclei
60. choroid; arachnoid
61. cleft
62. pineal
63. dopamine
64. decussate
65. wallerian; Schwann
66. eyes; tongue; XI

Teach People about Pathophysiology

Compare your answers with these sample answers.

67. Both doctors are correct. The difference is based on how different parts of the brain are connected to the rest of the body. The nerves that come down from the primary motor area of the brain cross over to the opposite side before they communicate to the nerves that tell the muscles what to do. So a stroke that affects the left arm and leg will be in the right side of the brain. On the other hand, the nerves that come from the cerebellum do not cross over, but rather stay on the same side. So an injury to the cerebellum that affects coordination on the left side of the body will be in the left side of the cerebellum.
68. Test face for pain, touch, and temperature, using a safety pin and hot and cold objects; test corneal reflex with a wisp of cotton; test motor function of face by asking her to clench her teeth, open her mouth against resistance, and move her jaw from side to side.
69. The names of spinal tracts provide the necessary information. The first part of the name tells where the tract begins. The second part of the name tells where the tract ends; that is where the axons synapse. So, the rubrospinal tract begins in the red nucleus and goes down the spinal cord; it is a motor tract. The spinothalamic tract begins in the spinal cord and goes to the thalamus in the brain; it is a sensory tract.
70. If his head leans to the side, that could compress a neck vein and increase the pressure in his brain.

307

Copyright © 2024 by Elsevier, Inc. All Rights Reserved.

Puzzle Out the Technical Terms

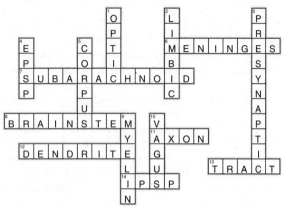

CHAPTER 16

Match the Definitions

1. E
2. C
3. F
4. A
5. B
6. D

Circle the Correct Words

7. conduction
8. norepinephrine; brown
9. increases
10. higher; lower
11. absence; rapid
12. glaucoma
13. transduction
14. phantom

Categorize the Sleep Disorders

15. Dyssomnia; B
16. Parasomnia; D
17. Dyssomnia; E
18. Dyssomnia; A
19. Dyssomnia; C

Order the Sleep Stages

20. A, E, D, B, C

Explain the Picture

21. C
22. Pain sensations from one side of the body go to the contralateral side of the brain. A brain injury in the sensory area on one side of the brain will cause a sensory defect on the opposite side of the body.
23. Paleospinothalamic and neospinothalamic
24. A-delta
25. In the substantia gelatinosa in the posterior (dorsal) horn of the gray matter of the spinal cord

Describe the Differences

26. Anosmia is the loss of the sense of smell, but ageusia is the loss of the sense of taste.

27. Conductive hearing loss occurs when sound waves cannot be transmitted through the middle ear, but sensorineural hearing loss occurs when there is a defective function of the organ of Corti or its central connections.
28. Fever is elevated body temperature caused by an increased hypothalamic set point, but hyperthermia is elevated body temperature without an increased hypothalamic set point.
29. Strabismus is deviation of one eye from the other when a person is looking at an object, but nystagmus is involuntary rhythmic movement of one or both eyes.
30. Presbycusis is loss of hearing for high-frequency sounds in older adults, but presbyopia is loss of accommodation of the lens of the eye, impairing near vision in older adults.

Complete the Sentences

31. hypothalamus; conservation
32. non-REM
33. REM
34. stye; sebaceous
35. REM
36. conjunctivitis
37. optic; increased
38. diplopia; ptosis
39. referred
40. central sensitization
41. sympathetic

Teach People about Pathophysiology

Compare your answers with these sample answers.

42. When you exercise, your body generates more heat. Leaving the sweat on your skin while you are exercising is beneficial because it evaporates, removing excessive heat from your body. That is a protection against heat illness. Think of being sweaty during exercise as a sign that you are taking steps to be stronger and healthier.
43. When our immune cells respond to the tissue injury of surgery, they secrete chemicals that we call endogenous pyrogens. These chemicals circulate to the hypothalamus and trigger fever, just like the exogenous pyrogens that you mentioned.
44. Do not worry because he is pale; that is a normal response to a cold body temperature. The body directs blood away from the skin to keep heat from leaving the body. That makes the skin look pale.
45. Glaucoma is too much pressure inside your eye. Although you cannot feel it, that excessive pressure slowly damages your eyes and eventually can cause blindness. You need to use the eyedrops to protect your vision.

Clinical Scenarios

46. Heat exhaustion; Lying flat, supine
47. Mr. Redd should be positioned flat because he has a decreased circulating blood volume; lying flat will increase perfusion of his brain.
48. He developed heat exhaustion from the interplay of several factors. He was producing heat with physical labor in a hot environment; thermoregulatory

Copyright © 2024 by Elsevier, Inc. All Rights Reserved.

mechanisms caused him to sweat profusely, but he was not able to replace the water and salt loss from the sweat, so he became dehydrated.

49. As Mr. Redd's body temperature began to rise, his hypothalamus triggered widespread cutaneous vasodilation. The combination of decreased circulating blood volume and widespread cutaneous vasodilation caused his blood pressure to decrease so that he was not able to perfuse his brain.

50. Tachycardia arose because Mr. Redd's arterial baroreceptors sensed his decreased blood pressure and stimulated his sympathetic cardioaccelerator nerves.

51. Mr. Redd needs to replace his sweat losses with water that has some sodium (salt) in it, such as salty broth or commercial electrolyte replacement fluid. He may tolerate room temperature fluid better than cold fluid at this point.

52. Employee heath personnel need to teach Mr. Redd to manage his sweat losses with water and some salt during his workday. They also need to teach Mr. Redd's supervisor the importance of frequent fluid replacement while working in a hot environment and be sure that appropriate fluids are provided in a convenient location.

53. Her injured tissue is inflamed and produces inflammatory mediators, some of which sensitize her nociceptors and some of which actually excite them to fire.

54. Glutamate

55. Increased activation of her sympathetic nervous system. (If you answered autonomic nervous system, remember that the autonomic nervous system has two branches, sympathetic and parasympathetic. The sympathetic system caused her clinical response to acute pain.)

56. Cool, clammy skin; dilated pupils; elevated blood glucose and free fatty acids

57. Non-nociceptive stimulation from touch can cause stimulate inhibitory interneurons in the dorsal horn of the spinal cord and decrease the sensation of pain. This is an example of segmental pain modulation.

58. Chronic peripheral neuropathic pain

59. Physiologic adaptation to persistent chronic pain occurs, so the sympathetic nervous system is not highly activated.

60. Neuropathic pain occurs when nerves are damaged. The injured nerves become hyperexcitable and fire in the absence of pain signals from the tissues. On the other hand, nociceptive pain occurs when the free nerve endings of primary pain afferents respond to stimuli from the tissues. In other words, nociceptive pain occurs when the nerves are intact.

CHAPTER 17

Match the Definitions
1. F
2. G
3. A
4. H
5. C
6. D

7. B
8. E

Circle the Correct Words
9. intention; ataxic
10. hyperventilatory; carbon dioxide
11. brainstem; nearby
12. greatly
13. vasogenic
14. upper; lower
15. spasticity
16. both upper and lower
17. abnormal movement
18. muscle; language

Categorize the Dysfunctions
19. Hypokinesia
20. Hyperkinesia
21. Hypertonia
22. Hyperkinesia
23. Hypokinesia
24. Hyperkinesia
25. Hyperkinesia
26. Hypertonia
27. Hyperkinesia
28. Hypertonia

Order the Levels of Consciousness
29. D, B, C, E, G, A, F

Explain the Pictures
30. Flexed; extended
31. Decorticate
32. Cerebral cortex
33. Extended; extended
34. Decerebrate
35. Brainstem

Describe the Differences
36. Hyperkinesia is excessive movement, but hypertonia is abnormally increased muscle tone.
37. Arousal is a state of being awake, but awareness involves content of thought.
38. Delirium is an acute confusional state caused by dysfunction of neurons and is potentially reversible; dementia is a confusional state caused by death of neurons and is not reversible.
39. Paralysis is loss of the voluntary motor function, but paresis is weakness (partial paralysis) of the voluntary motor function.
40. Paraplegia is paralysis of both lower extremities, but hemiplegia is paralysis of the upper and lower extremities on one side of the body.

Complete the Sentences
41. postures
42. emotion
43. hydrocephalus
44. stops

Copyright © 2024 by Elsevier, Inc. All Rights Reserved.

45. herniate
46. dominant; involuntary
47. flaccidity; spasticity
48. cerebelli
49. brainstem
50. prefrontal
51. vegetative

Compare the Demyelinating Disorders

Characteristic	Multiple Sclerosis	Guillain-Barré Syndrome
Location of the Demyelinated Axons	Central nervous system	Peripheral
Pathogenesis of the Demyelination	Genetic predisposition; T cells autoreactive against myelin enter the brain; autoreactive B cells produce autoantibodies; microglial activation and inflammation destroy myelin sheaths, denuding axons	Often triggered by an infection; T cells autoreactive against myelin infiltrate into nerves; macrophages destroy myelin sheaths, denuding axons
Signs and Symptoms	Quite variable, depending on the location of lesions; diplopia, motor decrements, urinary and bowel dysfunction	Ascending flaccid paralysis, from the feet upward; respiratory muscle weakness may occur; possible sensory changes
Usual Clinical Course	Remissions and exacerbations, with decreasing baseline; or steadily declining course	Return of the motor function, descending from the neck to toes; some people have residual weakness
Cells that Produce Myelin during Remyelination	Oligodendrocytes	Schwann cells

Clinical Scenarios

52. Neuritic (amyloid) plaques and neurofibrillary tangles. The plaques are collections of fragments of amyloid-beta protein that accumulate extracellularly in the brain, disrupt neural transmission, and cause death of the neurons. Neurofibrillary tangles are collections of chemically altered tau proteins detached from microtubules that occur intracellularly, disrupt transport processes within the neurons, and also contribute to neuronal death.
53. Many years, even decades
54. Her hippocampus, an area of the brain important for memory and learning
55. Alzheimer disease is progressive, and so far we do not have a way to stop it. The damage is spreading to other parts of her brain, like the part responsible for judgment. We have some resources to help you modify her environment to keep her safe, if you would like them.
56. Forward-flexed (stooped) posture; narrow-based, short-stepped (shuffling) gait that becomes faster as the person walks (festination); loss of postural righting reflexes; muscle rigidity; postural hypotension caused by altered autonomic function and medication side effect; impaired proprioception
57. An extrapyramidal disorder. Motor manifestations are a result of death of dopaminergic neurons that innervate the basal ganglia (the nigrostriatal pathway), causing a deficiency of dopamine and thus altered neurotransmission in pathways that facilitate and inhibit movement.
58. Soft speech is a characteristic of Parkinson disease, in part caused by bradykinesia and muscle rigidity that reduce airflow during speech, but also caused by altered sensory perception of the effort expended in vocal production.
59. People who have Parkinson disease, such as Mr. Armstrong, have an expressionless face because of muscle rigidity and loss of associated movements caused by their disease. The nonverbal cues that convey emotions are less visible to us. He has a broken hip and says he is in pain; his heart rate, respiratory rate, blood pressure, and blood glucose are elevated, all of which often accompany acute pain. I am sure he needs the pain medication now.
60. Our eyes have muscles attached to them that control how the eyes move. Normally, both eyes are coordinated so that we see only one image because our nerves tell our eye muscles how to work together. The places where the nerves tell the muscles what to do are called *neuromuscular junctions.* Myasthenia gravis involves abnormal antibodies that change the neuromuscular junctions so that they do not work as well. Therefore, your eye muscles become less coordinated and you see double.

Answer Key

Copyright © 2024 by Elsevier, Inc. All Rights Reserved.

61.

Assessment Finding	Myasthenic Crisis	Cholinergic Crisis
Muscle weakness and twitching, often starting within an hour after taking prescribed anticholinesterase medication		X
Increasing muscle weakness, especially after using the muscles, with no twitching	X	
Diarrhea and intestinal cramping		X
Increased saliva and tears		X
Extreme difficulty breathing	X	X
Severe difficulty swallowing	X	
Constricted pupils		X
Heart beating slowly		X
Heart beating fast	X	

CHAPTER 18

Match the Definitions
1. D
2. C
3. B
4. A

Circle the Correct Words
5. dura mater
6. contrecoup; coup
7. venous
8. Infection
9. stretching and tearing
10. mobile

11. unilateral
12. ischemic; hypertension
13. inflammation; impair
14. cervical
15. viruses
16. metastatic; generalized
17. migraine

Categorize the Neural Injuries
18. Primary
19. Secondary
20. Primary
21. Primary
22. Tertiary
23. Secondary

Complete the Chart

Function Below the Level of a Complete Spinal Cord Lesion	During the Period of Spinal Shock	After Return of Reflexes
Reflexes	Absent (areflexia)	Present, hyperactive
Motor	Flaccid paralysis	Spastic paralysis
Sensory	Absent	Absent
Bladder	Atonic	Reflex emptying
Bowels	Atonic	Reflex emptying

Copyright © 2024 by Elsevier, Inc. All Rights Reserved.

Match the Clinical Manifestations

24. C
25. D
26. A
27. B

Draw Your Answers

28.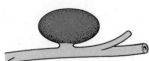

29.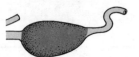

Describe the Differences

30. A brain contusion is a focal bruise that occurs when blood leaks from an injured blood vessel, but a concussion is a diffuse traumatic brain injury.
31. Although both of these conditions can occur after spinal cord injury, mass reflex involves flexor muscle spasms, profuse diaphoresis, piloerection, and automatic bladder emptying, but autonomic dysreflexia involves massive reflex firing of the sympathetic nerves below the level of injury, causing severe hypertension and other sympathetic nervous system manifestations.

Complete the Sentences

32. status epilepticus
33. epidural (or extradural)
34. consciousness; amnesia
35. excitotoxicity
36. vasogenic; low
37. cerebrovascular
38. pulposus
39. artery
40. tension
41. abscess
42. focus

Teach People about Pathophysiology

Compare your answers with these sample answers.

43. I know you are worried about Calvin's safety. See how Calvin is responding less and less to you when you try to talk with him? The bleeding above the surface of his brain is squeezing his brain and causing it to function poorly. It can damage his brain unless surgery is done to relieve the pressure.
44. Your brother and your friend have different types of injuries. Your friend has damage to the nerves that go from his spine to his leg muscles. Nerves are like electrical wires that send signals. Your friend's muscles do not get any signals, so they just lie there "flabby-like," as you said, and he cannot move them. Your brother has damage to different nerves: the ones that go down his spine from his brain. That is why he

cannot tell his legs to move. However, the nerves that go from his spine to his leg muscles are still working. His legs are spastic because his muscles are getting messages to contract, but those messages are no longer initiated or coordinated by his brain.
45. Multiple sclerosis damages the insulating myelin on nerve cells, and they do not work well. The signs and symptoms of multiple sclerosis are different in different people because the damage can occur many different places in the brain and spinal cord.
46. Severe headache and neck stiffness
47. We have several different kinds of cells in our brains. As you may know, the brain cells that transmit messages are called *neurons*. The neurons are not making your husband's brain tumor. We have other brain cells called *astrocytes* because they are somewhat star-shaped. The astrocytes are the ones that are reproducing out of control and becoming the tumor. "Oma" means *tumor,* so his tumor made of astrocytes is called an *astrocytoma.*

Clinical Scenarios

48. Right hemiparesis
49. Left side
50. Ischemic stroke
51. Atrial fibrillation is a risk factor for embolic ischemic stroke because blood clots formed in the left atria can embolize to the brain.
52. Cigarette smoking, obesity, high blood pressure, type 2 diabetes mellitus, and family history of cardiovascular and cerebrovascular disease all are risk factors for thrombotic ischemic stroke because they promote development of atherosclerosis. Rupture of an atherosclerotic plaque in a cerebral artery can trigger formation of a thrombus that occludes the artery.
53. Different areas of the brain control different functions. When a stroke damages part of the brain, that function is impaired. Your husband's stroke damaged the area of his brain that controls voluntary movement of his right arm and leg. His grandfather's stroke damaged another area of his brain: the area that controls speech.
54. Although the signs and symptoms of a TIA do go away, TIAs are a big risk factor for having another stroke. The same changes in your blood vessels that cause TIAs also cause strokes. That is why it is important to protect your blood vessels by taking your blood pressure and other medications, managing your diabetes and your weight, and working to stop smoking. I know these changes are challenging, but they help protect you from another stroke. Your doctor wants to know if you have a TIA so that she can help you.
55. Autonomic dysreflexia
56. Greatly elevated blood pressure and bradycardia
57. Uncontrolled reflex activation of sympathetic neurons below the level of injury increases blood pressure by increasing peripheral vascular resistance. Baroreceptor response above the level of injury causes the bradycardia.

Copyright © 2024 by Elsevier, Inc. All Rights Reserved.

58. The extremely high blood pressure could burst an intracerebral artery, causing a hemorrhagic stroke.

59. Sensory stimulation from a distended bladder or rectum, pressure ulcer, and wrinkles or foreign objects under the paralyzed portion of the body

60. Autonomic dysreflexia does not occur with T10 injury because so much of the sympathetic nervous system (SNS) still has supraspinal control with a T10 injury. For autonomic dysreflexia to occur, most of the SNS supraspinal control must be lost.

61. Your husband had a seizure, but that does not mean he has epilepsy. His seizure was caused by low blood sugar. Epilepsy is more than one seizure that does not have a clear underlying cause and meets other criteria. Your husband had one seizure, and we know that his low blood sugar caused it.

62. Generalized seizure. Focal seizures originate in one hemisphere, but generalized seizures involve both hemispheres from their onset.

63. Initial extensor muscle contraction with excessive muscle tone

64. Alternating flexion contraction and relaxation of muscles

65. He is in a postictal state.

66. Extreme muscle contraction during his seizure

CHAPTER 19

Match the Definitions
1. F
2. E
3. A
4. B
5. D
6. G
7. C

Circle the Correct Words
8. reduced; may not manifest
9. working; hypoactive
10. prenatal
11. mood
12. increased
13. hippocampus
14. pH
15. raphe nuclei; locus ceruleus
16. intrusive; increased; decreased
17. repetitive; ritualized

Categorize the Clinical Manifestations of Schizophrenia
18. Positive
19. Negative
20. Positive
21. Negative
22. Positive
23. Positive
24. Negative

Match the Assessments
25. D
26. A
27. B
28. E
29. C

Complete the Sentences
30. glutamate
31. excess; positive; deficit; negative
32. alogia
33. major
34. decreased; increased
35. agoraphobia
36. environmental
37. norepinephrine; serotonin
38. neurotrophic
39. ADHD

Teach People about Pathophysiology
Compare your answers with these sample answers.

40. The doctor is using the word *negative* to describe some symptoms of schizophrenia. Negative symptoms are things that we normally expect to see that are not happening. An example is David's not coming out of his room to talk with other people.

41. A hallucination is a false sensation, such as seeing, hearing, smelling, tasting, or feeling things that are not really there. A delusion is a persistent false belief, such as believing that someone is trying to poison you or that a person on television is talking personally to you.

42. One hypothesis about the neurobiology of schizophrenia is that too much dopamine effect on some neural pathways causes positive symptoms and too little dopamine effect in some other neural pathways causes the negative and cognitive symptoms of schizophrenia. Antipsychotic drugs block dopamine receptors and can decrease the positive symptoms of schizophrenia, but they also block dopamine receptors in other dopamine pathways. When these drugs block dopamine receptors in the basal ganglia, they cause the Parkinson-like side effects you are noticing.

43. Any of these changes that are different from Mr. Tennyson's usual behavior: no eye contact; mention of seeing, hearing, or smelling things in the room that the nurse cannot see; expressions of fear of being poisoned or controlled; speech incoherent or extremely rapid; deteriorated personal hygiene; not answering questions; difficulty paying attention.

44. People who are having a panic attack are very anxious, with intense sympathetic nervous system arousal, such as fast, pounding heart, shaky hands, and shortness of breath. On the other hand, people who are manic usually are euphoric and talk non-stop, very

Copyright © 2024 by Elsevier, Inc. All Rights Reserved.

fast, and loud. They skip rapidly from one topic to another and often announce grand plans that display poor judgment.

Clinical Scenarios

45. Delusion
46. The early brain defect can remain fairly undetected until further brain development requires adaptive use of the brain structures and overt dysfunction occurs.
47. A delusion is a persistent false belief, and no amount of reasoning will remove it. He will not believe you, no matter how much you show him his picture. Let's talk about some useful things that you could do for him.
48. Most antipsychotic medications decrease the positive symptoms but tend to make the negative ones worse. With effective medication, Mr. Trainor's delusion of being Julius Caesar and his sometimes-incoherent speech should diminish. His social withdrawal and poor personal hygiene may worsen.
49. Progressive loss of cortical tissue will continue, which can worsen negative and cognitive symptoms despite antipsychotic medications.
50. Major depression; dysphoric mood; insomnia; loss of appetite
51. Likely he has an underlying genetic vulnerability to depression that interacted with the stressor of having a myocardial infarction to cause the depression.
52. Reduction in the effects of brain monoamine neurotransmitters (serotonin, norepinephrine, dopamine)
53. Chronically elevated cortisol levels are found during major depression; this predisposes him to infection because chronically high cortisol level causes immunosuppression.

CHAPTER 20

Match the Definitions

1. C
2. D
3. A
4. B

Circle the Correct Words

5. folate
6. cerebellum; defect of neural tube closure
7. static
8. gait and bladder control; myelomeningocele
9. brain; 1 year
10. motor
11. epilepsy
12. 6

Characterize the Disorders

13. B, 2
14. E, 4
15. D, 5
16. A, 3
17. C, 1

Describe the Differences

18. A meningocele is a form of spina bifida in which the meninges protrude but the spinal cord remains in the spinal canal, but myelomeningocele is a form of spina bifida with protrusion of both the spinal cord and meninges through the skin.
19. Pyramidal cerebral palsy is spastic because it involves the pyramidal (corticospinal) pathways, which are upper motor neurons. Extrapyramidal cerebral palsy is non-spastic because it involves damage to basal ganglia or other brain areas that influence involuntary movement and coordination.

Complete the Sentences

20. hemorrhagic
21. aqueduct; hydrocephalus; cerebrospinal
22. bacteria
23. B; birth
24. enzyme; amino; tyrosine
25. retinoblastoma
26. pica; lead
27. brain tumor
28. location
29. closure

Teach People about Pathophysiology

Compare your answers with these sample answers.

30. Your baby is not paralyzed. He has meningitis, which means that his meninges (the membranes that surround his brain and spinal cord) are inflamed. Have you seen an inflamed finger or ankle? The inflamed part is painful when you try to move it. Baby Hector will not bend his neck because that would stretch his inflamed meninges and would be too painful. Straightening his legs also stretches his meninges, so that is why he cried. He will be more willing to move as his meningitis resolves.
31. What you described is normal. Little babies have that cute rooting reflex. As their nervous system matures, the reflex goes away. That normally happens at age 4 months when they are awake, so your baby is developing normally. See how he responds to your smile and your voice?
32. Hydrocephalus does mean having too much fluid in the brain, a special fluid called *cerebrospinal fluid*. The pictures you saw of hydrocephalus were little babies who developed hydrocephalus before the bones that form the skull had fused together. When babies are born, the pieces of their skull have not yet fused together, so there is room for their brains to grow. Remember when Jeannie was a baby and she had a fontanel? As she developed, her fontanel went away because her skull bones fused together and became solid. Infants who develop hydrocephalus that is not treated do get great big heads because their skulls can expand from the excess fluid. But when children whose skulls are solid, such as Jeannie, develop hydrocephalus, their skulls

Copyright © 2024 by Elsevier, Inc. All Rights Reserved.

cannot expand, and the excess fluid inside makes increased pressure that can cause brain damage. That is why the doctors need to work quickly to help Jeannie.

CHAPTER 21

Name the Hormones

1. Gland: pineal; One hormone: melatonin
2. Gland: hypothalamus; Six hormones: corticotropin-releasing hormone (CRH), thyrotropin-releasing hormone (TRH), growth hormone-releasing hormone (GHRH), somatostatin, gonadotropin-releasing hormone (GnRH), prolactin-releasing factor (PRF)
3. Gland: pituitary; Seven hormones from anterior: adrenocorticotropic hormone (ACTH), melanocyte-stimulating hormone (MSH), thyroid-stimulating hormone (TSH), growth hormone (GH), luteinizing hormone (LH), follicle-stimulating hormone (FSH), prolactin; Two hormones from posterior: antidiuretic hormone (ADH), oxytocin
4. Gland: thyroid; Three hormones: T_4, T_3, calcitonin
5. Gland: adrenal; Three hormones from cortex: aldosterone (mineralocorticoids), cortisol (glucocorticoids), adrenal androgens; Two hormones from medulla: epinephrine, norepinephrine
6. Gland: pancreas (islets); Four hormones: insulin, glucagon, amylin, somatostatin
7. Gland: parathyroid; One hormone: parathyroid hormone

Match the Definitions

8. C
9. E
10. D
11. B
12. A

Circle the Correct Words

13. a nerve tract; portal blood vessels
14. short; free
15. up-regulate; increases
16. cell membrane
17. proteins
18. GH
19. Lipid; DNA; nucleus
20. ACTH; cortex
21. insulin-like growth factors; somatomedins
22. medulla
23. increases; fight or flight response
24. gastrointestinal tract; decrease
25. decrease; increase
26. increase; inhibit; numerous
27. negative

Match the Functions

28. C
29. A
30. B

31. E
32. D

Explain the Picture

33. Anterior pituitary
34. B. Thyrotropin-releasing hormone (TRH); C. Thyroid-stimulating hormone (TSH)
35. D. +; E. –; F. +; G. –
36. Both will increase because the cells that secrete them no longer receive negative feedback from thyroid hormones.
37. Without the normal action of thyroid hormones on the target tissue, the metabolic rate will decrease and cells will produce less heat. Therefore, an individual is likely to gain weight and become intolerant to environmental cold.

Categorize the Hormones

38. Steroid
39. Peptide
40. Amine
41. Peptide
42. Peptide
43. Steroid
44. Peptide
45. Peptide
46. Steroid
47. Peptide
48. Amine

Complete the Sentences

49. posterior; anterior
50. cholesterol
51. vasopressin
52. receptors
53. cAMP
54. hypothalamus
55. thyroid
56. glucagon; amylin
57. thyroid; calcium
58. growth; growth factor

Describe the Differences

59. Direct effects of a hormone are changes in cell function that occur specifically from stimulation by a particular hormone, but permissive effects are less obvious hormone-induced changes that facilitate the maximal response or functioning of a cell.
60. Autocrine action is a hormone acting on the cell that produced it, but paracrine action is a hormone acting on a nearby cell that it reaches through the interstitial fluid.
61. Negative feedback occurs when the end result of hormone action on target cells suppresses secretion of that hormone, but positive feedback occurs when the end result of hormone action on target cells increases secretion of that hormone.

Copyright © 2024 by Elsevier, Inc. All Rights Reserved.

Teach People about Physiology

Compare your answers with these sample answers.

62. Urine insulin does not give us information about blood insulin levels because most insulin is destroyed in the body by enzymes and is not excreted in the urine.

63. A second messenger, like cGMP, is a substance released into a cell when the first messenger reaches the cell and signals it, but cannot enter the cell. The second messenger travels inside the cell and triggers cellular chemistry to happen, creating the clinical effects of that first messenger. For example, hormones and other signaling molecules that are small proteins cannot enter cells; they signal the cell from outside, which often causes a second messenger to be released. This is a normal process.

64. Although ADH is released from the posterior pituitary, it is synthesized in areas of the hypothalamus. Apparently the tumor damaged that portion of the hypothalamus, so they cannot make enough ADH.

65. We do make thyroid hormones every day, but then we store large amounts of those hormones in the thyroid glands. So when your new drug stops your thyroid gland from making new thyroid hormones, you still have a lot of stored thyroid hormones that will be released each day. Only after the stored ones are used up will we see the full drug effect.

66. Your blood calcium is abnormally high because your cancer cells make a substance similar to normal parathyroid hormone. Parathyroid hormone normally raises the blood calcium, but a negative feedback system decreases its production when calcium levels start to rise in the blood. The substance your cancer cells make acts like parathyroid hormone and raises blood calcium, but it is not controlled by negative feedback, and therefore your cancer cells are making too much of it.

67. Some hormones, such as ADH and ACTH, are water soluble and do not need carrier proteins in the blood. Thyroid hormones and steroid hormones are not water soluble, so they need carrier proteins.

68. Renin acts on a substance called *angiotensinogen,* which normally circulates in the blood. It converts it to angiotensin I. Then enzymes in the capillaries of the lungs convert angiotensin I to angiotensin II, which stimulates the cortex of the adrenal glands to secrete the hormone aldosterone. Aldosterone circulates to the kidneys and causes them to put more salt and water back into the blood. That kidney action increases the blood volume and can increase the blood flow in the kidney blood vessels.

CHAPTER 22

Match the Definitions

1. B
2. D
3. E
4. A
5. C

Sort the Disorders

6. SIADH; diabetes insipidus
7. Primary hyperthyroidism; primary hyperthyroidism
8. Cushing disease; secondary hyperthyroidism; secondary hypothyroidism

Circle the Correct Words

9. high
10. hypersecretion; hyposecretion
11. increased
12. 2; adipokines
13. 2
14. hypothyroidism
15. 1; cytotoxic T lymphocytes
16. amylin; glucagon
17. destruction of capillaries; damage to medium-sized and large arteries

Explain the Picture

18. Cushing
19. Cortisol excess causes lipolysis and altered fat distribution.
20. Bruising easily is part of Cushing disease because having too much cortisol causes proteins to break down and makes the small blood vessels very fragile.
21. ACTH. ACTH excess causes hyperpigmentation because excessive MSH is formed as an alternate cleavage product of the same hormone precursor. MSH stimulates production of melanin, a skin pigment.

Describe the Differences

22. A primary endocrine disorder is caused by a problem in the gland that secretes a hormone whose action is directed toward other tissues rather than to another gland, but a secondary endocrine disorder is caused by a problem with a gland that secretes a hormone whose target tissues are another gland that it stimulates or suppresses.

23. Thyrotoxicosis is the effects of having too much thyroid hormone, as seen with hyperthyroidism, but thyrotoxic crisis is the effects of dangerously high levels of thyroid hormone, with high fever, extreme tachycardia, and potential death from heart failure or cardiac dysrhythmias.

24. Neurogenic diabetes insipidus is caused by a problem in the hypothalamus or posterior pituitary that decreases ADH release, but nephrogenic diabetes insipidus is caused by a problem in the kidney itself that causes insensitivity to ADH.

25. Acromegaly occurs with hypersecretion of growth hormone in adults, but gigantism occurs with hypersecretion of growth hormone in children and adolescents whose epiphyseal plates have not yet closed, so their long bones are able to grow.

Answer Key

Copyright © 2024 by Elsevier, Inc. All Rights Reserved.

Match the Clinical Manifestations

26. F
27. E
28. A
29. H
30. I
31. G
32. J
33. C
34. B
35. D

Complete the Sentences

36. pituitary
37. pheochromocytomas
38. nephrogenic
39. panhypopituitarism
40. anterior; prolactinomas; galactorrhea
41. immune
42. myxedema; decreased
43. goiter; TSH
44. diabetic ketoacidosis
45. stones
46. disease; syndrome

Teach People about Pathophysiology

Compare your answers with these sample answers.

47. People who have type 2 diabetes make a little insulin, which goes to the liver and reduces the formation of ketoacids. People who have type 1 diabetes have severe insulin deficiency, and they have excessive fat breakdown and make ketoacids faster than the body can remove them.

48. A child who has too much growth hormone grows tall like a giant, but if an individual already is an adult before developing too much growth hormone, then the effects are different because the long bones have already stopped growing. Adults with growth hormone excess develop an enlarged jaw, forehead, and tongue, and large hands and feet, as you noticed with your wife.

49. Your parathyroid glands make parathyroid hormone and send it out into the blood. The parathyroid hormone circulates in the blood to your bones and changes them. The action of the parathyroid hormone takes a little calcium out of the bones. Because your body is making too much parathyroid hormone, too much calcium came out of your bones and made them weaker than they should be.

50. That does seem strange, doesn't it? However, there is a very good reason. Your nurses are monitoring for a complication of thyroid surgery that they can detect that way and get treated quickly if it occurs. During thyroid surgery, sometimes the parathyroid glands are injured because they are located right by the thyroid. With parathyroid gland injury, the blood calcium decreases and makes nerves and muscles jumpy and crampy. We can detect low blood calcium in the early stages with the blood pressure cuff as they are doing, so the nurses are taking good care of you.

51. Diabetes insipidus is different from diabetes mellitus, the sugar problem. Diabetes insipidus is a problem with a hormone called *antidiuretic hormone,* or *ADH.* ADH tells your kidneys to concentrate your urine. Diabetes insipidus occurs when the kidneys do not receive enough ADH signals. You may have noticed that the nurses are emptying your urine catheter bag very frequently. Your kidneys are making a lot of very dilute urine because ADH is not telling them to concentrate the urine.

52. Fat cells make signaling chemicals and release them into the blood. Some of these signaling chemicals cause your body to be resistant to the action of insulin, the hormone that normally moves sugar into cells. This makes your blood sugar too high. Insulin resistance is part of the problem in type 2 diabetes. If you lose weight, you will have less insulin resistance.

53. Your adrenal gland does not make enough cortisol and aldosterone, two hormones that normally help maintain your circulating blood volume. Without the normal action of these hormones, your blood volume gets too low. When you stand up, gravity pulls your blood downward, and if your blood volume is too low, your brain does not get enough blood to bring it the oxygen it needs. This makes you lightheaded.

54. His immune system killed the cells in his pancreas that normally make the hormone insulin.

Clinical Scenarios

55. Insulin resistance and pancreatic beta cell dysfunction
56. gastroparesis; autonomic neuropathy; microvascular
57. Diabetes is a sugar problem, but it affects many parts of the body. When blood sugar is high, it damages the tiny blood vessels that nourish our nerves and damages the nerves themselves too. Over time, some of the nerves stop working. The nerves that carry pain signals from your dad's heart have stopped working, so he did not feel any pain when he had his heart attack.
58. Diabetes speeds up the processes that cause hardening of the arteries, so the heart muscle gets less blood supply. The hardened, narrow arteries are likely to develop a clot, which cuts off the blood supply to the heart muscle and causes a heart attack.
59. Retinal cells are highly metabolic and need a good blood supply. Vision loss from diabetic retinopathy is progressive. Initially, microvascular disease from hyperglycemia causes thickening of the retinal capillary basement membranes, vein dilation, microaneurysm formation, and hemorrhages. Progression of retinal ischemia causes infarcts with scarring. Eventually, new blood vessels and fibrous tissue form within the retina or optic disc.
60. All of these factors can contribute to development of gangrene after a minor foot injury: diabetic neuropathy (lack of pain from injury); diabetic retinopathy (more difficult to examine feet); tissue hypoxia from capillary closure in microvascular disease and accelerated atherosclerosis in macrovascular disease;

317

Copyright © 2024 by Elsevier, Inc. All Rights Reserved.

Answer Key

impaired immune function and delayed healing from chronic hyperglycemia; glucose in tissues provides culture medium for pathogens.

61. He is at risk for diabetic nephropathy, which is manifested first by microalbuminuria.
62. Polyuria, hypotension, tachycardia, lethargy, confusion, stupor, coma
63. Weight loss with increased appetite
64. Oral temperature increased, resting heart rate increased (tachycardia)
65. Excessive thyroid hormones increase metabolic rate, thus increasing heat production.

66. Graves disease involves autoantibodies against TSH receptors called *thyroid-stimulating immunoglobulins (TSIs)*. The TSIs stimulate TSH receptors on the thyrocytes, causing the thyroid gland to secrete excess T_3 and T_4.
67. Exophthalmos. Fibroblasts located behind the eye have TSH receptors. Stimulation of these receptors by the TSI autoantibodies causes enlargement of the ocular muscles, accumulation of fat, and edema that push the eyeballs forward.
68. The autoantibodies against TSH receptors (TSIs) stimulated hyperplasia of her thyroid tissue, causing a goiter.

69.

Assessment Findings	Diabetic Ketoacidosis (DKA)	Type 1 Diabetes (without DKA)
Consumed an entire case of soda in one day and was asking for more		X
Became very sleepy and hard to awaken	X	

70. Cushing syndrome; fat redistribution; protein catabolism

CHAPTER 23

Match the Definitions
1. C
2. E
3. D
4. F
5. G
6. H
7. B
8. A

Circle the Correct Words
9. adipocyte hypertrophy
10. more
11. subcutaneous; visceral
12. orexigenic; anorexigenic
13. inhibit; stimulates
14. does not
15. proinflammatory; 2
16. glycogenolysis and gluconeogenesis

Categorize the Types of Adipose Tissue
17. Beige
18. Brown
19. Beige
20. Brown
21. White
22. Brown
23. White
24. White

Describe the Differences
25. Adipogenesis is formation of new fat cells, but adipocyte hypertrophy is enlargement of pre-existing fat cells.
26. Orexigenic neurons promote eating, but anorexigenic neurons inhibit eating.
27. Anorexia nervosa involves severe continued restriction of energy intake and a distorted body image, but bulimia nervosa involves recurrent episodes of severe overeating and compensatory behaviors such as self-induced vomiting or laxative overuse.
28. Bulimia nervosa involves recurrent episodes of severe overeating and compensatory behaviors such as self-induced vomiting or laxative overuse, but binge eating disorder involves recurrent episodes of severe overeating without the compensatory behaviors.
29. In short-term starvation, the body responds with glycogenolysis and gluconeogenesis with only a small amount of protein catabolism, but in long-term starvation, the body responds with lipolysis and eventually proteolysis, which can cause death.

Complete the Sentences
30. iron
31. non-shivering; brown
32. triglycerides
33. 30; exceeds
34. 25
35. arcuate; hypothalamus
36. portal
37. adipokines; macrophages
38. refeeding syndrome
39. anorexia

Answer Key

Copyright © 2024 by Elsevier, Inc. All Rights Reserved.

Choose Increase or Decrease

40. Increases
41. Decreases
42. Increases
43. Increases
44. Decreases
45. Increases
46. Increases

Teach People about Pathophysiology

47. You are correct about the normal action of leptin. However, obesity involves leptin resistance. With leptin resistance, cells do not respond to leptin, so that its normal action does not occur.
48. You noticed an important difference. Estrogen tends to cause fat to deposit on the surface of the body. Young women have higher estrogen and tend to develop what we call *peripheral obesity*. Men tend to deposit fat on the inside of the belly, so they have a different body shape. We refer to that deeper fat distribution as *visceral obesity*.
49. The term *obesogen* is used for a chemical from the environment that helps obesity develop. These obesogens stimulate formation of fat cells and may influence appetite and the rate that we burn fat for energy.
50. Overeating once a year is not an eating disorder. The overeating of an eating disorder occurs at least once a week for several months and is accompanied by a sense of lack of control over the eating.
51. The name *tumor necrosis factor alpha* may sound like it comes from cancer, but it does not. It is a chemical messenger that causes inflammation. In obesity, the fat tissue has more immune cells that usual and those immune cells make tumor necrosis factor alpha, which goes into the blood. The higher than normal blood levels of tumor necrosis factor alpha in obesity contribute to development of obesity-related diseases such as type 2 diabetes, heart disease, and cancer.

CHAPTER 24

Match the Definitions

1. B
2. C
3. E
4. A
5. D

Circle the Correct Words

6. occurs only during fetal life; begins at puberty
7. 1 year
8. childbirth
9. low
10. estradiol
11. LH and FSH; anterior; GnRH
12. progesterone
13. low; high; low

Order the Steps

14. B, D, C, A, E

Explain the Pictures

15. Y; testes
16. ovaries; wolffian (mesonephric)
17. The müllerian ducts join and become the uterus, fallopian tubes, cervix, and upper two-thirds of the vagina.
18. male; female
19. Both Bartholin and Cowper glands secrete substances that enhance the motility and viability of sperm.
20. A = menstruation; B = proliferative phase; C = secretory phase; D = ischemic phase; E = menstruation
21. Secretory phase
22. Progesterone
23. Estrogen
24. Ovulation

Describe the Differences

25. Puberty is the onset of sexual maturation, but adolescence is the stage of human development between childhood and adulthood and includes social, psychological, and biological changes.
26. Menarche is the beginning of menstruation, but menopause is the cessation of menstruation.

Complete the Sentences

27. 23
28. clitoris
29. endometrium; basal
30. fundus
31. corpus luteum
32. androgens (or androstenedione); testosterone
33. luteal
34. fallopian tube

Teach People about Physiology

Compare your answers with these sample answers.

35. As women age, the character of the vagina changes. The lining gets thinner. The secretions become fewer and less acidic, which makes a more favorable environment for microorganisms to grow and cause infection. So you are more vulnerable to infection now that you are older.
36. Yes, those fringes, or fimbriae to use their technical name, have an important purpose. See how they are near the ovary? When an ovary releases an egg, those fringes move and create a current that draws the egg into the fallopian tube so that the egg can travel down the tube toward the uterus. Do you want to know where the egg gets fertilized?
37. Yes, there is a good reason. Because of the hormonal changes during the menstrual cycle, your breasts are likely to be the fullest and most tender right before menstruation, and less tender afterward. A mammogram right after your menstrual period will be more comfortable for you.

Copyright © 2024 by Elsevier, Inc. All Rights Reserved.

38. Heat is bad for developing sperm. That is why the testicles hang outside the body, to keep them cool so that they can make sperm. If you sit in the hot tub, you will get your testicles too hot, which can decrease your sperm count and reduce your chances of having a baby.

39. Any person who has a vagina, uterus, fallopian tubes, and functioning ovaries can become pregnant if they engage in vaginal intercourse.

CHAPTER 25

Match the Definitions
1. E
2. D
3. H
4. A
5. G
6. I
7. B
8. C
9. F

Circle the Correct Words
10. luteal; emotional
11. acid
12. chronic pain of; duct
13. obesity; pelvic
14. estrogen; excessive
15. transformation; columnar
16. asymptomatic; bleeding
17. estrogen; progesterone
18. standard deviations
19. are not; fibrocystic disease
20. vaginismus

Categorize the Disorders
21. Disorder of orgasm
22. Disorder of desire
23. Disorder of sexual pain
24. Disorder of sexual pain

Explain the Pictures
25. In Figure A (ductal carcinoma in situ), the proliferating cells have not crossed the basement membrane, but in Figure B (advanced breast cancer), they have crossed it and invaded other breast tissues.
26. No, DCIS does not always progress to invasive cancer.
27. Figure B
28. Painless
29. Lymphatics (or axillary lymph nodes)
30. Within the same tumor, breast cancer often is heterogeneous. Tumors evolve. The cancer cells can vary in their multiple mutations; the tumor also includes macrophages and fibroblasts that are recruited to the tumor, become part of its microenvironment, and drive development of heterogeneity of the cancer cells.

Categorize the Risk Factors
31. Genetic
32. Environmental/lifestyle
33. Reproductive
34. Environmental/lifestyle
35. Hormonal
36. Environmental/lifestyle
37. Environmental/lifestyle
38. Hormonal
39. Familial

Describe the Differences
40. Primary dysmenorrhea is associated with excessive endometrial prostaglandins in ovulatory cycles, in the absence of pelvic disease, but secondary dysmenorrhea is associated with pelvic disease.
41. Primary amenorrhea is the absence of menstruation by a specific age, but secondary amenorrhea is the absence of menstruation for a time equivalent to three or more cycles in women who have previously menstruated.
42. Endometriosis is the presence of functioning endometrial tissue outside the uterus, but adenomyosis is the presence of endometrial tissue within the uterine myometrium.

Complete the Sentences
43. vaginosis
44. 13
45. GnRH
46. endometriosis
47. hypothalamus; anterior; FSH; estrogen
48. salpingitis; oophoritis; pelvic inflammatory
49. dermoid
50. human papilloma; cervical
51. galactorrhea; prolactin; pituitary

Teach People about Pathophysiology
Compare your answers with these sample answers.

52. Gonorrhea can lead to pelvic inflammatory disease and scar the fallopian tubes. This scarring can prevent the sperm from meeting and fertilizing the ovum.
53. With fibrocystic breast disease, there is extra connective tissue that is like scar tissue, and little fluid-filled sacs form in the breast. You are correct that it is not cancer.
54. Normally, friendly bacteria live in the vagina; they keep the yeast organisms from multiplying. Antibiotics get rid of the bacteria that cause a bladder infection, but they also get rid of the friendly bacteria in the vagina. That provides an opportunity for the yeast to grow.
55. A follicular cyst occurs when the dominant follicle fails to rupture or one or more of the non-dominant follicles fail to regress. The causes are not well understood but most likely involve altered levels of the hormones involved in the ovarian cycle.

Copyright © 2024 by Elsevier, Inc. All Rights Reserved.

56. Some of the cells that normally are part of the lining of the uterus have migrated into places in your body where they do not belong. That tissue responds to your hormonal cycles and bleeds when you are menstruating. Because the blood is trapped inside your body, it causes inflammation and pain.

57. Women who have uterine cancer often develop vaginal bleeding as you did, and their cancer gets diagnosed and treated in the early stages. However, women who have ovarian cancer usually do not have symptoms that can call attention to the cancer, so their cancer gets diagnosed and treated late, sometimes after it has spread to other organs.

Clinical Scenarios

58. pelvic inflammatory disease (PID); bacteria; lower
59. The most common infecting organisms in PID are bacteria; bacterial infections usually cause fever.
60. PID includes infection of the uterus, fallopian tubes, and ovaries.
61. Dyspareunia
62. Dyschezia
63. Dyspareunia and dyschezia occur with PID because Jodie has widespread inflammation in her pelvic organs, which sensitizes pain receptors.
64. Jodie already has indicated that she experiences increased pain when she jumps or tries to walk briskly.
65. Potential complications of PID that Jodie may experience in the future include infertility, ectopic pregnancy, and pelvic adhesions with chronic pelvic pain.
66. PCOS involves at least two of these conditions: irregular ovulation, elevated levels of androgens, or polycystic ovaries shown on ultrasound. Mrs. Orrins has all of them: menstrual periods five times per year, elevated testosterone, hirsutism and acne, and polycystic ovaries.
67. Increased
68. Increased
69. Women with PCOS are more likely to experience sleep apnea than women who do not have PCOS.
70. Obesity is common with PCOS. In addition, weight gain tends to exacerbate the signs and symptoms.

CHAPTER 26

Match the Definitions
1. K
2. I
3. H
4. J
5. C
6. A
7. B
8. D
9. F
10. E
11. G

Circle the Correct Words
12. estrogen
13. rise
14. squamous cell carcinoma; adenocarcinoma
15. mumps
16. ischemia and necrosis
17. inner layers; periphery
18. by ascending the urinary tract; pyelonephritis
19. erection

Describe the Differences
20. In phimosis, the foreskin cannot be retracted over the glans penis, but in paraphimosis, the foreskin is retracted and cannot be returned to its normal position over the glans.
21. Delayed puberty comes abnormally late (no clinical signs of puberty by age 14), but precocious puberty comes abnormally early (sexual maturation before age 9).
22. Although both are scrotal masses, a varicocele consists of abnormally dilated veins within the spermatic cord, and a hydrocele is a collection of fluid within the tunica vaginalis.

Complete the Sentences
23. erectile dysfunction
24. testicular
25. chemical epididymitis
26. androgen
27. estrogens
28. erection, emission, ejaculation
29. estrogen/testosterone
30. sexually
31. prostate

Teach People about Pathophysiology
Compare your answers with these sample answers.

32. As you know, your prostate gland is enlarged. The prostate gland surrounds the urethra, the tube through which the urine flows when you empty your bladder. When your prostate gland got bigger on the outside, it also grew on the inside, squeezing your urethra, so it is narrower. It is like stepping on a garden hose and compressing it but not totally squashing it flat. Not as much water will flow through the narrow hose. With your enlarged prostate, the urine has to flow through a more narrow tube, so it takes longer to empty your bladder.
33. Unlike most other cancers, many prostate cancers grow very slowly. So it actually is possible to watch them rather than do surgery to remove them.
34. No, you do not have gonorrhea. Nongonococcal means that some other microorganism, not the one that causes gonorrhea, caused your urethritis. It could be *Chlamydia* or another organism.
35. That procedure with the flashlight is called *transillumination,* and it is a standard way of diagnosing a hydrocele. The light shines through the skin differently if there is fluid inside or if there is a solid mass inside. It sounds like he definitely knows how to help you.

Copyright © 2024 by Elsevier, Inc. All Rights Reserved.

36. Undescended testicles are associated with increased risk for testicular cancer. Testicular cancer can spread to nearby lymph nodes; he was feeling your groin lymph nodes to see if they are enlarged.

CHAPTER 27

Circle the Correct Words
1. receptive
2. men
3. secondary; on the palms of the hands and soles of the feet
4. Women; buboes
5. anogenital cancer; genital warts
6. parasite; adheres to
7. uncircumcised
8. highly; virus
9. whether or not they have

Characterize the Sexually Transmitted Infections
10. *Chlamydia trachomatis;* gram-negative intracellular bacterium
11. *Neisseria gonorrhoeae;* gram-negative diplococcus
12. Herpes simplex virus; enveloped, linear, double-stranded DNA virus that has a latent stage in neurons
13. *Treponema pallidum;* anaerobic spirochete
14. Human papillomavirus; non-enveloped, circular, double-stranded DNA virus that has numerous strains

Order the Steps
15. B, E, D, A, C

Explain the Picture
16. Scabies
17. A parasitic itch mite, *Sarcoptes scabiei*
18. The mite burrows through the skin, depositing its eggs.
19. Pruritus, especially at night
20. By any form of skin-to-skin contact and by fomites such as infested bedding

Describe the Differences
21. A chancre is a painless ulcer with indurated (hard) edges, but a bubo is a painful, swollen abscessed lymph node.
22. Condylomata acuminata are genital warts caused by HPV, but condylomata lata are flat lesions characteristic of syphilis.
23. "Crabs" are pubic lice that attach to hair and bite the skin for nourishment, but scabies are mites that burrow into the skin to lay eggs.

Complete the Sentences
24. epithelial
25. epididymitis; pelvic inflammatory disease
26. eye; days
27. secondary
28. donovanosis
29. skin; lymph

30. B
31. vesicles
32. less; shorter

Teach People about Pathophysiology
Compare your answers with these sample answers.

33. Yes, it is possible. Women can have gonorrhea without symptoms, but they still can pass on the infection. Some women have symptoms of gonorrhea, but many do not.
34. There are different types of HPV. Some of them cause warts, but others can cause cancer. The HPV shot can help protect you against cancer of the cervix, which you may know is the opening of the uterus, the organ where a baby develops.
35. A fomite is not an insect. It is an inanimate (non-living) object such as a towel, kickboard, pool floats, or other object that someone else with the infection has used. The other way to transmit this infection is by skin-to-skin contact with someone who has it.
36. Normally, a woman has some helpful bacteria that live in her vagina. Having enough of these helpful bacteria is important because they keep the non-helpful bacteria from growing there. Bacterial vaginosis occurs when the balance between the helpful bacteria and non-helpful bacteria changes and too many of the non-helpful bacterial are growing. This makes the fishy smell that caused you to go to your nurse practitioner.
37. Usually, a chancre heals without making a scar. We can talk about how to keep the area clean, so other bacteria do not infect it as well.
38. The medicines we have do not get rid of herpesvirus, but they reduce the symptoms of an outbreak. The herpesvirus hides in the nerves when it is not active. It travels down the nerves again and can cause repeated outbreaks, like you are experiencing. Would you as to talk about factors that seem to increase the risk for having an outbreak?

Case Scenario
39. They have similar manifestations, and they may coinfect a woman.
40. Although you do not have any symptoms, you have an infection of your cervix. As you know, the cervix is the entry to the uterus. The *Chlamydia* organism can spread up into the uterus and into other parts of your reproductive organs, causing painful pelvic inflammatory disease, also called PID. You may have heard of PID. We want to prevent that.
41. In women, *Chlamydia* first infects the cervix and/or the urethra.
42. Chlamydia enters host cells and reproduces inside them in a two-part cycle. An "elementary body" that survives outside cells enters the host epithelial cells and becomes metabolically active. It reproduces inside the cells, which eventually rupture, releasing more elementary bodies that then infect more cells.

Copyright © 2024 by Elsevier, Inc. All Rights Reserved.

43. Yes, PID can cause infertility. The infection can cause scarring in the fallopian tubes, the tubes through which the eggs travel and get fertilized by sperm. If these tubes scar shut, then a woman cannot become pregnant.

44. Chlamydia is quite common. In fact, it is the most common reportable sexually transmitted infection caused by bacteria in the United States. So many other people have had this infection.

45. Chlamydial conjunctivitis and chlamydial pneumonia

CHAPTER 28

Match the Definitions
1. D
2. F
3. E
4. A
5. B
6. C

Classify the Cells
7. Agranulocyte
8. Agranulocyte
9. Agranulocyte
10. Granulocyte
11. Agranulocyte
12. Granulocyte
13. Granulocyte

Match the Functions
14. C
15. F
16. D
17. E
18. G
19. B
20. A

Circle the Correct Words
21. do not have; multi-lobed
22. granulocytes; bands
23. blood cells; bone marrow
24. red; yellow
25. four; four; ferrous Fe^{2+}
26. hepcidin; transferrin; ferritin; hemosiderin
27. inhibit; trigger

Categorize the Lymphoid Organs
28. Secondary
29. Primary
30. Secondary
31. Secondary
32. Secondary
33. Primary

Order the Steps
34. F, C, A, E, D, B

Explain the Pictures
35. Exposure of platelets to subendothelial collagen causes the platelets to adhere to this injured area.
36. The platelets on the right have become activated.
37. Strands of fibrin. Fibrin comes from the action of thrombin on fibrinogen, an inactive precursor that circulates in the blood until the clotting system is activated.
38. Platelets have actin and myosin filaments in them that enable them to contract. This contraction of aggregated platelets expels the serum from inside the clot.
39. Erythropoietin
40. kidney; bone marrow
41. Erythropoiesis (production of more erythrocytes)
42. Tissue hypoxia from the decreased oxygen content of arterial blood
43. Steps 7-9: When more erythrocytes are present in blood, they carry more oxygen, which relieves tissue hypoxia and thus decreases release of erythropoietin.

Describe the Differences
44. A leukocyte is a white blood cell of any type, but a lymphocyte is a special type of white blood cell with specific immune functions.
45. Plasma is the liquid portion of blood with its dissolved substances, but serum is plasma minus the clotting factors.
46. A multipotent stem cell can differentiate into many different types of cells, but a hematopoietic stem cell can differentiate only into the various types of blood cells.
47. A reticulocyte is an immature erythrocyte that has a nucleus, mitochondria, and ribosomes, but an erythrocyte is fully mature and does not have any of these organelles.
48. Ferritin is a protein that binds and stores iron, but apoferritin is ferritin that does not have iron attached.

Name the Progenitors
49. Myeloid
50. Lymphoid
51. Myeloid
52. Myeloid
53. Lymphoid
54. Myeloid
55. Myeloid
56. Lymphoid
57. Myeloid

Complete the Sentences
58. clotting
59. albumin; neutrophils
60. reversibly; spleen
61. thrombocytes; megakaryocytes; bone marrow
62. erythrocytes; platelets
63. thromboplastin; extrinsic
64. fibrin; plasminogen; liver
65. older

Copyright © 2024 by Elsevier, Inc. All Rights Reserved.

Categorize the Substances

66. Antithrombotic
67. Promotes clotting
68. Antithrombotic
69. Antithrombotic
70. Promotes clotting
71. Promotes clotting
72. Antithrombotic
73. Antithrombotic
74. Antithrombotic

Teach People about Pathophysiology

Compare your answers with these sample answers.

75. Those red cells are not in your body any more. Red blood cells live only about 4 months, so the ones that were transfused are gone, and your body has made new red cells.
76. Yes, reticulocytes are immature red blood cells, but they continue to mature in the bloodstream. Your increased reticulocyte count tells us that your bone marrow is making new red cells.
77. Red blood cells need iron to make hemoglobin. They use hemoglobin to carry oxygen from your lungs to the rest of your body. All parts of your body need oxygen to keep functioning. If there is not enough iron in your diet, your red blood cells will not be able to carry enough oxygen.
78. If a person has a spleen, immune cells in the spleen called *macrophages* remove the old red blood cells and recycle their parts. If a person does not have a spleen, like your brother, immune cells in the liver take over that job. Those liver immune cells are called *Kupffer cells,* and they are a type of macrophage.
79. Red blood cells contain a lot of hemoglobin, a substance that enables them to carry oxygen. When red blood cells die, their hemoglobin is taken apart, and a piece of the hemoglobin is changed chemically into bilirubin. Normally, bilirubin travels in the blood to the liver, where it is changed chemically again. So if the man in the mystery story had a lot of red blood cells die suddenly, it makes sense that he would have a lot of bilirubin in his blood.
80. Platelets store these proteins and other substances in granules. That way they can release them very rapidly.
81. Blood clots have a substance called *fibrin* in them, and our bodies make protective enzymes that chop up the fibrin to dissolve the clot. D-dimer is a fibrin degradation product, which means that it is a tiny piece of a fibrin clot that a protective enzyme is trying to remove. If D-dimer is elevated in your blood, it can indicate that there is a clot.
82. When a blood vessel is healing, we make special protective chemicals that dissolve the clot slowly and break it up into very tiny pieces. That way there are no large pieces of clot to cause problems.

CHAPTER 29

Match the Definitions

1. E
2. G
3. A
4. F
5. C
6. B
7. D

Match More Definitions

8. C
9. H
10. G
11. F
12. B
13. D
14. A
15. E

Circle the Correct Words

16. decreases; turbulent
17. macrocytic
18. alcohol
19. macrocytic
20. highest; decreases
21. iron metabolism; anemia of chronic disease
22. deficiency
23. relative; secondary absolute
24. alloimmune; intravascularly
25. large
26. clotting
27. parasite invasion; hypersensitivity
28. late; early
29. production; bone marrow; decreases
30. leukocytosis; leukopenia
31. Localized; generalized
32. immature

Categorize Anemias by the Appearance of the Erythrocytes

33. Microcytic-hypochromic
34. Normocytic-normochromic
35. Macrocytic-normochromic
36. Normocytic-normochromic
37. Macrocytic-normochromic
38. Normocytic-normochromic

Categorize Anemias by Their General Causes

39. Increased erythrocyte destruction
40. Impaired erythrocyte production
41. Impaired erythrocyte production
42. Increased erythrocyte destruction
43. Increased erythrocyte destruction
44. Impaired erythrocyte production
45. Impaired erythrocyte production
46. Impaired erythrocyte production

Copyright © 2024 by Elsevier, Inc. All Rights Reserved.

Describe the Differences

47. Leukemias are cancers of blood-forming cells, but lymphomas are cancers of lymphatic tissue.
48. A lymphocytic leukemia arises from the lymphoid cell line that normally produces B and T lymphocytes and natural killer cells, but a myelogenous leukemia arises from the myeloid cell line that normally produces granulocytes, monocytes, erythrocytes, and platelets.
49. Splenomegaly is enlargement of the spleen, but hypersplenism is overactivity of the spleen.

Explain the Pictures

50. Normocytic
51. Normochromic
52. Hypochromic
53. Glossitis
54. Koilonychia
55. Iron deficiency anemia
56. Pallor but not jaundice. Jaundice occurs with massive hemolysis, not with anemia caused by decreased erythrocyte production.
57. This question can have several correct answers, such as excessive menstrual bleeding, chronic gastrointestinal blood loss, or any other situation in which iron intake is less than iron loss.
58. Heparin-induced thrombocytopenia
59. Platelet factor 4 (PF4)
60. Heparin
61. The PF4-heparin complex
62. After the HIT antibodies bind the PF4-heparin complex, the Fc (nonspecific) end of the antibodies binds to platelet Fc receptors, activating the platelets, which release substances that promote clotting.
63. In the veins of the lower extremities, although arterial clots also may occur in the lower extremities or elsewhere in the body

Match the Abnormalities

64. B
65. C
66. A

Complete the Sentences

67. -chromic; -cytic
68. recessive; iron
69. iron
70. vera; erythrocytes
71. lymphocytes; bone marrow; chemicals; radiation
72. cytokines; iron
73. intrinsic; immune
74. spleen; macrophages
75. hapten
76. eight; bilirubin
77. B; virus; lymphadenopathy
78. Burkitt; B; jaw; virus
79. acute myelogenous leukemia; chronic lymphocytic leukemia
80. infection
81. multiple myeloma
82. fatigue (or anemia); infection; bleeding
83. rupture
84. Hodgkin lymphoma

Locate the Defect

85. Hemoglobin synthesis defect
86. Membrane defect
87. Hemoglobin synthesis defect
88. Enzyme pathway defect

Teach People about Pathophysiology

Compare your answers with these sample answers.

89. Red blood cells do come from bone marrow, but the bone marrow needs to be stimulated to produce them. Normal kidneys make a messenger called *erythropoietin* that goes in the blood to bone marrow and stimulates it to make red blood cells. With chronic kidney disease, the kidneys do not make enough of this messenger, and the bone marrow does not make enough red blood cells. That is why you have anemia.
90. Ordinarily, red blood cells do not cause clotting, but your body is making so many red blood cells that your blood is too thick, and that makes it more likely to clot.
91. As you know, anemia means that you do not have enough red blood cells. Red blood cells are needed to carry oxygen to our muscles and other areas of the body. With anemia, your body does not have quite enough oxygen, and you feel tired.
92. Your body accumulates too much iron, which can damage your liver. Red blood cells have iron in them, so removing some blood on a regular basis removes iron from your body and protects your liver.
93. When your bone marrow became unable to make new blood cells, you already had some red cells, white cells, and platelets circulating in your blood. These cells have a typical life span before the body removes them. Red blood cells have the longest life span; they live about 4 months. So your white cells and platelets decreased in your blood before your red cells did.
94. When your husband bled so much, he lost red blood cells, which made him anemic. At the same time, he also lost fluid, which decreased his blood pressure. He became lightheaded because he did not have enough blood bringing oxygen to his brain. After he was given fluid, his blood volume became more normal, so he is not lightheaded any more, but he still does not have enough red blood cells.
95. The penicillin in your daughter's blood attached to her red blood cells. Then her body made antibodies that attached to the red blood cells and marked them for destruction. The marked red blood cells were destroyed in an organ called the *spleen*. The spleen normally removes worn-out red blood cells, but when the antibodies marked your daughter's red blood cells because of the penicillin, too many of them were destroyed.

Copyright © 2024 by Elsevier, Inc. All Rights Reserved.

96. Arterial thrombi are composed primarily of platelet aggregates held together by strands of fibrin, but venous thrombi are composed primarily of erythrocytes, greater amounts of fibrin, and fewer platelets.

97. Normally we have clotting factors that circulate in our blood and make our blood clot when we need to stop bleeding. However, your husband's blood made so many little clots that it used up most of his clotting factors. Now he is bleeding because he does not have enough clotting factors left.

98. In general, there are two types of problems that can cause a bleeding disorder. One is a problem with the platelets, and the other is a problem with the clotting factors that normally circulate in blood. Because your platelets are fine, they probably are looking at your clotting factors. I encourage you to ask your doctors what they are testing.

99. ITP stands for some technical words: *immune thrombocytopenic purpura*. I can explain what that means. *Immune* means that your immune system has started destroying your platelets. Sometimes people use the word *idiopathic* instead of immune because we do not know exactly why the immune system starts destroying platelets. *Thrombocytopenic* means that your body has too few platelets in the blood. Platelets normally keep people from bleeding inappropriately. Those red dots in your skin are tiny little bleeding spots because you do not have enough platelets. *Purpura* refers to those purple blotches on your skin where a little blood has oozed into your skin. So ITP means that for some unknown reason, your immune system is destroying a lot of your platelets and that you have little spots and discolored areas due to bleeding in your skin. ITP is not contagious because it is an immune system problem; it is not caused by virus or bacteria.

100. Your symptoms are similar because you both have too few platelets in your blood. However, the reasons that you and your son have too few platelets are different. The cancer drugs suppressed your bone marrow, so your bone marrow is not producing enough platelets. Your son's bone marrow is producing enough platelets, but his immune system is attacking them, so they have a shorter survival time.

101. Von Willebrand disease is a coagulation disorder, which means that he will start bleeding if it is out of control. Look for bleeding gums after oral hygiene, oozing or bleeding from injection or catheter sites, bruising after very little pressure, or nosebleeds.

102. Bence Jones proteins are pieces of antibodies that are excreted in the urine in multiple myeloma. They are important because they help establish the diagnosis of multiple myeloma and because they can damage the kidneys.

103. Plasma cells are mature B lymphocytes, a type of immune system cell. Their normal function is to secrete antibodies. In plasma cell myeloma, malignant plasma cells secrete entirely too much of one kind of antibody.

104. In acute leukemia, such as the ALL that Knut has, leukemia cells in the bone marrow crowd out the normal cells that make red blood cells, so the bone marrow is not able to make enough red blood cells. As you may know, red blood cells normally carry oxygen to all parts of the body. With too few red blood cells, the muscles and other tissues do not get enough oxygen, which makes Knut tired.

105. You had a different kind of anemia. Menstruating women can develop iron deficiency anemia from losing iron in menstrual blood every month; iron tablets replace the lost iron and cure the anemia. However, your father has anemia from a different cause. His leukemia cells are crowding out the cells that normally make red blood cells in the bone marrow, so he cannot make enough red blood cells. Giving him iron will not help because the cell factories are not working.

106. When you have a sore throat, there is inflammation, and the immune cells that respond to inflammation become activated. They release chemicals that make the lymph nodes where they accumulate get swollen and painful. In Hodgkin lymphoma, the immune cells are gathering in a large number in lymph nodes, which makes them swell dramatically, but the immune cells are not activated, and they do not release the inflammatory chemicals that would cause pain.

107. When the body makes white blood cells, they go through several stages. As they mature, we say that they differentiate. A well-differentiated white blood cell is one that is mature. That is a difference between acute and chronic leukemia. In acute leukemia, which you do not have, the white cells are poorly differentiated, which means that they are immature. In chronic leukemia, the kind you have, the white cells are well differentiated, which means that they are mature, although they do not function normally.

Clinical Scenarios

108. Normally, dietary vitamin B_{12} is released from foods in the stomach and binds to intrinsic factor, a substance secreted by gastric parietal cells. The vitamin B_{12}–intrinsic factor complex binds to receptors in the ileum, which enables vitamin B_{12} absorption.

109. Mrs. Swenson developed autoantibodies that triggered destruction of parietal cells in her stomach, so the production of intrinsic factor decreased or stopped. Without the intrinsic factor, dietary vitamin B_{12} cannot be absorbed. Because vitamin B_{12} is necessary for erythropoiesis, she developed anemia.

110. Numbness and tingling are classic manifestations of pernicious anemia because vitamin B_{12} is necessary for normal nerve function. Nerve demyelination and damage from insufficient vitamin B_{12} are progressive and often not reversible.

111. Cobalamin must be continued (at longer intervals) after her vitamin B_{12} blood level is normal because she still cannot absorb dietary vitamin B_{12}.

Copyright © 2024 by Elsevier, Inc. All Rights Reserved.

112. Disseminated intravascular coagulation
113. Extensive clotting consumes clotting factors and platelets, leading to hemorrhage.
114. In DIC, there is widespread exposure of the pre-existing tissue factor to the blood plus increased expression of tissue factor caused by proinflammatory cytokines. The tissue factor activates the clotting cascade through the extrinsic pathway, causing widespread (disseminated) clotting.
115. Activated protein C is an endogenous anticoagulant. The lack of its anticoagulant function contributes to the widespread clotting in DIC.
116. Widespread clotting in DIC causes inadequate tissue perfusion and ischemia. Ms. Day is at risk for failure of the kidneys, liver, lungs, and other organs, depending on where clots develop.
117. Is the swelling in his neck tender? Has he had recent unintentional weight loss? Fever? Night sweats? Fatigue? Any other symptoms?
118. Not painful. The lymphadenopathy of Hodgkin lymphoma is painless because it is due to accumulation of a mass of white blood cells. If it were enlarged because of inflammation, it would be painful, but inflammation is not the reason for the enlargement.
119. Reed-Sternberg cells
120. Blood tests in Hodgkin lymphoma do not show large numbers of circulating malignant cells because the cells are confined to the lymph nodes, as indicated by the term *lymphoma*.
121. Many other B or T lymphocyte or natural killer cell lymphomas (collectively called *non-Hodgkin lymphomas*) can cause cervical lymphadenopathy. Note: If your answer was simply non-Hodgkin lymphoma, be sure you understand that the term does not denote one specific lymphoma, but rather it is a name for a group of different lymphomas.

CHAPTER 30

Match the Definitions
1. E
2. F
3. A
4. C
5. D
6. B

Draw Your Answers
7.
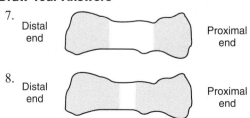

8.
Distal end — Proximal end

9.
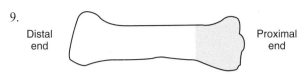

Circle the Correct Words
10. adolescence; higher
11. 2; growth
12. aspirin; hemolytic
13. recessive; heterozygous; homozygous
14. 6 to 12 months of age; is not
15. hemorrhagic

Order the Steps
16. D, A, C, E, B, F, H, G

Describe the Differences
17. The most common form of adult hemoglobin is composed of two alpha and two beta polypeptide chains, but embryonic and fetal hemoglobins are composed of two alpha and two gamma polypeptide chains.
18. Children who have hereditary spherocytosis experience persistent hemolysis because their erythrocytes have a membrane defect that makes them fragile, but children who have G6PD deficiency do not have hemolysis unless they are exposed to certain drugs or other oxidative stressors that trigger a hemolytic crisis.
19. Hemoglobin A_1 is normal adult hemoglobin with two alpha chains and two beta chains, but hemoglobin S, associated with sickle cell disease, has a valine instead of a glutamic acid at particular point on the beta chains.
20. People who have sickle cell anemia have two copies of the mutated gene (are homozygous) and produce only hemoglobin S, but people who have sickle cell trait have one mutated gene (are heterozygous) and produce a mixture of hemoglobin A and hemoglobin S.

Interpret the Table
21. The fetal intrauterine environment is hypoxic, which stimulates fetal erythropoietin production and drives vigorous erythropoiesis.
22. Reticulocytes are immature erythrocytes. Their high levels in the cord blood reflect the very active erythropoiesis of fetal life.
23. The normal WBC count is much higher in an infant than in a school-aged child. Without this knowledge, a health care provider might mistake the normally high WBC count in infancy for an indication of infection.

Complete the Sentences
24. liver
25. aplastic
26. lungs
27. sequestration; hypovolemic shock
28. Cooley; alpha
29. bleeding; joints

Copyright © 2024 by Elsevier, Inc. All Rights Reserved.

30. lymphocytic; failure
31. infection; hypermetabolism
32. thrombosis (or clotting)
33. painless; virus
34. lymphoid

Match the Hemophilias
35. C
36. A
37. B

Teach People about Pathophysiology
Compare your answers with these sample answers.

38. As you know, your son's hemoglobin has an abnormal structure. One of the amino acids in the protein chains is different from normal. When the inside of his red blood cells becomes dehydrated or too acidic or is without oxygen for too long, then the abnormal hemoglobin polymerizes into long strands. These long strands of hemoglobin change the shape of the red blood cell and force it to sickle.
39. When a lot of red blood cells are destroyed in a short period of time, as in a hemolytic crisis, the hemoglobin inside them cannot be processed fast enough, and a hemoglobin breakdown product called *bilirubin* accumulates. When bilirubin enters the body tissues that we can see, it makes them look yellow. People who do not have enough red blood cells often look pale, as you expected, but if they have a lot of rapid hemolysis, what we see is the yellow color we call jaundice.
40. As you know, Archer's red blood cells are fragile and break easily. When they break, the hemoglobin inside gets changed chemically in the body, and some of the parts are put in the bile. That can make the bile more concentrated, and then it is likely to start forming gallstones.

Case Scenarios
41. Mrs. Scott developed antibodies against Rh-positive red cells from her first pregnancy. Her antibodies will cross the placenta. If the fetus is Rh-positive, the maternal antibodies will cause hemolysis in the fetus.
42. Mrs. Scott did not have antibodies against Rh-positive red cells when she first became pregnant. Very few fetal erythrocytes cross the placental barrier into the maternal circulation during a normal pregnancy. However, large numbers of fetal erythrocytes do enter maternal circulation when the placenta detaches at childbirth. Mrs. Scott formed the antibodies against Rh-positive red cells after Jacob was born.
43. Baby Ashley's liver and spleen were enlarged because she had hemolysis during her fetal life and erythropoiesis increased at those extramedullary sites.
44. Baby Ashley became jaundiced after she was born because she has Rh-positive red cells and her mother's antibodies against Rh-positive red cells were causing hemolysis. Her immature liver was unable to conjugate the large amounts of bilirubin that result from

hemolysis. Buildup of bilirubin in the blood and tissues causes jaundice.
45. During fetal life, unconjugated bilirubin is excreted through the placenta.
46. Kernicterus is accumulation of bilirubin in neural tissues. It causes severe neurological damage. Baby Ashley has high risk for kernicterus if she does not receive treatment.
47. Jim's platelet count was low because he developed antiplatelet antibodies that bound to his platelets, causing their destruction by phagocytic immune cells. His bone marrow was not able to make new platelets fast enough to replace those that were being destroyed.
48. His erythrocyte count should have been normal because in primary immune (idiopathic) thrombocytopenic purpura, the autoantibodies are specific for platelets.
49. Platelets are necessary for hemostasis. When the platelet count is low, small leaks in capillaries cannot be plugged, and blood seeps into the skin tissues, causing the areas of bruising known as purpura.

CHAPTER 31

Match the Definitions
1. C
2. F
3. H
4. A
5. B
6. D
7. E
8. G

Choose the Correct Words
9. three; tricuspid; two; mitral
10. more; more
11. vasoconstriction
12. 70%; small
13. myosin, calcium
14. more; less
15. thinner; more; veins only
16. media; smooth muscle and elastic fibers
17. constricts
18. stiffening

Match the Functions
19. Right pulmonary artery; B
20. Superior vena cava; D
21. Pulmonary valve; E
22. Tricuspid valve; K
23. Chordae tendineae; G
24. Inferior vena cava; H
25. Interventricular septum; L
26. Mitral valve; J
27. Aortic valve; A
28. Left pulmonary veins; I
29. Left pulmonary artery; F
30. Aorta (aortic arch); C

    Copyright © 2024 by Elsevier, Inc. All Rights Reserved.

Select the Faster Ones

31. SA node
32. AV node
33. Sympathetic nerve firing
34. Stimulation of cardiac β_1 receptors
35. Changes in autonomic nerve activity
36. Blood flow in an arteriole

Categorize the Effects

37. Vasoconstriction
38. Vasoconstriction
39. Decrease
40. Increase
41. Decrease
42. Increase
43. Increase
44. Vasodilation
45. Vasodilation
46. Vasoconstriction
47. Vasoconstriction

Order the Steps

48. D, B, E, C, A

Explain the Picture

49. Atrial depolarization
50. Contract (atrial systole)
51. From SA node through the atrium, AV node, His-Purkinje system, to ventricular myocardium
52. Contracting (ventricular systole)
53. Q wave
54. To prevent backward flow of blood into the atria when the ventricles contract

Describe the Differences

55. The endocardium is the innermost layer of the heart, but the epicardium is the outermost layer of the heart.
56. Systole is contraction of the muscular wall of a cardiac chamber, but diastole is relaxation of it.
57. Angiogenesis is the growth of new capillaries, but arteriogenesis is a new artery branching off from a preexisting artery.
58. Laminar flow has concentric layers of molecules that move parallel to the vessel wall, but turbulent flow has eddy currents that move in whorls, creating more resistance to flow and a less beneficial effect on the endothelium.

Complete the Sentences

59. semilunar; three
60. left; right
61. epicardium
62. coronary; right
63. anterior descending; circumflex
64. acetylcholine; cholinergic; norepinephrine; adrenergic
65. calcium
66. intercalated
67. autoregulation
68. thoracic; subclavian
69. vasorum
70. ultrasound; intravenously; magnetic; medium (dye)

Calculate the Answers

71. 60 mmHg
72. 100 mmHg
73. 3.5 L/min
74. 60%

Sort the Laws

75. Frank-Starling law of the heart
76. Laplace's law
77. Poiseuille's law

Teach People about Physiology

Compare your answers with these sample answers.

78. The muscle walls are different thicknesses because the two ventricles need to do different amounts of work. Remember that the right ventricle sends blood to the lungs? The lungs are a low-pressure system, and the right ventricle does not have to work very hard to pump blood into the lung blood vessels. Now, think about the work that the left ventricle has to do. It has to pump the blood out to the rest of the body: head, arms, legs, trunk, everywhere except the lungs. The left heart has to work harder because that is a high-pressure system, so it needs to have a thicker muscle.
79. LAD means left anterior descending, which is a branch of the left coronary artery. A blockage in the LAD is concerning because this artery supplies blood to much of the interventricular septum and to portions of both ventricles.
80. Troponin is a relaxing protein. You may remember that binding of myosin and actin creates myocardial contraction. When troponin combines with tropomyosin, another relaxing protein, the two of them prevent myosin and actin from binding for a moment, and the myocardium relaxes.
81. Hearts have special cells that actually generate the heartbeat automatically. So even though the nerves are not attached when a heart is transplanted, the heart still continues to beat. If that function continues normally, no pacemaker is needed.

CHAPTER 32

Match the Definitions

1. G
2. D
3. A
4. B
5. C
6. E
7. F

Copyright © 2024 by Elsevier, Inc. All Rights Reserved.

Circle the Correct Words

8. edema and ulceration
9. pulmonary; systemic
10. compresses; venous distention
11. resistance; increase
12. less
13. no; lifestyle modifications
14. runs between the layers of the wall
15. HDL; LDL
16. an abnormal immune response; streptococci or other organisms
17. a chronic; compress

Identify the Acronyms

18. DVT; deep vein thrombosis
19. LDL; low density lipoprotein
20. STEMI; ST elevation myocardial infarction
21. CAD; coronary artery disease
22. CHD; coronary heart disease
23. PAD; peripheral arterial disease
24. MVP; mitral valve prolapse

Explain the Pictures

25. Atherosclerosis
26. Diapedesis into the artery wall
27. Tunica intima
28. Lipid (specifically, oxidized LDL)
29. Foam cell or foamy macrophage
30. Lipids (specifically, oxidized LDL)
31. Migrating into the tunica intima
32. A collagen cap
33. Figure 2 (figure on the right)
34. Fatty streak formation

Categorize the Clinical Manifestations

35. Left heart failure
36. Right heart failure
37. Right heart failure
38. Left heart failure
39. Left heart failure
40. Left heart failure
41. Left heart failure
42. Right heart failure

Describe the Differences

43. A thrombus is a blood clot attached to the endothelium in a blood vessel or cardiac chamber, but an embolus is a blood clot or other bolus of matter that circulates in the blood.
44. Primary hypertension has no known cause, but secondary hypertension is caused by another disease process, such as renal disease.
45. Myocardial hibernation involves persistently ischemic myocardium that undergoes metabolic adaptation to survive until perfusion is restored, but myocardial stunning involves temporary loss of contractile ability after perfusion has been restored.
46. In dilated cardiomyopathy, the cardiac chambers are enlarged (have increased diastolic volume), and the myocardium has decreased contractility, but in restrictive cardiomyopathy, the cardiac chambers have decreased diastolic volume because the myocardium is rigid and non-compliant.
47. Valvular stenosis is narrowing of a valve, which impedes the forward flow of blood, but valvular regurgitation is incomplete closure of a valve, which allows blood to leak backward through the valve.

Name the Risk Factors

48. **H** I S T O R Y
49. P O L **Y** G E N I C
50. **P** O T A S S I U M
51. A G **E**
52. **R** E N I N
53. O B E S I **T** Y
54. M A G N **E** S I U M
55. S **N** S
56. **S** O D I U M
57. C **I** G A R E T T E S
58. A L C **O** H O L
59. I N T **O** L E R A N C E

Complete the Sentences

60. thromboembolus
61. stasis
62. hypertrophy; myocardial infarction
63. malignant; brain
64. orthostatic; 20; 10; falls
65. bacterial; fat
66. atherosclerosis; atherosclerosis
67. ischemia; infarction
68. adiponectin
69. demand; supply
70. scar
71. reperfusion
72. polyarthritis; erythema; pharynx
73. high-output
74. Prinzmetal; vasospasm
75. unstable

Match the Consequences

76. C
77. D
78. B
79. A

Teach People about Pathophysiology

Compare your answers with these sample answers.

80. What goes on in your head affects your blood vessels and your heart and can raise your blood pressure. In the short term, stress activates your sympathetic nervous system, causing your blood vessels to squeeze tighter and your heart to beat faster. This raises your blood pressure quickly. And, in the long term, your body's responses to stress make your blood vessel lining not work as well, so your blood pressure stays high all the time. The stress in your head can be quite hard on your body. Would you like to hear a little about what stress management involves?

Copyright © 2024 by Elsevier, Inc. All Rights Reserved.

81. An aneurysm is a place in the wall of an artery that is weaker than normal, so that the blood pushes it outward like a balloon. Your partner's aneurysm is in their aorta, a large artery that has a lot of blood flowing through it. They want to operate to fix the aneurysm before it ruptures. If it ruptures, your partner could bleed to death in a short time. Repairing the area of the aneurysm will reduce the risk for it rupturing.

82. The three big causes of clot development are stasis of blood, increased clotting ability, and injury to the inside of a blood vessel. Stasis of blood means that the blood is not moving, such as when it pooled in your legs during your long car ride. Increased clotting ability means that the blood clots more easily than usual, such as when influenced by the estrogen in contraceptives or hormone supplements. And injury to the inside of a blood vessel means that the lining is rough, such as occurs from cigarette smoking.

83. Even though a heart attack affects the heart and a stroke affects the brain, they are related because the underlying problem is a problem called *atherosclerosis*. Some people call atherosclerosis "hardening of the arteries." As you may know, arteries are blood vessels that carry oxygen and nutrients to the heart, the brain, and other body parts. The lining of the arteries is supposed to be smooth, so the blood can travel easily. When a person has atherosclerosis, the linings of the arteries get thickened and rough. Sometimes a clot develops and stops the blood flow. If that happens in the heart, the person can have a heart attack. If that happens in the brain, the person can have a stroke. Did your doctor talk with you about ways to manage your diet and exercise to reduce your own risk for having a heart attack or stroke?

84. When we exercise, the heart needs to pump more blood than when we are not exercising, to bring oxygen to our muscles. As you know, you have a narrow valve in your heart. This narrow valve limits the amount of blood that your heart can pump out to the rest of your body. When you are not exercising, your heart is able to pump out enough blood to meet your needs. However, when you exercise, this narrow valve prevents your heart from pumping the extra blood to your muscles and the rest of your body. You get so tired because your muscles are not receiving the extra oxygen they need. And you can get faint when your heart is not able to pump enough blood to your brain.

85. As you may know, your heart muscle contracts to pump blood around your body, and then it relaxes to fill with blood that it will pump out in the next contraction. *Heart failure with reduced ejection fraction* means that your heart has difficulty emptying when it contracts to pump out the blood. Heart failure with *preserved* ejection fraction means that a heart does not fill properly when it relaxes.

86. Big, strong muscles need more oxygen than normal-sized ones. Abnormally big, strong heart muscles may not get enough oxygen through the little blood vessels that serve the heart muscle. When a portion of the heart muscle needs more oxygen than the blood vessels are able to provide, the stage is set for a heart attack to occur.

87. It may or may not be a heart attack. The chest pain and other symptoms he had could be caused by a heart attack or by a blood vessel in his heart squeezing shut temporarily. So they call it "acute coronary syndrome" until they can determine the difference. Meanwhile, they do emergency procedures that can help his heart no matter which of the two problems it is.

88. Your grandma is not having an emergency. Let me explain. You probably saw a TV show on which somebody had *ventricular* fibrillation, and it was an emergency. That is a different kind of fibrillation. Your grandma has *atrial* fibrillation. Fibrillation means a muscle is quivering or contracting in a disorganized fashion. Some little muscles at the top of your grandma's heart quiver from time to time and get disorganized, but the rest of your grandma's heart can work without them. Would you like me to draw you a picture of atrial fibrillation?

Clinical Scenarios

89. Ask him about the following: family history of heart disease; personal history of hyperlipidemia, hypertension, diabetes, or atherosclerotic disease in other vascular systems (e.g., history of stroke or peripheral vascular disease); history of cigarette smoking; habitual amount of physical activity; usual diet; and any recent stressors.

90. He may have peripheral vascular disease due to atherosclerosis.

91. An ECG taken now may be completely normal because his pain (and his transient ischemia) has resolved. It may reveal evidence of previous myocardial infarction.

92. Stable angina is the angina pain from myocardial ischemia that occurs predictably with exertion and is relieved with rest or nitroglycerin.

93. Yes, you are remembering well. Some people experience angina pain in the back, jaw, or shoulder, or down their left arm. The chest pain that you experienced is the classic type of angina, but people now realize that myocardial ischemia can cause atypical symptoms also.

94. Cutting down on saturated fat is a great idea because it will reduce one of the risk factors for atherosclerosis. Remember that atherosclerosis in your coronary arteries is the underlying reason for your angina. LDL cholesterol from the saturated fat accumulates in the inner layer of blood vessels and is an important part of an atherosclerotic plaque. If you eat less saturated fat, you reduce your risk. Would you like me to arrange a meeting with a dietitian to help you plan specific ways to eat less saturated fat?

95. He had extracellular fluid volume (ECV) excess. Evidence includes the pulmonary edema and his

Copyright © 2024 by Elsevier, Inc. All Rights Reserved.

underlying congestive heart failure, which is known to cause ECV excess. Treatment with diuretics and low-sodium diet are appropriate for ECV excess. He also has hypertension; low-sodium diet also reduces blood pressure.

96. They heard the adventitious sounds caused by fluid in the alveoli.
97. He likely had bilateral ankle edema caused by increased capillary hydrostatic pressure.
98. He most likely had a bounding pulse.
99. He needs to monitor for increasing ECV excess in order to take action before pulmonary edema arises. A sudden weight gain of 2 pounds (1 kg) indicates gain of 1 liter of fluid.
100. Sodium holds water in the extracellular fluid, thus expanding the ECV. He needs to reduce his ECV rather than expand it.

Puzzle Out the Technical Terms

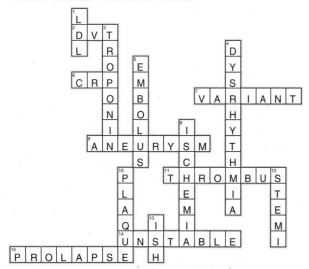

CHAPTER 33

Identify the Acronyms
1. ASD; atrial septal defect
2. PDA; patent ductus arteriosus
3. VSD; ventricular septal defect

Circle the Correct Words
4. shunt
5. difference between, systemic
6. cyanotic
7. left-to-right
8. cyanosis
9. rarely
10. close spontaneously

Characterize the Congenital Heart Defects
11. E, 2
12. H, 3
13. D, 1
14. C, 3
15. B, 2
16. G, 1
17. A, 1
18. F, 3

Describe and Explain the Differences
19. In fetal life, blood flows through the ductus arteriosus from the pulmonary artery to the aorta, allowing blood to bypass the fetal lungs; if the ductus arteriosus does not close after birth, blood flows through it in the opposite direction—from the aorta to the pulmonary artery, sending oxygenated blood through the lungs again. In fetal life, the uninflated lungs are a very high-pressure system, so blood flows from the very high-pressure pulmonary artery into the aorta, which has a lower pressure; after birth, inflation of the lungs makes them a very low-pressure system, so blood flows from the higher pressure aorta into the lower pressure pulmonary artery.
20. Clinical manifestations of a congenital heart defect that causes a moderate right-to-left blood shunt are caused by hypoxemia and cyanosis; they include poor feeding, poor weight gain, dyspnea on exertion, fatigue, and exercise intolerance. By contrast, clinical manifestations of a congenital heart defect that causes a moderate left to right blood shunt are caused by pulmonary overcirculation or acyanotic heart failure; they include poor feeding, failure to thrive, dyspnea, tachypnea, orthopnea, and frequent respiratory infections. The reason for the difference in the clinical manifestations is the type of blood that goes out the aorta: with a right-to-left shunt, that blood is not fully oxygenated; with a left-to-right shunt, the blood in the aorta is fully oxygenated, but an extra volume of blood passes through the lungs, causing extra work for the heart.

Complete the Sentences
21. 90
22. murmur
23. atrioventricular; trisomy 21 (Down)
24. hypoplastic
25. right; left; extrauterine
26. truncus arteriosus
27. Kawasaki; coronary
28. renal
29. kidneys
30. hypertension
31. high; low
32. cyanotic

Teach People about Pathophysiology
Compare your answers with these sample answers.

33. The aorta is a big blood vessel that brings blood from the heart to the rest of the body. That scary word *coarctation* simply means that there is a narrow part in the aorta in the location where there was a passageway before your baby was born. The narrow part

Copyright © 2024 by Elsevier, Inc. All Rights Reserved.

of the aorta makes the blood pressure high in your baby's arms and low in his legs, so that is why the nurses are measuring blood pressure in his leg. His leg is fine; the nurses are monitoring the effects of his heart problem.

34. When your baby cries or when she tries to nurse, she needs more oxygen because she is using her muscles. The defects in her heart make less oxygen in her blood, so she does not have enough oxygen when she uses her muscles. The blue color tells us that her muscles need more oxygen than her blood is carrying. She does not nurse very long because her muscles need more oxygen and get tired, not because she does not

like you. See how her fingers start to curl around your finger when you put it in her hand?

35. Before a baby is born, the ductus arteriosus is a normal blood vessel; you are remembering well. The ductus is supposed to close after birth. The word *patent* means that the ductus arteriosus still is open; because of that, some blood moves abnormally through it between two blood vessels.

36. Your baby has only one heart defect. An atrial septal defect is an abnormal opening between the two top parts of the heart. Blood flowing through that opening is turbulent and makes a sound we call a murmur. Would you like to listen to it through my stethoscope?

Work with the Clinical Scenario

37.

Assessment Findings	Cyanotic Congenital Heart Defect	Acyanotic Congenital Heart Defect
Poor feeding, diaphoresis with feeding, but no change in color of the nailbeds or mucous membranes		X
Episodes of bluish nailbeds and mucus membranes with crying	X	
Cardiac murmur	X	X
Severe acidosis on the first day of life	X	

38. coarctation of the aorta; lower extremity perfusion; ductus arteriosus

CHAPTER 34

Match the Definitions
1. I
2. A
3. H
4. E
5. F
6. G
7. B
8. C
9. D

Order the Steps
10. E, C, G, B, D, A, F, I, H

Match the Functions
11. B
12. D
13. A
14. C

Circle the Correct Words
15. two; three
16. coughing
17. lower

18. veins; arteries
19. has
20. oxygenated; left
21. $Paco_2$
22. brainstem
23. constrict; dilate
24. external
25. fully; $[(760 - 47) \times 0.209]$
26. PaO_2
27. Bohr
28. FEV_1; SaO_2
29. microbiota

Explain the Picture
30. PaO_2
31. SaO_2
32. Peripheral
33. Left; increased affinity of hemoglobin for oxygen enables erythrocytes to load up with oxygen in the lungs.
34. Right; decreased affinity of hemoglobin for oxygen enables erythrocytes to release oxygen in the tissues.
35. Decreased pH, increased $PaCO_2$, and increased heat from cellular metabolism
36. Left
37. Left shift of the oxyhemoglobin dissociation curve increases the affinity of hemoglobin for oxygen, causing less oxygen to be released at the tissues.

Copyright © 2024 by Elsevier, Inc. All Rights Reserved.

Describe the Differences

38. A terminal bronchiole is a conducting airway, but a respiratory bronchiole is a gas-exchange airway.
39. Type I alveolar cells provide the structure of alveoli, but type II alveolar cells secrete surfactant.
40. The visceral pleura covers the lungs, but the parietal pleura lines the thoracic cavity.
41. PaO_2 is the partial pressure of oxygen in the arterial blood, but PAO_2 is the partial pressure of oxygen in the alveoli.
42. Ventilation is movement of air into and out of the lungs, but respiration is exchange of oxygen and carbon dioxide during cellular metabolism.

Complete the Sentences

43. upper
44. macrophages
45. respiratory; alveolar; alveoli
46. alveolocapillary
47. 500
48. irritant
49. downward; increases; negative
50. elastic
51. decreased; increases; increasing
52. 0.8; less
53. Pao_2

Match the Zones

54. C
55. B
56. A

Teach People about Physiology

Compare your answers with these sample answers.

57. The main air tube branches into two air tubes, one that goes to the right lung and one that goes to the left lung. The air tube that goes to the right lung is a little larger and does not angle as much as the left one. That makes it easier for foreign bodies such as a peanut to enter the right side.
58. Cilia are tiny hair-like structures that beat rhythmically and move a layer of mucus upward toward your throat. That mucus layer traps dust and microorganisms that could make you sick and carries them away from your lungs.
59. A small amount of the blood carried by the pulmonary veins is deoxygenated blood from the bronchial circulation, which is part of the systemic circulation. The bronchial circulation nourishes tissue in the conducting airways and does not participate in gas exchange.
60. When a small bronchiole gets blocked, the alveolar partial pressure of oxygen decreases in the alveoli that airway serves. It is not useful to perfuse alveoli that are not ventilated, so the pulmonary arterioles constrict in that area, sending the blood to other alveoli that are well ventilated. That makes the lungs more efficient.

61. To calculate oxygen content of blood, you need the PaO_2, hemoglobin, and SaO_2.
62. Carbon dioxide diffuses across membranes much more easily than oxygen. That makes it possible to excrete enough CO_2 from the lungs even when a lung problem decreases diffusion of oxygen into the blood.

Puzzle Out the Technical Terms

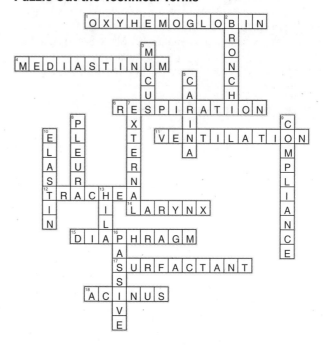

CHAPTER 35

Match the Definitions

1. D
2. E
3. A
4. B
5. C
6. F

Circle the Correct Words

7. $PaCO_2$
8. effusion
9. decreased
10. swallowing; pneumonitis
11. dullness; crackles; pink and frothy
12. exudative; transudative
13. non-productive; low-grade
14. restrictive; obstructive
15. expiration
16. chronic
17. cigarette smoking; vague
18. biologics

Categorize the Causes

19. Hyperventilation
20. Hypoventilation

Copyright © 2024 by Elsevier, Inc. All Rights Reserved.

21. Hypoventilation
22. Hyperventilation
23. Hypoventilation
24. Hyperventilation
25. Hypoventilation

Order the Steps
26. E, B, D, A, G, C, H, F

Explain the Picture
27. asthma
28. No, not the first antigen exposure, as demonstrated by the presence of antigen-specific antibodies (IgE)
29. The IgE is produced by plasma cells (mature B lymphocytes) that have become committed to a specific antigen.
30. The Fc (constant fragment) end of IgE binds to Fc receptors in the mast cell plasma membrane. This allows the Fab (antigen-binding fragment) end to be available to bind antigen.
31. The mast cell degranulates when the antigen binds to the IgE located on the mast cell membrane. Mast cell degranulation releases inflammatory mediators that cause inflammation, bronchoconstriction, and increased secretion of mucus.

Describe the Differences
32. Dyspnea is a feeling of breathlessness, but orthopnea is a feeling of breathlessness when lying flat.
33. Chylothorax is lymph in the pleural space but hemothorax is blood in the pleural space.
34. Absorption atelectasis is alveolar collapse caused by gases being absorbed from alveoli that are obstructed, but compression atelectasis is alveolar collapse caused by external pressure on the alveoli.
35. In a communicating pneumothorax, the pressure of the air in the pleural space is the same as barometric pressure because the air drawn into the pleural space during inspiration is forced back out during expiration, but in tension pneumothorax, the pressure of the air in the pleural space exceeds barometric pressure because air enters during inspiration but cannot exit during expiration.

Match the Breathing Patterns
36. C
37. E
38. D
39. B
40. F
41. A

Complete the Sentences
42. paroxysmal nocturnal dyspnea
43. inward; flail
44. air
45. bronchiectasis; sputum
46. connective (or fibrotic); decreased
47. remodeling
48. mucus; constriction
49. status asthmaticus
50. α_1-antitrypsin; proteolytic enzymes
51. chronic bronchitis; mucus; productive
52. barrel; dyspnea
53. right; hypertension
54. hoarseness
55. bronchogenic carcinoma; hormones

Teach People about Pathophysiology
Compare your answers with these sample answers.

56. Your grandpa has a chronic lung disease called *emphysema*. Some of the lung structures inside his chest have been destroyed, so he has to use his respiratory muscles extra hard to move air in and out of his lungs.
57. ARDS means acute respiratory distress syndrome or adult respiratory distress syndrome. Do you know what inflammation is? If you skin your knee, it gets red and swollen because it is injured, and we call that inflammation. Your uncle has a lot of inflammation inside his lungs, which is making them stiff, so that it is difficult to breathe. That is why he is in the hospital where they are taking care of him.
58. Your cousin may not cough up blood. He breathed in the germs that cause tuberculosis, but his protector white blood cells probably are attacking and surrounding them, so they cannot hurt his lungs badly enough to make him cough blood. It is important for him to take his tuberculosis medicine every day to help get rid of the germs so that he will not cough up blood.
59. When he was working in the coal mine every day, your grandpa breathed in a lot of coal dust. The coal dust went into his lungs, and over the years, his body made scar tissue. Have you seen a scar develop after someone gets a cut? That is what happened deep inside your grandpa's lungs. More and more scar tissue formed until his lungs got very stiff and it became hard for him to breathe.
60. Your relatives were exposed to different kinds of materials in their occupations. Silica is inorganic, which means that it did not come from a living material. On the other hand, mold is organic, which means that it is a living material. Long-term exposure to both of these materials causes buildup of scar tissue in the lungs, which we know as pulmonary fibrosis. However, the actual process that causes this fibrosis is different. Exposure to inorganic materials causes the disease process known as pneumoconiosis; exposure to organic materials causes the disease process known as hypersensitivity pneumonitis.
61. Normally, blood that goes through the lungs and picks up oxygen empties into the left side of the heart, which pumps the blood to the rest of the body. If the left heart is not able to pump out the blood effectively, blood will

Copyright © 2024 by Elsevier, Inc. All Rights Reserved.

back up into the blood vessels in the lungs. This makes too much pressure in those lung blood vessels, so some water moves out of the blood vessels and into the lung spaces. He had difficulty breathing because some of his lung spaces had water in them instead of air.

62. The airway obstruction from mucus and the eventual airway damage cause hypoxemia in chronic bronchitis. Over time, hypoxemia causes increased erythrocyte production, so these patients get polycythemia.

Clinical Scenarios

63. empyema; pleural space.
64. Empyema fluid usually originates as leakage of lymphatic drainage from sites of bacterial pneumonia.
65. Mrs. Beeson is short of breath because the accumulated empyema fluid is compressing her left lung or at least preventing it from expanding, which interferes with ventilation and gas exchange.
66. Mrs. Goh, age 46, emigrated from Southeast Asia 25 years ago. She is admitted to the hospital with low-grade fever, shortness of breath, and a cough producing discolored sputum. Further evaluation reveals that she has had an unintentional weight loss of 15 pounds in the past 4 months. Examination of her sputum is positive for *Mycobacterium tuberculosis*. Her diagnosis is active tuberculosis (TB) disease.
67. Tuberculosis is transmitted through the air, contained in droplet nuclei created when a person who has untreated active tuberculosis coughs.
68. A tubercle is an accumulation of white blood cells, mostly derived from neutrophils, macrophages, and lymphocytes, around microorganisms that phagocytes are unable to remove effectively.
69. Yes, Mrs. Goh should have had a positive tuberculin skin test when she had latent TB disease. This test indicates that her immune system has encountered the TB bacillus and reacted to it. It does not distinguish between latent infection and active disease.
70. Mrs. Goh likely developed some sort of immuno-compromise. Although there are many possibilities, common causes of immunocompromise include immunosuppressive drugs (for example prednisone or cancer chemotherapy), AIDS, or conditions such as chronic alcoholism or liver disease.
71. Bacterial pneumonia because she has exudate in her alveoli, a productive cough, and a substantial fever and chills, which characterize a bacterial pneumonia. Viral pneumonia usually is mild and self-limited and does not produce a substantial alveolar exudate.
72. Cigarette smoking compromises the upper airway defenses. Bacteria reach the lung, causing inflammation. Bacteria, white blood cells, cytokines, and exudate flood the alveoli, causing V/Q mismatching that leads to hypoxemia.
73. Phagocytic cells, such as macrophages, will clear much of the consolidated exudate.

74. Smoking paralyzes the cilia, can cause squamous metaplasia, can trigger chronic inflammation in the bronchi, and increases the production of mucus. These effects of smoking all compromise the upper airway defenses, making her more vulnerable to pneumonia.
75. Ms. Silber developed a pulmonary embolism from a deep venous thrombosis in the lower extremity that had the fracture.
76. Although ventilation (V) continues with a pulmonary embolism, the pulmonary embolus stops perfusion (Q) in pulmonary blood vessels, creating ventilation-perfusion (V/Q) mismatch.
77. You could not move your broken leg because it is in a cast, so the blood did not flow very fast in it. Slow-moving blood clots rather easily, which allowed a blood clot to form in one of your deep leg veins. When the clot broke loose, it traveled in the blood to your lungs and got stuck in one of the blood vessels in your lungs. As you probably know, the blood needs to travel through the lungs to pick up oxygen. When the clot blocked blood flow in your lung, you needed more oxygen. That is why you became short of breath and were breathing so fast. [Note: If you used technical terms such as *immobility, stasis of blood, thrombus, embolus, perfusion,* or *ventilation* in your answer without explaining them, remember that you need to use language suitable for a layperson, and try your answer again.]

CHAPTER 36

Match the Definitions
1. D
2. C
3. A
4. B
5. F
6. E

Circle the Correct Words
7. atelectasis; surfactant
8. collapse inward; compliant
9. barking
10. bacterial; 2 to 6
11. inspiration
12. unilateral; tonsillitis
13. viral
14. atypical; not
15. follows; progressive; hypoxemia
16. days or weeks after; multiple organs

Categorize the Respiratory Disorders
17. Upper airway infection
18. Lower airway infection
19. Upper airway infection
20. Lower airway infection

Answer Key

Copyright © 2024 by Elsevier, Inc. All Rights Reserved.

21. Upper airway congenital malformation
22. Upper airway infection
23. Upper airway infection
24. Upper airway infection

Explain the Picture

25. D
26. A
27. Obstruction in area E will alter the nature of the cough.
28. Stridor
29. Stridor is inspiratory in area B and expiratory in area C.
30. Area A

Complete the Sentences

31. respiratory distress syndrome
32. croup; virus; subglottal
33. adenotonsillar
34. surfactant; hyaline
35. bronchopulmonary dysplasia; development
36. respiratory syncytial virus; rhinorrhea; increased
37. pneumonitis
38. asthma

Teach People about Pathophysiology

Compare your answers with these sample answers.

39. The respiratory virus that your baby has makes the lining of the airways (little air tubes) swell. Your baby has tiny little airways, so if their lining swells, there is not much room at all for the air to pass through. He is breathing fast because he needs more oxygen than can travel though his swollen little airways. That is why we are watching him and taking good care of him. His big sister has bigger airways, so they will not swell shut if their lining swells a little from a virus. She may have had a different virus, too. There are a lot of different viruses and hers just caused a runny nose.

40. What you described is normal for a baby. A baby's ribs are flexible, not rigid like an adult's ribs. When a baby inhales, air is drawn in, and so is the chest wall. This is normal for a little baby like yours.

41. Croup is swelling inside the neck that makes a little child cough, make strange noises when breathing, and have difficulty breathing. It must have been scary to see and hear that with your little brother. Little children are the ones who get croup. You are too grown up to get croup.

42. Resistance to airflow is inversely proportional to the fourth power of the radius. So, if the radius decreases to half of its baseline value, resistance to airflow will be 16 times greater. Thus, a little bit of edema in an infant's little airway can cause severe airway obstruction.

43. Snoring is common with a condition called *obstructive sleep apnea.* This is an important cause of being sleepy during the day, as Jason is.

44. Usually when a baby is born, adrenalin and other hormones triggered during labor cause surfactant release in the baby's lungs. These hormones are not released as much during an elective C-section, so the baby tends to have less surfactant. As you know, RDS is caused by not having enough surfactant in the lungs.

45. I understand that you are concerned about Howie. The good news is that SIDS happens only in children who are less than 12 months old. Howie will not develop SIDS because he has grown past the vulnerable age. You will feel more rested and enjoy Howie more during the day if you do not wake yourself up every 2 hours all night.

46. We really do need to remove it now. If it stays in your airways, you could get an infection there. Or it could cause more irritation and swelling that could block your breathing. Your wheezing tells us that your airway already is narrowed now, so we need to pay attention.

47. Dog germs do not cause asthma. Your little sister got asthma because she probably has an allergy in her breathing tubes. When she plays with dogs, she breathes in little bits from the dog hairs that trigger her asthma. Apparently, you do not have an allergy in your breathing tubes, so those little bits from the dog hairs do not make you cough and have trouble breathing.

Clinical Scenarios

48. The admitting nurse did not make a mistake. When a child has acute epiglottitis, examination of the throat can trigger laryngospasm, which blocks breathing and may be fatal.

49. epiglottis; preventing him from swallowing

50. Turbulent airflow through a partially obstructed airway causes stridor. Darrell's airway was partially obstructed by his swollen epiglottis.

51. The epiglottis is a little flap that normally covers the opening to our airway when we swallow. The epiglottis sends the food or liquid to our stomach when we eat or drink and keeps it from going toward our lungs. *Epiglottitis* means that the epiglottis is inflamed and swollen. Darrell's epiglottis was swollen and blocking his breathing. That is why we put the tube down his throat so that he can breathe.

52. Darrell is unable to swallow, so he was given intravenous antibiotics.

53. Acute epiglottitis that is treated appropriately usually resolves after a few days.

54. CF is an autosomal recessive disorder, which means that a person must have two CF genes in order to have CF. Each of your parents has only one CF gene, so they do not have CF. You inherited one CF gene from each of your parents, which gives you two CF genes.

55. CFTCR means *cystic fibrosis transmembrane conductance regulator,* a protein that transports chloride

337

Copyright © 2024 by Elsevier, Inc. All Rights Reserved.

ions across epithelial cell membranes. A defect in this gene causes cystic fibrosis by creating an abnormal CFTCR that works ineffectively.

56. Factors that contribute to the recurrent respiratory infections in CF include the very thick dehydrated mucus from abnormal CFTCR function that impedes normal mucociliary clearance of bacteria; chronic infection with bacteria that form biofilms; and eventual development of bronchiectasis, which makes pouches where mucus collects and bacteria grow.

57. Chronic infiltration of neutrophils in CF contributes to inflammation through secretion of oxidants (which promote inflammation) and neutrophil elastase and other proteases (which damage tissue and contribute to development of bronchiectasis).

58. Biofilms in the airways in CF enable bacteria to evade the immune system and resist antibiotics.

59. Digital clubbing

60. The CFTCR defect in CF also causes digestive secretions, especially those from the pancreas, to be abnormally thick, which impedes absorption of nutrients.

CHAPTER 37

Match the Definitions
1. C
2. D
3. A
4. F
5. G
6. B
7. E
8. I
9. H
10. J

Circle the Correct Words
11. cortex
12. pores; epithelium
13. external; pudendal
14. protein; concentrate
15. excretion
16. glomerular filtration rate
17. increase; decreases; increases
18. low; high; reabsorption
19. uromodulin; distal; infection
20. increases; concentrate
21. loop of Henle; vasa recta
22. activate; parathyroid hormone
23. glomerular filtration rate; effective renal plasma flow

Locate the Structures
24. Renal cortex
25. Renal medulla
26. Renal cortex
27. Renal cortex
28. Renal medulla
29. Renal medulla
30. Renal medulla
31. Renal cortex
32. Renal cortex
33. Renal cortex

Order the Steps
34. A, E, G, B, F, H, J, D, I, C

Match the Functions
35. C
36. E
37. B
38. A
39. D

Explain the Picture
40. Proximal convoluted tubule
41. Mitochondria provide ATP for the active transport processes that enable the reabsorption function of these cells.
42. Microvilli increase the surface area for reabsorption.
43. The cell from the thick ascending limb of the loop of Henle

Match the Mechanisms
44. B
45. C
46. A

Describe the Differences
47. The urethra carries urine from the bladder to the exterior of the body, but a ureter carries urine from the kidney to the bladder.
48. The principal cells secrete potassium and reabsorb sodium and water, but the intercalated cells reabsorb potassium and secrete hydrogen ions.
49. Tubular secretion moves substances from the peritubular capillaries into the renal tubular lumen, but tubular reabsorption moves them from the renal tubular lumen into the peritubular capillaries.

Complete the Sentences
50. hilum
51. microvilli
52. nephron; juxtamedullary
53. mesangial
54. renal plasma flow
55. sympathetic; vasoconstrict
56. favor; oppose
57. renalase
58. erythropoietin; erythropoiesis
59. clearance
60. increases; chronic
61. increases; catabolism

Finish the Descriptions
62. In the spinal cord, the sensory neurons activate parasympathetic motor pathways that cause the bladder muscle to contract. Inhibition of the sympathetic innervation of the internal urethral sphincter accompanies this process. Unless this reflex is inhibited voluntarily, micturition occurs.

Answer Key

Copyright © 2024 by Elsevier, Inc. All Rights Reserved.

63. Renal afferent arterioles constrict, which prevents an increase in filtration pressure. This protects the glomeruli from damage and maintains renal excretion.

64. In the blood, renin converts angiotensinogen to angiotensin I, which angiotensin-converting enzyme changes to angiotensin II, a vasoconstrictor. Angiotensin II also stimulates secretion of aldosterone from the adrenal cortex. Aldosterone circulates to the kidneys, where it increases reabsorption of sodium and water and excretion of potassium.

Teach People about Physiology

Compare your answers with these sample answers.

65. The walls of the ureters have special muscles that contract in rhythmic waves we call peristalsis. This is similar to the way that digested food moves through the intestines. Peristalsis moves the urine to the bladder regardless of body position.

66. The arterial blood that is not filtered at the glomerulus enters another capillary bed before it leaves the kidney. That capillary bed is the peritubular capillaries that surround the renal tubules; it is important in allowing the tubules to reabsorb and secrete substances to produce the proper composition of the urine. After the peritubular capillaries, the blood goes into the renal venous system and back into the systemic veins.

67. Remember that these refugees come to us with protein malnutrition. Our kidneys need urea from the normal breakdown of protein in order to concentrate the urine. If there is not enough protein in the body, there will not be enough urea, and the kidneys will not be able to do their maximal job of concentrating the urine.

68. That number is correct. We do not urinate out our body fluids because the kidney tubules that receive that filtered fluid put about 99% of the fluid back into the blood. So we only urinate out what the kidneys have selected for excretion, and we keep the rest of the fluid in our bodies.

69. The basic change is a decrease in the number of nephrons as people age. Among other changes, that decreases the ability to concentrate the urine. Thus, you make a larger urine volume at night than you used to make, and you wake up to urinate. Some changes in bladder function with age may contribute to nocturia as well.

CHAPTER 38

Match the Definitions
1. C
2. A
3. D
4. B

Circle the Correct Words
5. damages
6. undergoes hypertrophy of existing glomeruli and tubules
7. calcium phosphate; uric acid
8. neurogenic bladder

9. bladder; painless
10. retrograde up the urethra; retrograde up a ureter
11. confusion
12. renal pelvis and tubules; pain; interstitium
13. histologic appearance
14. irreversible; chronic kidney disease
15. the glomerular filtration rate

Categorize the Causes
16. Intrarenal
17. Intrarenal
18. Prerenal
19. Intrarenal
20. Prerenal
21. Postrenal
22. Postrenal

Order the Steps
23. D, A, C, E, B

Identify the Examples
24. D
25. A
26. B
27. C

Describe the Differences
28. Cystitis is inflammation of the urinary bladder, but pyelonephritis is inflammation of a kidney.

29. The urine in acute glomerulonephritis contains erythrocytes, red cell casts, white cell casts, and varying degrees of protein, which usually is not severe, but the urine in nephrotic syndrome contains massive amounts of protein and lipids and either a microscopic amount of blood or no blood.

30. Azotemia is accumulation of nitrogenous wastes in the blood, manifested as elevated BUN and often creatinine as well, but uremia is a syndrome that includes azotemia and numerous other clinical manifestations such as fatigue, anemia, and pruritus.

Complete the Sentences
31. calculi; calcium
32. prostate; pelvic organs
33. carcinomas; epithelium
34. uroepithelium; micturition (or urination)
35. interstitial
36. immune
37. diabetes
38. 50
39. 400

Match the Clinical Manifestations
40. D
41. F
42. A
43. C
44. B
45. G
46. E

Copyright © 2024 by Elsevier, Inc. All Rights Reserved.

Complete the Table

Normal Renal Function	Result of Impaired Function in the Uremic Syndrome
Excrete nitrogenous wastes	Azotemia (elevated BUN and plasma creatinine)
Excrete potassium ions	Hyperkalemia
Excrete metabolic acids	Metabolic acidosis
Excrete phosphate	Hyperphosphatemia and hypocalcemia
Activate vitamin D	Hypocalcemia, secondary hyperparathyroidism, renal osteodystrophy
Secrete erythropoietin	Anemia
Excrete sodium and water	Extracellular fluid volume excess, hypertension, potential for pulmonary edema

Teach People about Pathophysiology

Compare your answers with these sample answers.

47. Casts are little molds of the inside of little tubes in your kidneys that help make urine. When you have a kidney infection, white blood cells go into the kidney to fight the infection. Some of them stick inside the little tubes and make these casts, which detach and go out in the urine. The casts do not injure you. They are the protective white blood cells. Having white blood cell casts in the urine is a sign that you have a kidney infection.

48. When you have a bladder infection, there is a risk for the infection going up into your kidneys. That risk increases during pregnancy because the urine tubes from the kidneys to the bladder are more relaxed during pregnancy. Chills and fever occur with a bacterial infection; if you develop a kidney infection, it likely will signal itself with chills and fever. If that happens, call the office so that the infection can be treated rapidly.

49. Yes, being tired does come from your kidney disease. You know that kidneys normally make urine. Kidneys also have another normal function: they release a hormone called *erythropoietin* that stimulates bone marrow to make new red blood cells. Red blood cells normally carry oxygen to all parts of your body. With your chronic kidney disease, your kidneys are not making enough of that erythropoietin hormone that stimulates red blood cell production. Without the proper signals, your bone marrow does not make enough red blood cells, and your muscles and other parts of your body do not get the oxygen you need. That makes you very tired. In addition, if the potassium is high in your blood, that can make your muscles weak, which can contribute to being tired.

50. I know it is difficult not to eat strawberries when they are in season, but there is a good reason for you to avoid them. Strawberries contain a lot of potassium. As you know, your kidneys cannot make enough urine. Normally, when we eat strawberries and other potassium-rich foods, our kidneys excrete the extra potassium in the urine, so it does not build up in the blood. Because your kidneys are not able to do that, if you eat strawberries, the potassium will build up in your blood and can cause your heart to beat irregularly or even stop. So it really is important for you not to eat a lot of strawberries.

51. Kidney damage can be in different amounts. The nephrons are the parts of your kidneys that help make urine. If you still have some functioning kidney tissue, but a lot of your nephrons are not working properly, your kidneys will lose their ability to concentrate urine. Normally, our kidneys concentrate the urine more at night, so we urinate less at night. However, you are making more urine than usual because your kidneys are not able to concentrate it. This is why you are getting up to urinate at night.

52. You do have a kidney stone. That kidney stone stuck in your ureter, and the urine backed up into your kidney, stretching part of the inside of your kidney. The enlarged kidney from accumulation of urine is called *hydronephrosis*.

53. Some of your glomerulus filters are damaged and let water and red blood cells through. However, many of your glomerulus filters are totally clogged up and are not letting the water through, so you are making less urine than usual.

54. His renal tubules are recovering, so he is making more urine, but he is not able to concentrate urine well because he is not fully recovered.

55. Diabetes damages the inside of the kidney slowly until it cannot function. In your husband's case, a lot of kidney cells died from the lack of blood flow, but if their scaffold is not damaged, they can grow back, and he does have a chance to recover.

56. The red blood cells are entering your kidneys through damaged glomeruli, where the blood is filtered in the kidneys at the very beginning of making urine. This means that they stay in the urine for a relatively long time; this enables the acid urine to react with them and cause a chemical change that gives a brownish color. The bladder is lower in the urinary tract, so the red

Answer Key

Copyright © 2024 by Elsevier, Inc. All Rights Reserved.

blood cells do not stay in the urine as long; bleeding from the bladder produces a pink- or red-colored urine.

57. Normally, glomerular membranes have a negative charge, which keeps negatively charged proteins like albumin out of the urine. In nephrotic syndrome, the glomerular membranes have lost their normal negative charges. This enables massive amounts of proteins to move into the renal tubules.

58. Stress incontinence is involuntary loss of urine control when there is more pressure in the abdomen, such as when coughing or laughing. Do you know someone who has developed stress incontinence?

59. There are many causes of anemia. Heavy menstruation takes iron from our bodies, and raisins help put it back. It sounds as if you did a good job with that. However, now your anemia has a different cause that raisins will not help. Your kidneys are not stimulating your bone marrow properly, so your bone marrow is not making enough red blood cells. Raisins can put more potassium in your blood than your kidneys can handle, so you should not eat them.

60. The location of the injury determines what bladder dysfunction will occur. Lesions in the sacral area of the spinal cord or peripheral nerves that innervate the bladder cause underactive, hypotonic, or flaccid bladder function, often with loss of bladder sensation. Lesions in the brain or spinal cord above the sacral area cause loss of coordinated neuromuscular contraction and overactive or hyperreflexive bladder function.

61. renal calculi; dehydration causing concentrated urine

62. The pain of a calculus moving down a ureter is rhythmic because a ureter engages in peristalsis, rather than simply being a passive tube.

63. Mr. Flores's supervisor needs to know the importance of keeping the workers hydrated in the heat and to make appropriate fluids available to them. Mr. Flores needs to remember to find an alternate fluid container and be sure to keep well hydrated in the future. Depending on the composition of his calculi, he might receive additional teaching to decrease his risk.

64. Pain with urination

65. Need to urinate more often than usual

66. Strong need to urinate immediately

67. Most bladder infections are caused by bacteria, such as *E. coli*, which ascends the urethra. Viral and fungal bladder infections do occur, but much less commonly.

68. Cystitis

CHAPTER 39

Match the Congenital Abnormalities

1. E
2. A
3. C
4. G
5. B
6. D
7. F

Circle the Correct Words

8. all of the; adolescence
9. third; increases; 2 years
10. high; increases
11. cystitis; decreases
12. non-specific; enuresis
13. difficult
14. 5; functional
15. idiopathic; absence
16. bladder outlet
17. autoimmune; glomerulus

Explain the Pictures

18. In picture B, the ureter travels straight through the bladder wall, whereas in picture A, it crosses at an oblique angle.
19. Picture A
20. Vesicoureteral reflux
21. When the bladder wall contracts, the ureter continues to be patent, and urine refluxes up the ureter, flowing back into the bladder as the bladder relaxes.
22. If bacteria reach the bladder, they are less likely to be flushed out, which increases the risk for cystitis. Reflux of infected urine up the ureter to the kidney predisposes to pyelonephritis.

Describe the Differences

23. In hypospadias, the urethral meatus is located on the ventral side of the penis, but in epispadias, it is located on the dorsal side of the penis.
24. A hypoplastic kidney is small with fewer nephrons but otherwise normal, but a dysplastic kidney contains abnormal tissue.
25. Primary incontinence occurs when a child has not developed bladder control beyond the age at which bladder control usually is achieved, but secondary incontinence occurs when a child who has been dry for at least 6 months becomes incontinent again.
26. Chordee is a congenital defect in which the penis bends ventrally, but penile torsion is a congenital defect in which the penile shaft is twisted.

Complete the Sentences

27. horseshoe
28. exstrophy
29. ureteropelvic junction; hydronephrosis
30. dysplasia
31. *PDK1*; cysts
32. nephroblastoma; kidney; abdomen
33. hypoalbuminemia; periorbital
34. nephrotic syndrome

Teach People about Pathophysiology

Compare your answers with these sample answers.

35. Yes, that foamy urine is part of her nephrotic syndrome. Her urine is foamy because it has a lot of protein in it. Usually that protein stays in the blood, but with nephrotic syndrome, the protein barrier in the kidneys is not working, and proteins go into the urine.

Copyright © 2024 by Elsevier, Inc. All Rights Reserved.

36. *Poly* means "a lot," and *cystic* refers to cysts, which are little sacs that are filled with fluid in polycystic kidney disease. So polycystic kidney disease is a condition in which a lot of little sacs form and fill up with fluid. As more and more cysts form, they compress the normal kidney tissue, so that it cannot function.

37. Normally, the amniotic fluid surrounding the developing baby helps the lungs develop. Part of that fluid comes from the developing baby's kidneys. When the developing baby's kidneys do not form correctly, there is less of that useful amniotic fluid. Thus the lungs do not develop well.

38. Tami, a likely explanation is that you have autosomal recessive polycystic kidney disease and that Mrs. Singleton has autosomal dominant polycystic kidney disease. These two genetic forms of polycystic kidney disease involve different gene mutations and have different clinical time courses.

39. Yes, it was not a direct infection. Instead, the *E. coli* produced a toxin that entered the blood and attached to some white blood cells. Those white blood cells carried the toxin to Molly's kidneys, where it caused a lot of damage. I am pleased to see that she is recovering now.

Clinical Scenario

40. No, the strep organism did not infect Shane's kidneys. What happened is that his immune system learned to defend against the strep organism, and after the strep was all gone, Shane's immune system attacked his kidneys and damaged them.

41. The smoky brown color is caused by hematuria; the red blood cells leak through spaces in the damaged glomeruli.

42. Shane's glomerular filtration rate decreased because of damaged glomeruli with thickened glomerular membranes. His kidneys retained sodium and water, increasing his vascular hydrostatic pressure, which promotes edema, especially in dependent areas like the ankles.

43. An immune complex is an antibody attached to an antigen. In acute poststreptococcal glomerulonephritis, immune complexes form or lodge in the glomeruli, which causes inflammation and glomerular damage.

CHAPTER 40

Match the Definitions

1. C
2. D
3. E
4. A
5. B

Match the Cells

6. D
7. A
8. B
9. C
10. G
11. H
12. E
13. I
14. F

Circle the Correct Words

15. stimulate; delay
16. liver; alkaline
17. its secretion
18. immunoglobulin A
19. peristalsis
20. delay; delay
21. microvilli; oligopeptides
22. small; initial; small
23. sterile; weeks
24. liver; bile
25. inactive; active; active
26. decrease; decrease; remain normal

Categorize the Stimuli

27. Increase
28. Decrease
29. Increase
30. Increase
31. Increase
32. Increase

Order the Steps

33. B, D, F, A, C, E

Explain the Picture

34. The liver
35. Liver lobule
36. Sinusoids
37. Branches of the hepatic portal vein and the hepatic artery
38. Central veins
39. The highly permeable endothelium that lines the sinusoids enables movement of nutrients, drugs, and other molecules into the hepatocytes, where they are metabolized.
40. The canaliculi, which empty into the bile ducts

Describe the Differences

41. The upper third of the esophagus has striated muscle, but the lower third has smooth muscle.
42. The visceral layer of the peritoneum covers the abdominal organs, but the parietal layer extends along the abdominal wall.
43. The antrum of the stomach is the lower portion, but the fundus is the upper portion.
44. A micelle is a water-soluble collection of bile salts and various forms of fat and cholesterol in the intestinal lumen, but a chylomicron is a water-soluble collection of triglycerides, cholesterol, and lipoproteins that circulates in the lymph and blood.

Copyright © 2024 by Elsevier, Inc. All Rights Reserved.

Match the Enzymes

45. E
46. F
47. D
48. B
49. C
50. A

Complete the Sentences

51. celiac; superior mesenteric
52. duodenum, jejunum, ileum
53. lacteal; fat (or lipid)
54. secretion; absorption
55. pyloric; Oddi
56. liver; iron
57. ileocecal; closed
58. transverse; descending; sigmoid
59. smooth; striated
60. round; falciform; abdominal
61. cholesterol; enterohepatic
62. enterokinase
63. submucosa; muscularis
64. enteric; myenteric

Teach People about Physiology

Compare your answers with these sample answers.

65. Mucus in the stomach protects the wall of the stomach from the acid and digestive enzymes that could damage it. The mucus forms a protective barrier.
66. Pepsin is sensitive to how acidic its environment is. In an acidic environment such as the stomach, pepsin is active, but in a less acidic (more alkaline) environment such as the intestine, pepsin does not function anymore.
67. Eating some vitamin C at the same time as the iron pill helps the iron enter the body (be absorbed) more easily. The vitamin C reduces ferric iron to ferrous iron, which is the form more easily absorbed.
68. The appendix is attached to the first portion of the large intestine. After the stomach, food travels into the small intestine and then the large intestine before the waste exits our bodies as a bowel movement. The appendix hangs off the initial part of the large intestine like a little pouch.
69. The gastrocolic reflex helps us have a bowel movement right after eating. When the stomach is stretched by food and partially digested food enters portions of the small intestine, the large intestine starts contracting more and moves its contents onward to become a bowel movement.
70. Bile is important and useful. It helps process dietary fats in the intestines so that the animal or the person gets the benefit from eating the fats. Bile is made by the liver and stored in the gallbladder until it goes into the intestines when the animal or person eats fats.

Puzzle Out the Technical Terms

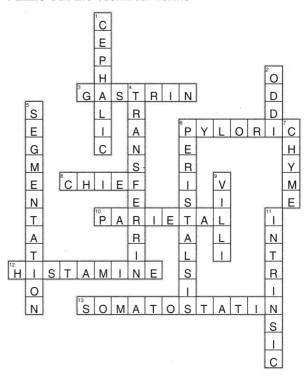

CHAPTER 41

Match the Definitions

1. D
2. F
3. B
4. J
5. A
6. H
7. C
8. G
9. E
10. I

Circle the Correct Words

11. decreased; lower; cough
12. sliding; is
13. vomiting; constipation
14. digestive enzymes; necrotic; peritonitis
15. a chronic; immune
16. adenocarcinomas; squamous cell carcinomas
17. intrahepatic; posthepatic
18. hypertension; vasodilation; bacterial
19. yellow; sclera of the eye

Categorize the Clinical Manifestations

20. Portal hypertension
21. Hepatocyte dysfunction
22. Hepatocyte dysfunction
23. Portal hypertension

Copyright © 2024 by Elsevier, Inc. All Rights Reserved.

24. Portal hypertension
25. Portal hypertension
26. Hepatocyte dysfunction

Order the Steps
27. D, B, F, A, E, C, G

Characterize the Types of Hepatitis

Characteristic	Hepatitis A Infection	Hepatitis B Infection	Hepatitis C Infection	Hepatitis D Infection	Hepatitis E Infection
Routes of transmission	Fecal-oral, parenteral, sexual	Parenteral, sexual	Parenteral	Parenteral, fecal-oral, sexual	Fecal-oral
Acute or chronic?	Acute	Acute or chronic; often chronic	Acute or chronic; often chronic	Chronic	Acute
Carrier state	No	Yes	Yes	Yes	No

Describe the Differences

28. GERD (gastroesophageal reflux disease) is reflux of acid and pepsin from the stomach to the esophagus that causes esophagitis, but NERD (non-erosive reflux disease) involves similar symptoms with no visible sign of esophagitis.
29. Type A chronic gastritis is caused by autoimmune damage primarily in the gastric fundus, but type B chronic gastritis is caused by non-immune mechanisms such as *H. pylori*, chronic use of alcohol and non-steroidal anti-inflammatory drugs, and occurs primarily in the gastric antrum.
30. Maldigestion is failure of the chemical processes of breaking down (digesting) nutrients that take place in the intestinal lumen or at the brush border of the intestinal mucosa of the small intestine, but malabsorption is the failure of the intestinal mucosa to transport the digested nutrients into the blood or lymph.
31. In alcoholic cirrhosis, the damage begins with the hepatocytes, but in biliary cirrhosis, the damage begins in the bile canaliculi and bile ducts.

Match the Disorders

32. B
33. G
34. D
35. F
36. A
37. E
38. C
39. I
40. H

Complete the Sentences

41. achalasia
42. hiatal hernia
43. alkalosis; acidosis
44. days
45. peptic; *pylori*
46. fat; lipase
47. muscle; colon
48. periumbilical; right lower

49. D
50. icteric; recovery
51. cystic; cholesterol
52. lipase; alcohol
53. alcohol; obesity; cirrhosis

Complete the Chart

Characteristics	Crohn Disease	Ulcerative Colitis
Family history	More common	Less common
Location of lesions	Entire GI tract, with the small and large intestines most common, skip lesions	Rectum and colon, continuous lesions
Nature of lesions	Involve entire thickness of intestinal wall	Involve the mucosal layer only
Fistulas and abscesses	Common	Rare
Narrowed lumen, possible obstruction	Common	Rare
Recurrent episodes of diarrhea	Common	Common
Blood in stools	Less common	Common
Clinical course	Remissions and exacerbations	Remissions and exacerbations

Match the Risk Factors

54. D
55. B
56. C
57. A

Answer Key

Copyright © 2024 by Elsevier, Inc. All Rights Reserved.

Teach People about Pathophysiology

Compare your answers with these sample answers.

58. With alcoholic hepatitis, the liver is inflamed, and there are necrotic cells because of the alcohol damage, so the person has signs and symptoms of acute inflammation and liver dysfunction. The liver often regenerates and recovers from hepatitis if the person stops drinking. With alcoholic cirrhosis, alcohol damage triggers overgrowth of connective tissue (fibrosis) that distorts the liver. Although hepatocytes regenerate, they are not connected properly to blood vessels or bile ducts, so the person has hepatocyte dysfunction. In addition, liver fibrosis obstructs the portal vessels that flow into the liver, causing pressure to rise in the portal system. Portal hypertension and hepatocyte dysfunction cause the signs and symptoms of cirrhosis. Cirrhosis usually is considered to be irreversible.

59. Barrett esophagus occurs in persons who have heartburn with GERD, but it is not the same as heartburn. The term describes physical changes that have occurred in the esophagus when there has been a lot of acid reflux. Normal esophagus cells do not live well in a location where there is a lot of acid and other substances from the stomach. If acid reflux occurs again and again, the body replaces the normal esophagus cells with another type of normal cell that can endure the acid. Barrett esophagus is not cancer, but it is a warning sign that a portion of the esophagus is at risk for cancer.

60. Some of the enzymes that the pancreas normally makes are inactive enzymes, and they are not activated until they reach the intestines where they digest food. However, in pancreatitis, those enzymes become activated inside the pancreas, so they start digesting the pancreas and cause damage and pain.

61. You both definitely have a lot of stress right now. Your wife is unconscious, but her body is experiencing a lot of physical stress that causes some physiologic changes. Stress ulcers are multiple little areas of injury in the lining of the stomach that occur in people who have injuries serious enough that they need to be in the ICU. Stress ulcers do not cause any pain, although they can bleed. We are taking the best care possible of your wife. Now let us talk about your stress. What ways do you have of managing it?

62. Some bile and secretions from your pancreas are going backward into your stomach remnant, where they are not supposed to go. They contain substances that damage the inside wall of your stomach remnant.

63. A healthy liver removes potentially harmful substances from the blood and changes them chemically so they are not harmful. When the liver does not work well, potentially harmful substances build up in the blood and can circulate to the brain. They change how the brain works, which causes the confusion and drowsiness you see in your partner.

64. The hepatocytes in a well-functioning liver synthesize albumin and put it into the blood. In cirrhosis, many of the hepatocytes have been destroyed or are not working well, so the liver is not able to synthesize enough albumin to keep the blood levels normal.

Clinical Scenarios

65. genetic predisposition; T-cell; microbiota
66. The nurse practitioner needed to check for appendicitis as a possible cause of Ms. Hawk's abdominal pain.
67. Active episodes of ulcerative colitis often involve bloody diarrhea; she already has developed iron deficiency anemia from blood loss.
68. Several gastrointestinal disorders cause diarrhea and crampy abdominal pain, including ulcerative colitis and Crohn disease. A colonoscopy provides a view of the colonic mucosa that assists with the diagnosis.
69. Although a positive family history is less common with ulcerative colitis than with Crohn disease, ulcerative colitis does have a genetic component that sets the stage for abnormal immune response that damages the bowel mucosa.
70. Inflammatory bowel disease is a risk factor for colon cancer, especially if people have had the condition for numerous years. It is important to detect colon cancer in the early stages, before it metastasizes, so that it can be treated successfully. Ms. Hawk's mother had colon cancer.
71. She needs to replace the salt and water that are being lost in the diarrhea. If she has continued diarrhea and does not replace the fluid and salt, she will develop clinical dehydration, the combination of extracellular fluid volume deficit and hypernatremia.
72. acute pancreatitis; ethanol metabolites; trypsin
73. lipase; amylase
74. hypocalcemia; tetany
75. Alcohol withdrawal

CHAPTER 42

Match the Definitions

1. D
2. C
3. A
4. B

Circle the Correct Words

5. other anomalies
6. feeding; hearing
7. B and C; no
8. a congenital; right; volvulus
9. dilation; collapse
10. over time; faltering growth
11. cystic fibrosis
12. acute infectious diarrhea

Categorize the Conditions

13. Congenital
14. Congenital

Copyright © 2024 by Elsevier, Inc. All Rights Reserved.

15. Acquired
16. Congenital
17. Congenital
18. Acquired
19. Acquired
20. Congenital
21. Acquired
22. Acquired

Order the Steps
23. C, A, D, B, E

Explain the Picture
24. Esophageal atresia
25. Excessive amount of amniotic fluid is associated with esophageal atresia because normally the fetus swallows amniotic fluid that then absorbs into the placental circulation. Because the esophagus is a blind pouch, this process cannot occur, and the volume of amniotic fluid increases.
26. Tracheoesophageal fistula
27. Air will enter the stomach, distending it; gastric secretions will regurgitate into the trachea and enter the lungs, causing inflammation by damaging the lung tissue.

Describe the Differences
28. Marasmus is severe acute malnutrition caused by deficiency of all nutrients, but kwashiorkor is severe acute malnutrition caused by deficiency of protein.
29. Physiologic jaundice occurs in the first week after birth and is not associated with underlying disease, but pathologic jaundice has higher bilirubin levels and is associated with disease.

Match the Risk Factors
30. C
31. A
32. D
33. B

Complete the Sentences
34. week
35. recessive; copper; liver
36. bile; hypertension
37. celiac; celiac sprue; T; epithelium
38. proteins (or albumin); fat
39. fat; edema
40. kernicterus
41. necrotizing enterocolitis; bowel; death
42. 12
43. pancreatic; mucus; sweat

Match the Signs and Symptoms
44. C
45. D
46. A
47. E
48. B

Teach People about Pathophysiology
Compare your answers with these sample answers.

49. Because they do not eat until after they are born, newborn babies normally have meconium in their intestines. Normal meconium moves easily through the intestines and comes out when the bowels move. The usual cause of having thick meconium as your baby does is lack of some digestive enzymes. That is why they are doing some tests, to determine what the problem is. Meanwhile, the enema should help to soften the thick meconium so it will move out as it should.
50. That little pouch on Travis's intestine has some cells inside it that normally belong in the stomach. Those cells are making acid and strong digestive enzymes like they are supposed to do in the stomach; however, the acid and enzymes are in the little intestinal pouch, where they damage the pouch wall. This damage makes an ulcer, which is an open sore that can bleed. This is why Travis was bleeding into his intestine and you saw the blood in his diaper.
51. The word *aganglionic* explains the problem with Diego's bowel. Normally there are collections of nerve cells called *ganglia* in the wall of the bowel. The nerves normally make the bowel muscles contract and move the bowel contents. Diego does not have all of the normal ganglia in a portion of his bowel wall, so the bowel contents do not move through it. The bowel contents accumulate behind that part of his bowel and distend it, making it big.
52. When the bowel contents stop moving, they get hard and stuck. We call that impacted. The hard mass does not move, but liquid can go around it, so that is why Diego had some watery diarrhea.
53. Normally, the small intestine has little projections, like tiny fingers, that are called *villi*. They stick into the liquid contents of the intestine and move the nutrients into the body. When the villi are flattened, as happened to Nina, there is less chance to take the nutrients into the body. Nina needs nutrients from her food so that she can grow. As long as you avoid gluten in her diet, her intestine will have a chance to repair itself and function more normally again.
54. Nina had diarrhea because the nutrients stayed in her intestine instead of moving into her body. Without the villi, the water in the intestine could not go back into her body, and those extra nutrients in her intestine kept more water in the intestine. This gave her the diarrhea.

CHAPTER 43

Match the Definitions
1. F
2. E
3. A
4. B
5. D
6. C

Copyright © 2024 by Elsevier, Inc. All Rights Reserved.

Match the Cell Functions

7. E
8. D
9. F
10. G
11. B
12. C
13. A

Circle the Correct Words

14. cancellous
15. canaliculi; lacunae
16. endochondral ossification; does
17. no; does not
18. myoblasts; myotubes
19. endurance; prevent fatigue; provide precision of movement
20. sarcoplasmic reticulum membranes; calcium
21. recruiting more muscle units
22. tension; length; tension

Categorize the Substances

23. Inhibits
24. Facilitates
25. Facilitates
26. Facilitates
27. Inhibits
28. Facilitates

Order the Steps

29. A, C, B
30. E, B, A, C, D
31. E, C, A, G, B, D, F, H

Explain the Pictures

32. articular; type II collagen
33. cancellous (spongy); red marrow
34. marrow; yellow marrow (fatty tissue)
35. compact; cortical
36. periosteum; connective
37. diaphysis
38. B and D
39. B
40. D
41. I band
42. A band
43. I band

Describe the Differences

44. Compact bone is solid, extremely strong, and highly organized, with its basic structural unit being the haversian system, but cancellous bone is less complex and forms an irregular meshwork composed of trabeculae that branch and unite with one another.
45. A diarthrosis is a freely movable joint, but a synarthrosis is an immovable joint, and an amphiarthrosis is a slightly movable joint.
46. Osteoid is the matrix of bone that is not yet mineralized, but bone is the fully mineralized structure.

47. A synovial joint is connected by a fibrous joint capsule that contains a fluid-filled space, but a symphysis is a cartilaginous joint in which bones are united by a pad of fibrocartilage, such as the intervertebral disks.

Complete the Sentences

48. bone morphogenic; osteoblasts
49. collagen; proteoglycans
50. subchondral; tidemark
51. fascia
52. myosin
53. motor unit
54. cross-bridge
55. debt; lactic
56. density; fracture
57. sarcopenia; II; I

Compare and Contrast the Muscle Fibers

Characteristic	Type I Fibers	Type II Fibers
Speed of Contraction	Slow	Fast
Intensity of Contraction	Low	High
Type of Metabolism	Oxidative	Glycolysis
Number of Mitochondria	Many	Few
Amount of Myoglobin	High	Low
Color	Red	White
Capillary Supply	Profuse	Intermediate to sparse

Teach People about Physiology

Compare your answers with these sample answers.

58. Osteocytes are osteoblasts that are terminally differentiated; in other words, they are fully matured and no longer build bone. They communicate with both osteoblasts and osteoclasts about when and where to form and resorb bone as well as other functions that keep bone functional.
59. The normal fluid in your knee joint, called *synovial fluid,* supplies nourishment to the cartilage. Synovial fluid is filtered from the blood, so it contains the nourishment your cartilage needs.
60. No difference; those terms refer to the same muscles. The term *striated* refers to the striped pattern that persons see when they look at skeletal muscle with a microscope.
61. You ask an important question! Muscles need increased intracellular calcium to contract, and then they need less calcium so that they can relax. The sarcotubular system releases calcium for muscle contraction and then takes it up and stores the calcium during muscle relaxation.

Copyright © 2024 by Elsevier, Inc. All Rights Reserved.

62. The term *lean body mass* is another way of saying *muscle mass*. So they are talking about bulking up their muscles.
63. Muscles take in creatine from the blood. They change some of it into phosphocreatine, which provides energy for muscle contraction. Our bodies normally make creatine, so you already have some creatine in your blood.

CHAPTER 44

Match the Definitions
1. B
2. E
3. F
4. A
5. C
6. D

Circle the Correct Words
7. shoulder; elevate the arm
8. sprain; strain
9. epicondyle
10. epicondylopathy
11. muscles; tendons; tendons; muscles
12. venous; pain
13. skeletal muscle; dark; creatine kinase; kidneys
14. bacteria; sequestrum
15. formation; destruction
16. break down; lysosomes
17. alcohol

Categorize the Characteristics
18. Osteoarthritis
19. Rheumatoid arthritis
20. Rheumatoid arthritis
21. Osteoarthritis
22. Rheumatoid arthritis
23. Rheumatoid arthritis
24. Rheumatoid arthritis
25. Osteoarthritis
26. Osteoarthritis
27. Rheumatoid arthritis

Order the Steps
28. B, E, H, F, G, D, C, A

Explain the Pictures
29. Ulnar drift
30. Rheumatoid arthritis
31. With loss of joint mobility, the individual uses the hands less, and muscles surrounding the joints atrophy.
32. In rheumatoid arthritis, the joints swell initially because of synovitis (inflammation of the synovial membrane) caused by autoimmune processes. The inflammation can spread to other joint structures.
33. Because rheumatoid arthritis is an autoimmune disease, the autoantibodies, autoreactive T lymphocytes, and other immune cells can cause damage and inflammation anywhere in the body that the autoantigens are located.
34. Osteoarthritis
35. Bouchard
36. Heberden
37. The primary cause is osteophytes (bone spurs) that develop around the margins of the joint.
38. Matrix metalloproteinases are elevated in osteoarthritis and are major contributors to the destruction of articular cartilage.

Match the Fractures
39. D
40. F
41. A
42. E
43. L
44. I
45. K
46. J
47. H
48. B
49. G
50. C

Describe the Differences
51. Delayed union is the healing together of fractured bone fragments that takes longer than usual after a fracture, but malunion is healing of a fracture with the bone in a non-anatomic position.
52. Dislocation is temporary displacement of a bone from its normal position in a joint, but subluxation is partial dislocation, so contact between the two joint surfaces is only partially lost.
53. Tendinitis is inflammation of a tendon, but tendinosis involves degradation of the collagen fibers in the tendon.
54. Rhabdomyolysis is rapid breakdown of skeletal muscle that causes release of intracellular contents, including myoglobin, but myoglobinuria is the presence of myoglobin in the urine.

Match the Pathophysiologies
55. D
56. F
57. E
58. A
59. B
60. C

Complete the Sentences
61. reduction; fixation
62. heterotopic ossification (or myositis ossificans)
63. D; rickets
64. skull; brain
65. metastatic; osteosarcoma
66. ground substance
67. tophi
68. weakness; fatigue

Copyright © 2024 by Elsevier, Inc. All Rights Reserved.

69. contracture
70. spindles
71. myalgic; postexertional
72. disuse
73. relaxation; contraction

Match the Tumor Characteristics

74. D
75. C
76. B
77. E
78. A

Teach People about Pathophysiology

Compare your answers with these sample answers.

79. No, *compound* does not mean infected. It means that there is an open connection between the broken bone and the external environment. This exposes your bone to microorganisms that are on your skin and outside your body, which is why your doctor is concerned about infection. The term *compound* simply means that the skin is broken with a wound that leads to the fracture site.
80. The sore on your ankle is infected with bacteria. It is likely that some bacteria moved inward from your sore and spread directly to your bone, where they made a new infection.
81. I know you are concerned about money for food for your family. Let me tell you something important about your leg bone. When bone is healing, it lays down soft fibers around the break, and then later it makes bone in that location. This takes time. You need the cast to stabilize the two ends of the bone together so that the repair will be solid. If we take off the cast too early, the repair is not completed, and the bone could collapse or break again where it was broken. I would like to call a social worker who can help you with resources for your family while you cannot work. Would you like to talk with her?
82. Those nodes on your knuckles are part of the osteoarthritis. They are bone spurs. Osteoarthritis involves thinning and loss of cartilage in joints, but it also involves excess bone growth in some locations that makes bony bumps. The technical name for those bony bumps is osteophytes, but most people just call them bone spurs.
83. They are looking for a particular substance, an enzyme called *alkaline phosphatase,* that certain types of bone cancers release into the blood. Knowing the amount of that substance in your blood will help them monitor the situation in your bones.

Clinical Scenario

84. Bone mass is decreased in osteopenia, but it is severely decreased in osteoporosis.
85. In osteoporosis, bone resorption occurs faster than bone formation.
86. Kyphosis in osteoporosis is caused by vertebral compression fractures.

87. Around age 30
88. It decreases.
89. In the first few years after menopause, bone mineral density decreases quite rapidly, and then it has a more gradual decline.
90. Estrogen normally stimulates production of osteoprotegerin (a protective factor) and decreases the production of RANKL (a factor that stimulates osteoclasts). Estrogen also exerts antiapoptotic effects on osteoblasts and proapoptotic effects on osteoclasts. With less estrogen effect after menopause, osteoclast activity increases.
91. Regular, moderate weight-bearing exercise can slow down bone loss in osteoporosis. It also increases muscle strength, thus reducing her risk for falls.

Puzzle Out These Technical Terms

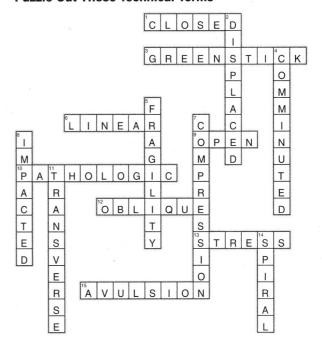

CHAPTER 45

Match the Definitions

1. D
2. E
3. F
4. A
5. B
6. C
7. J
8. G
9. H
10. I

Circle the Correct Words

11. 20s; continues after
12. well; years
13. ends; midshaft

349

Copyright © 2024 by Elsevier, Inc. All Rights Reserved.

14. twisting; almost always
15. Septic arthritis; joint; joints
16. head of the femur
17. tibial tubercle

Explain the Picture
18. axial
19. appendicular
20. The bones in question 15 (the appendicular skeleton)
21. B; Diaphysis; A; Epiphyses
22. D
23. Adolescents
24. F
25. Recurrent interruption of the blood supply to the femoral head causes the ossification center to become necrotic and collapse; then it is remodeled gradually by live bone.

Describe the Differences
26. With intramembranous formation, the bone arises from aggregation of cells that mature into osteoblasts in the vascularized fetal mesenchyme, but with endochondral formation, the bone forms from cartilage.
27. Osteosarcoma is a malignant bone tumor, but osteochondroma is a benign bone tumor.
28. Osteomyelitis is bacterial infection of bone and bone marrow, but septic arthritis is bacterial infection within a joint.
29. Septic arthritis is bacterial infection within a joint, but juvenile idiopathic arthritis is an autoimmune disease that causes inflammation of joints, mostly the large joints.

Complete the Sentences
30. acetabulum; waddling
31. asymmetric
32. structural
33. D; mineralized (or ossified)
34. osteochondroses
35. Ewing; pain
36. rhabdomyosarcoma; striated (or skeletal); mass

Teach People about Pathophysiology
Compare your answers with these sample answers.

37. Babies normally are born with bowlegs. Bowlegs still are normal at age 20 months. In fact, bowlegs are normal up to age 30 months. If your son still has bowlegs when he is older than 30 months, then that would be the time to consult a doctor. Most likely he will grow out of the bowlegs as he develops normally.
38. Osteogenesis imperfecta is a genetic disease involving defective collagen synthesis, which causes bones to be extremely brittle and break very easily. That is why it is called *brittle bone disease.*
39. Your tibia was growing rapidly, but there was not enough blood supply to part of it, so that part of the bone died. Often the bone will grow back when a person rests for several weeks. You really need to rest

your knee until the doctor says you can start using it again.
40. Children who are not yet walking and present with a long bone fracture have a greater than 75% chance of that fracture being caused by abuse. Tibial fractures are common in such cases. When abuse is suspected, radiographs must be taken to evaluate for head trauma, other fractures, and fractures in different stages of healing.
41. An infant's bone has blood vessels that perforate the growth plate; this makes it easy for bacteria that have infected a bone to reach the joint. In older children, the arterioles end beneath the epiphyseal plate.

Clinical Scenario
42. Duchenne muscular dystrophy; dystrophin
43. pelvic girdle; anterior tibial and peroneal
44. Duchenne muscular dystrophy is inherited as an X-linked recessive condition or occurs from a sporadic mutation that silences the dystrophin gene on the short arm of the X chromosome.
45. Normally, the protein dystrophin helps anchor the actin cytoskeleton of skeletal muscle fibers to the basement membrane so that the fibers do not become damaged by the repeated stress of contraction.
46. Tommy's lower extremity and lower back muscles are weak. When he gets up from the floor, he pushes up with his hands and then uses his hands to climb up his legs until he is upright. That is the Gower sign.
47. CPK and the other enzymes are normally inside muscle fibers. When muscle fibers die in Duchenne muscular dystrophy, they spill their contents into the interstitial area, and these enzymes leak into the blood.
48. Tommy's calf muscles enlarged because fat and connective tissue have accumulated within them as his muscle fibers die. Because his muscles are degenerating, his calves are weak, even though they are enlarged.
49. Duchenne muscular dystrophy is a progressive degenerative disease. The shoulder girdle muscles will become involved, and he will have increasing disability. Most people who have the disease die in their mid-20s from respiratory infection and respiratory muscle weakness, although treatment continues to extend life for others.

CHAPTER 46

Match the Definitions
1. C
2. G
3. I
4. F
5. H
6. A
7. B
8. J
9. E
10. D

Copyright © 2024 by Elsevier, Inc. All Rights Reserved.

Circle the Correct Words

11. dermis
12. dermis
13. sympathetic; dermal
14. thinner; less; fewer
15. is not
16. virus; herald patch; pregnancy
17. skin; women
18. edema; inflammation
19. bacterium; tick
20. central; frontotemporal
21. ice crystals; distal to proximal

Categorize the Disorders

22. Bacterial infection
23. Fungal infection
24. Autoimmune
25. Bacterial infection
26. Fungal infection
27. Autoimmune
28. Fungal infection
29. Autoimmune
30. Autoimmune
31. Autoimmune

Order the Layers and Note their Functions

Latin Name of Epidermal Layer	Function of Epidermal Layer
Stratum corneum	Barrier of dead keratinocytes that protects against microorganisms and excessive water loss
Stratum granulosum	Enables keratinocytes to form granules of proteins that protect against water loss
Stratum spinosum	Enables keratinocytes to enlarge and move upward
Stratum basale	Formation of new keratinocytes

Explain the Pictures

32. Raised? Yes; Extends into dermis? Yes; Lesion: Cyst
33. Raised? Yes; Extends into dermis? No; Lesion: Vesicle
34. Raised? Yes; Extends into dermis? No; Lesion: Wheal
35. Raised? Yes; Extends into dermis? Yes; Lesion: Papule
36. Raised? No; Extends into dermis? No; Lesion: Macule
37. The lesion would need to be larger; a bulla is a vesicle with a diameter larger than 1 cm.
38. The lesion would need to be larger; a patch is a macule with a diameter larger than 1 cm.
39. 33
40. 32

Describe the Differences

41. A furuncle is an infection of a hair follicle that extends to the surrounding tissue, but a carbuncle is a collection of infected hair follicles that forms a draining abscess.
42. Apocrine sweat glands are fewer in number, have little known function, and are located in the axillae, scalp, face, abdomen, and genital areas, but eccrine sweat glands are more abundant, have thermoregulatory function, and are distributed over the body, with the greatest numbers in the palms of the hands, soles of the feet, and forehead.
43. A keloid is an elevated scar that extends beyond the border of the injury, but a hypertrophic scar is an elevated scar that stays within the border of the injury.
44. Acne vulgaris is the typical acne that is common in adolescence, but acne rosacea is a chronic, readily exacerbated, inflammatory skin disease that develops primarily in middle age.

Match the Functions

45. C
46. D
47. A
48. E
49. F
50. B

Complete the Sentences

51. dermatitis
52. contact; IV; delayed (or T-cell mediated)
53. stasis; seborrheic
54. keratinocytes; epidermal; exacerbations (or flare-ups)
55. itching
56. rhinophyma
57. pemphigus; autoantibodies
58. gastrointestinal tract
59. simplex; HSV-1; HSV-2
60. human papilloma; cancer
61. sun; Kaposi sarcoma

Match the Tumors

62. B
63. A
64. G
65. D
66. C
67. E
68. H
69. F

Teach People about Pathophysiology

Compare your answers with these sample answers.

70. Vitiligo is not contagious. Your husband has those light spots in his skin because the cells that normally make skin color are not making the pigment that gives skin its color.
71. Cells called *melanocytes* live in the skin where hair is formed. They make the pigments that color our hair.

Copyright © 2024 by Elsevier, Inc. All Rights Reserved.

As we age, we have fewer of these pigment-creating cells, so our hair gets gray or white.

72. Psoriasis is not a fungal infection. It is not an infection at all, and it is not contagious. These silvery scaly patches on your skin are caused by excessive growth of skin cells, probably involving signals from immune cells. You can go ahead and hug your son because he will not get psoriasis from your touch.

73. We need a good flow of blood to keep our skin and the tissues beneath it healthy. Pressure injuries develop when the skin and the area beneath it do not get enough blood flow because the pressure of the body flattens the blood vessels. Without proper blood flow, the tissue dies, and an open sore can develop. This happens especially over bony areas like the heels and the sacrum (the bone right above the buttocks).

74. There is no difference. *Wheals* is the technical word for a raised area of the skin that looks like hives or mosquito bites. You are correct in calling them hives. Did they tell you to stop taking the penicillin?

75. I think there is another reason that your aunt does not smile at you. Scleroderma makes the skin of the face very hard and tight, like a stiff, hard plastic mask. This makes it very difficult for persons to smile or move their faces when they talk. Let's find a way for you to visit with your aunt and see what she really feels.

Clinical Scenario

76. herpes zoster; varicella-zoster virus
77. sensory; postherpetic neuralgia
78. It was not her first exposure to the virus. The first exposure causes chickenpox. The virus then ascends to a dorsal root ganglion, where it is dormant until it is reactivated.
79. The shingles lesions follow the distribution of the sensory nerve that the virus has infected. The virus would need to be present in both dorsal root ganglia in that dermatome to cross the midline.
80. Mrs. Maxwell is experiencing multiple stressors and therefore probably is somewhat immunosuppressed. The virus often reactivates when an individual becomes immunosuppressed.
81. Postherpetic neuralgia

CHAPTER 47

Match the Definitions
1. C
2. A
3. D
4. B

Circle the Correct Words
5. epidermal; immune
6. highly; staphylococci; vesicles; crust
7. circulates to
8. exanthema subitum; nonpruritic; after; infants
9. grow; shrink
10. do not

Categorize the Infections
11. Fungal
12. Bacterial
13. Fungal
14. Viral
15. Viral
16. Fungal
17. Viral
18. Viral

Explain the Picture
19. Sebum (sebaceous gland secretions)
20. Adolescents and young adults (ages 12 to 25)
21. Comedones (or comedos, but comedones is the technical version)
22. A whitehead
23. Hormone: androgens; Bacterium: *Cutibacterium acnes* (former name was *Propionibacterium acnes*)

Describe the Differences
24. Atopic dermatitis is associated with a history of allergy and an impaired epidermal barrier to allergens, but diaper dermatitis is an irritant contact dermatitis initiated by prolonged exposure to urine and feces.
25. Rubeola is measles, but rubella is German measles, a milder viral disease.
26. Variola is smallpox, but varicella is chickenpox.
27. Hand, foot, and mouth disease is caused by a virus, but scabies is caused by a parasite that infests the skin.

Complete the Sentences
28. IgE; asthma
29. Tinea corporis; puppies
30. proteases
31. herpes zoster; shingles
32. veins; arteries
33. bedbugs; lice; nits
34. sweat
35. neonatorum; weeks
36. pediculosis

Match the Clinical Manifestations
37. D
38. A
39. F
40. E
41. B
42. C

Teach People about Pathophysiology
Compare your answers with these sample answers.

43. Impetigo is quite different from chickenpox. A virus causes chickenpox, but impetigo is a bacterial infection of the skin.
44. In chickenpox (varicella), the rash begins as pruritic macules that soon become vesicles, burst, and scab over. Often, all three forms of the lesions are visible at the same time. With measles (rubeola), the rash remains macular, usually is not pruritic, and is preceded

Copyright © 2024 by Elsevier, Inc. All Rights Reserved.

by fever. Characteristically, chickenpox rash begins on the trunk, scalp. or face and measles rash begins on the head and spreads to the trunk. They both spread to the extremities.

45. Molluscum contagiosum is caused by a pox virus that stimulates the epidermal cell proliferation that makes that strange structure. This condition is not dangerous and it usually goes away without treatment within 6 to 9 months.

46. Although rubella is a mild illness, if a pregnant woman gets rubella early in pregnancy, it causes the developing baby to have serious birth defects or even die before birth.

47. When the nurse practitioner looked in Donny's mouth, she probably saw some white spots surrounded by red rings called *Koplik spots* that are characteristic of measles. Along with his fever and other symptoms, Donny had a classic case of measles right before the rash appears.

Clinical Scenario

48. The linear lesions are burrows made by the scabies mite in which it lays eggs.

49. The itching probably is due to immune system response to the larval stage of the scabies mite.

50. The major complication is secondary infection of the lesions damaged further by scratching.

51. Scabies is transmitted by direct contact and also through mites or eggs living on clothing or bed linen that was contaminated recently.

52. Flea bites are very different from the scabies that Angie has. Instead of the lines that you see with scabies, flea bites tend to occur in clusters. The bites are raised and have a small red puncture in the middle.

CHAPTER 48

Match the Definitions

1. B
2. D
3. A
4. C

Circle the Correct Words

5. increasing
6. decreases; decreases; acidosis
7. glucose; fuel for survival
8. 10; gluconeogenesis
9. protein; colloid osmotic
10. second; first
11. does not; urine output
12. hypermetabolic; hypercoagulability

Categorize the Causes

13. Hypovolemic
14. Cardiogenic
15. Septic
16. Cardiogenic
17. Neurogenic
18. Anaphylactic
19. Hypovolemic
20. Cardiogenic
21. Hypovolemic
22. Neurogenic
23. Anaphylactic
24. Septic

Select the Order

25. B
26. B
27. B
28. A
29. A
30. A
31. A
32. B
33. B
34. A
35. B

Describe the Differences

36. Bacteremia is the presence of viable bacteria in the blood, but sepsis is a life-threatening organ dysfunction caused by a dysregulated host response to infection

37. Sepsis is a life-threatening organ dysfunction caused by a dysregulated host response to infection, but septic shock is sepsis that is complicated by persistent hypotension refractory to fluid therapy.

38. A first-degree burn destroys the epidermis only, but a second-degree burn destroys both the epidermis and at least part of the dermis.

Match the Specific Clinical Manifestations

39. C
40. E
41. D
42. A
43. B

Complete the Sentences

44. vasogenic
45. vasodilation; hypovolemia; distributive
46. cardiogenic shock
47. multiple organ dysfunction syndrome; MODS
48. subcutaneous tissue
49. capillary seal
50. neutrophils; 100
51. general (or nonspecific); lungs

Teach People about Pathophysiology

Compare your answers with these sample answers.

52. Shock means that the heart and blood vessels are not able to supply enough blood to all parts of the body, which causes widespread dysfunction of the cells and tissues that make up the body.

53. The responses are different in these two types of shock because they involve different pathophysiology. In

Copyright © 2024 by Elsevier, Inc. All Rights Reserved.

cardiogenic shock, the heart itself is impaired, and the low cardiac output triggers a compensatory release of catecholamines, by way of sympathetic nerve stimulation. This increases systemic vascular resistance. However, in neurogenic shock, the heart is functional, but the blood vessels have undergone widespread vasodilation due to lack of sympathetic nerve stimulation. This inactivity of the sympathetic system causes decreased systemic vascular resistance, which is the primary problem.

54. Both of those terms are correct descriptions of your burns. "Partial thickness" means that the burn did not reach the deepest layer of the skin. "Second degree" is another way to describe the same type of burn.

55. Activated neutrophils cause a lot of inflammation in MODS. They release reactive oxygen species that damage the endothelium and other tissues, causing damage to cell and organelle membranes as well as DNA integrity. Activated neutrophils also secrete enzymes that dissolve protein, chemicals that activate platelets, and other chemicals that cause maldistribution of blood flow. All of this damage may cause cells to die by necrosis and thus contributes to organ dysfunction.

Clinical Scenario

56. Approximately 32%
57. His head should not blister because he sustained full-thickness burns there.
58. His superficial partial-thickness burns should be the most painful because the pain sensors are intact in those areas. Pain sensation is somewhat diminished in the areas of deep partial-thickness burns and should be absent in the full-thickness burn areas because the pain sensors were destroyed.
59. Mr. Eisner is at high risk for hypovolemia, and even hypovolemic shock, because of evaporative fluid loss from the burned area and from increased capillary permeability that causes fluid shift into the interstitial areas.
60. He would be expected to have concurrent hypovolemia and edema due to shift of vascular fluid into the interstitial areas. Edema of his face is likely to impair his breathing unless he is intubated.
61. The areas of deep partial-thickness burns have the greatest risk for scarring.
62. If he survives, Mr. Eisner will need skin grafts on the areas of full-thickness burns because otherwise they will not heal. All of the skin structure has been destroyed in those areas, so there are no cells to initiate regrowth.

CHAPTER 49

Match the Definitions

1. B
2. C
3. A

Circle the Correct Words

4. systolic
5. consciousness; breathing; color
6. mottling
7. hypovolemic
8. hypothermia; bradycardia
9. sensitive
10. microvasculature; oxygen free radicals
11. 100; 180; lower
12. vasodilation; high; vasoconstriction; low
13. is not
14. Scald; flame

Categorize the Causes

15. Hypovolemic
16. Distributive
17. Obstructive
18. Distributive
19. Obstructive
20. Hypovolemic
21. Distributive
22. Cardiogenic

Describe the Differences

23. With compensated shock in children, systolic blood pressure is adequate for age, and there are signs of inadequate tissue perfusion, but with hypotensive shock, systolic hypotension is associated with the inadequate tissue perfusion.
24. Primary multiple organ dysfunction syndrome (MODS) is the simultaneous failure of at least two organs that occurs soon (3 to 7 days) after a single cause, but secondary MODS typically occurs later and the organ dysfunction may be sequential.
25. The ebb phase of metabolism after a burn injury typically occurs for the first few (3 to 5) days and is characterized by reduced oxygen consumption, impaired circulation, and cellular shock, but the flow phase of metabolism begins after the ebb phase and is a hypermetabolic state, characterized by increased oxygen consumption and elevated catecholamines, glucocorticoids, and glucagon that raise blood glucose and increase caloric requirements dramatically.
26. SIRS is a systemic response to inflammation with specific clinical criteria that occurs with or in the absence of infection, but sepsis is SIRS caused specifically by infection.

Complete the Sentences

27. distributive
28. obstructive; embolism
29. hypoxia; collapse; terminal
30. heart rate
31. sepsis (or SIRS)
32. procoagulant
33. cardiovascular
34. burn
35. foot
36. infection; bacteria

Answer Key

Copyright © 2024 by Elsevier, Inc. All Rights Reserved.

Teach People about Pathophysiology

Compare your answers with these sample answers.

37. The key to defining shock is the acute circulatory dysfunction that results in inadequate delivery of oxygen and nutrients to the tissues, not just locally, but throughout the body. In children, that can happen when systolic blood pressure is normal, low, or even high, but mean arterial pressure typically is low.

38. The temperature of the skin gives us important information about shock. In some kinds of shock, like the ones you have seen on television, the skin is cool. This happens when damage to the heart causes shock, for example. In this case, warm blood does not flow to the skin, so the skin gets cool. But your son has a different type of shock. His shock is caused by injury to his spinal cord, and warm blood still reaches his skin, so his skin is warm.

39. SIRS means systemic inflammatory response syndrome, which indicates that Devon has some changes caused by inflammation. Examples of those changes are fever, heart beating fast, breathing fast, and changes in the white blood cells in the blood.

40. Little children who are burned need a lot more IV fluid, proportionately, compared to adults. A young child of Carly's age cannot concentrate urine as effectively as an adult can to conserve fluid. Burned skin allows a lot of fluid to escape from the body, so we need to replace that fluid.

41. A burn does not bleed initially, so we need to continue our assessment to find the source of the bleeding, which will be an additional injury.

42. It can take a year or two for a scar to mature fully. In addition, Austin will grow, and his body will change size, so his scars need to be watched all the time he is growing to be sure that they do not start constricting his body and limiting his ability to function.

Clinical Scenario

43. hypovolemic shock; volume resuscitation
44. poor tissue perfusion; disappear
45. With diarrhea for 3 days, Kiley's output of sodium and water was greater than her intake, causing her to become dehydrated and hypovolemic. Her low blood volume was not sufficient to deliver enough oxygen and nutrients to meet the metabolic needs of her tissues, even with compensatory mechanisms operating.

46. Two compensatory mechanisms are at work: (1) fluid shift from interstitial into the vascular space to help maintain the circulating volume and (2) increased stimulation of the sympathetic nervous system (SNS), which increases the heart rate (thus the increasing cardiac output) and causes vasoconstriction (thus increasing systemic vascular resistance). Because blood pressure equals cardiac output times the systemic vascular resistance, activation of the SNS raises blood pressure. In Kiley's case, the activated SNS maintains a normal range blood pressure in the face of significant hypovolemia.

47. Kiley's tachycardia indicates the activation of her sympathetic nervous system, a compensatory mechanism that is helping to maintain her blood pressure in the normal range.

48. The compensatory activation of Kiley's sympathetic nervous system causes cutaneous vasoconstriction, which helps to maintain her blood pressure but reduces the flow of warm blood to her skin, making it cool.

49. Fluid replacement will be intravenous because rapid vigorous replacement is indicated.

50. With effective treatment, Kiley's extremities should become less mottled and warmer to touch, her capillary refill should become more brisk, her peripheral pulse stronger. She should become less lethargic, and her fontanel should become less depressed. Her eyes should appear less sunken. Although infants have immature kidneys and are not able to concentrate urine maximally to conserve fluid during dehydration, Kiley's urine output may increase as she improves.

51. Kiley's fluid intake of water and sodium should have been increased immediately when she developed diarrhea, to balance her increased output. The babysitter needed appropriate education, a way to contact the parents who were camping, and the phone number of the pediatrician, to consult for guidance.

Copyright © 2024 by Elsevier, Inc. All Rights Reserved.